DATE DUE

Psychodynamic Treatment of
Anorexia Nervosa and Bulimia

Psychodynamic Treatment of Anorexia Nervosa and Bulimia

Edited by

CRAIG L. JOHNSON, Ph.D.

THE GUILFORD PRESS
New York ∴ London

This book is dedicated to Laura and Ben.

Printed in the United States of America

This book is printed on acid-free paper.

Last digit is print number: 9   8   7   6   5   4   3

Library of Congress Cataloging-in-Publication Data

Psychodynamic treatment of anorexia nervosa and bulimia / edited by
    Craig L. Johnson.
        p.   cm.
    Includes bibliographical references and index.
    ISBN 0-89862-550-5
    1. Anorexia nervosa—Treatment.   2. Bulimia—Treatment.
3. Psychodynamic psychotherapy.   4. Feminist therapy.
    [DNLM: 1. Anorexia Nervosa—psychology.   2. Anorexia Nervosa—
therapy.   3. Bulimia—psychology.   4. Bulimia—therapy—
psychotherapy.   WM 175 P9747]
    RC552.A5P8   1991
    616.85'26—dc20
    DNLM/DLC
    for Library of Congress   90-13867
                                                                   CIP

Contributors

WILLIAM N. DAVIS, Ph.D. Center for the Study of Anorexia and Bulimia, New York, New York

AMY BAKER DENNIS, Ph.D. Center for the Treatment of Eating Disorders and National Anorexic Aid Society, Columbus, Ohio; Midwestern Educational Resource Center, Bloomfield Hills, Michigan

CRAIG L. JOHNSON, Ph.D. Department of Psychology, Laureate Psychiatric Clinic and Hospital, Tulsa, Oklahoma; Department of Psychiatry, Northwestern University Medical School, Chicago, Illinois

LAURA LYNN HUMPHREY, Ph.D. Department of Psychiatry, Northwestern University Medical School, Chicago, Illinois; Northwestern Memorial Hospital, Chicago, Illinois

ANN KEARNEY-COOKE, Ph.D. Private Practice, Cincinnati, Ohio

HOWARD D. LERNER, Ph.D. Department of Psychiatry, University of Michigan, Ann Arbor, Michigan

SUSAN SANDS, Ph.D. Department of Psychiatry and Behavioral Medicine, Stanford University, Stanford, California; The Wright Institute, Berkeley, California; Private Practice, Berkeley, California

RANDY A. SANSONE, M.D. Department of Psychiatry, Laureate Psychiatric Clinic and Hospital, Tulsa, Oklahoma; Department of Psychiatry, College of Medicine, University of Oklahoma, Tulsa, Oklahoma

JOHN A. SCHNEIDER, Ph.D. Department of Psychiatry, Stanford University School of Medicine, Stanford, California; Department of Psychiatry, School of Medicine, University of California—San Francisco, San Francisco, California; Private Practice, Berkeley, California

CATHERINE STEINER-ADAIR, Ph.D. The Project on the Psychology of Women and the Development of Girls, Harvard University, Cambridge, Massachusetts; Middlesex Family Associates, Lexington, Massachusetts

STEVEN STERN, Ph.D. Department of Psychiatry and Behavioral Sciences, Northwestern University Medical School, Chicago, Illinois

MICHAEL STROBER, Ph.D. Department of Psychiatry, School of Medicine, University of California—Los Angeles, Los Angeles, California; UCLA Neuropsychiatric Institute and Hospital, Los Angeles, California

ALAN SUGARMAN, Ph.D. San Diego Psychoanalytic Institute, San Diego, California; Department of Psychiatry, University of California—San Diego, San Diego, California

WILLIAM JAMES SWIFT, M.D. Department of Psychiatry, Medical School, University of Wisconsin—Madison, Madison, Wisconsin

DAVID L. TOBIN, Ph.D. Program Director, Eating Disorders Program, Department of Psychiatry, The University of Chicago, Chicago, Illinois

SUSAN C. WOOLEY, Ph.D. Department of Psychiatry, University of Cincinnati College of Medicine, Cincinnati, Ohio

Preface

Over the last decade clinicians working with eating-disordered patients have increasingly recognized that despite the homogeneity of the demographics, behavior, and cognitions among these patients, the disturbed eating behavior can serve a variety of different biological, interpersonal, and intrapsychic adaptations. The homogeneity of clinical presentation within the group prompted early efforts to find parsimonious, if not simple, explanations for the symptoms. The early treatment literature in the field reported almost exclusively on brief treatment (6 weeks to 3 months) either psychopharmacological or variations of cognitive—behavioral interventions. While this treatment literature showed that approximately two-thirds of the patients treated responded favorably in a short period of time, the follow-up periods have been too short to know how lasting the treatment effects are. Despite the favorable outcomes from brief treatment for many patients, it is clear that approximately one-third of the eating-disordered patients did not respond to briefer interventions.

Recent research has indicated that approximately one-third of the patients who present with disordered eating also have significant personality disorders or Axis II co-morbidity. It is my clinical impression that this subgroup of patients account for most of the poor outcome in the brief treatment literature. They are difficult to treat and usually require longer-term, informed individual psychotherapy. This book was designed to address the challenges of the more difficult to treat eating-disordered patient. My approach to recruiting authors was to invite established, psychodynamically oriented clinicians who have been doing longer-term treatment, to comment on their clinical experience. I believe the book makes a useful contribution to our continuing search for effective treatment interventions for this group of patients.

Contents

·I·

ASPECTS OF THE SELF AND QUESTIONS OF TECHNIQUE

∴ *1* ∴

Bulimia: A Displacement from Psychological Self to Body Self

ALAN SUGARMAN
*San Diego Psychoanalytic Institute
and University of California, San Diego*

Several years ago, my own clinical experience with bulimic women, as well as others' research about the prognostic importance of body image distortion in such women (Garfinkel, Moldofsky, & Garner, 1977), led me and a colleague to suggest that these women used their bodies as transitional objects (Sugarman & Kurash, 1982). At that time we stated,

> Specifically, the failure to adequately separate both physically and cognitively from the maternal object during the practicing subphase leads to a narcissistic fixation on one's own body at the expense of reaching out to other objects in the wider world through the use of external transitional objects. This arrest in the area of transitional objects has profound consequences as regards self–other boundary differentiation, individuation, and the capacity for symbolization. (p. 58)

But problems exist with those early formulations that I would like now to address. Some (Goodsitt, 1983; Taylor, 1987; Woodall, 1987) have quibbled with the use of the term "transitional object," preferring to retain what they interpret Winnicott (1953) to have meant in his poetic but vague introduction of the concept. Although one might take issue with the need to reify such concepts, our own failure at that time to have delineated adequately a developmental line of transitional phenomena

3

(Sugarman & Jaffe, 1989) certainly added to the confusion. More serious was our overly simplified emphasis, as we chose to address only the cognitive and object relations lines of development and their contribution to bulimic symptomatology. This heuristic choice to emphasize only these lines of development made the subsequent formulation sound as though these women were concretely re-enacting early developmental experiences. It failed to acknowledge explicitly that the symptom is a compromise formation, born out of intrapsychic conflicts; it also leads to distorted self- and object representations that cannot be viewed as veridical images of early experiences of the self or other (Schwartz, 1988). Furthermore, we failed to make explicit that the formulations presented arose out of clinical work with hospitalized bulimics, the most disturbed segment of the bulimic spectrum. The body may not have the same psychodynamic significance for those women whose character structures are more neurotically organized.

This chapter is an attempt to expand these early and insufficient formulations into a more comprehensive perspective on why the body is used as an arena in which these women can enact their numerous neurotic conflicts as well as their far less numerous developmental deficiencies. In order to clarify this complex and multidetermined phenomenon, it is necessary first to understand the role of the body self in the intrapsychic economy of the mind.

IMPORTANCE OF THE BODY SELF

Freud (1923/1961), of course, was all too aware of the body as the foundation for the personality when he stated that the ego was "first and foremost a body ego" (p. 26). With this statement he meant to convey that the sense of self originates in early bodily sensations and proprioceptive stimulation. In particular, the shift from sensations arising within the body to sensations arising from the sensory receptors on its external surface gives rise to reality testing and a greater sense of self–other differentiation (Frosch, 1964; Lichtenberg, 1978; Mahler & McDevitt, 1982). Still others have emphasized the body's unique position both as the source of perception and as an object that can be perceived. This aspect of the body as a "perceiving perceptible" (Merleau-Ponty, 1962), or its "double touch phenomenon" (Hoffer, 1950), is a key contributor to the fledgling self-representations that begin to comprise the individual's representational world (Sandler & Rosenblatt, 1962). This ability both to perceive and to be perceived

> elicits two sensations of the same quality and these lead to the distinction between the self and the non-self, between body and what subsequently

becomes environment. In consequence, this factor contributes to the processes of structural differentiation. Delimitation between the self-body and the outer world, the world where the objects are found, is thus initiated. (Hoffer, 1950, p. 19)

Even Piaget's emphasis on earliest experience being sensorimotor implies that the earliest sense of self is a somatic one. Rudimentary experiences of self and other emerge out of the action patterns that characterize earliest infancy. As "good enough" mothering occurs, the infant begins to differentiate subtle inner experience; a tenuous sense of agency emerges as somatic communication leads to the needed response from the mother. Early misattunement caused either by the mother's failure to respond appropriately (Robertson, 1962; Edgcumbe, 1984) or a child's constitutional impairment in communicating its needs so that they can be gratified (Dowling, 1977) leads to a disrupted early sense of agency, a deficient body self, and ultimately a distorted self-representation. Cause–effect relationships around the most vivid and important of the developing infant's experiences, its somatic ones, fail to be established. But if the early fit between infant and environment is good, the ensuing body representation will be vital and competent, as will be the self-representation of which the body self eventually becomes one component.

Thus, one's earliest experience of self is centered solely around somatic experiences (Sugarman & Jaffe, 1988, 1990). There is no sense of self separate from body self. The body self is the seat of interactions with important others in the environment, drive experiences, affects, and early ego forerunners (such as perception, motility, stimulus barrier, and nascent intentionality). At this earliest stage of self, all these various functions and processes exist in a relatively undifferentiated matrix in which self remains undifferentiated from the object.

DIFFERENTIATION OF THE BODY SELF

As "hatching" from the symbiotic orbit occurs and the toddler engages the separation–individuation process (Mahler, Pine, & Bergman, 1975), numerous processes converge to foster a differentiation between body self and self-representation that parallels the ongoing differentiation between self- and object representations. Differentiation of ego and id (Hartmann, 1939), and drive differentiation and early neutralization (Jacobson, 1964), accompanied by a cognitive shift to preoperational thinking (Piaget, 1937; Wolff, 1960; Sugarman & Jaffe, 1990), promote a representation of self that is somewhat more symbolic and comprehensive. Maturation in these different developmental lines eventually leads to evocative object constancy and a mental representation of self that is less locked into the spatial and temporal context in which the world of love objects is encountered via bodily action. A genuine representational world (Sandler & Rosenblatt, 1962) emerges in which the self-representation is relatively distinct from the object representation and the body self is one of several facets of the toddler's self-representation, which expands to include other key elements, such as self-as-child, self-as-daughter, and self-as-girl. (Numerous other differentiations within the self-representation also occur. The ones I describe here are particularly relevant in the genesis of bulimia.) The mother–child relationship is crucial in facilitating this shift, as the mother's ability to recognize and verbalize the child's somatic communications raises them to a verbal, symbolic level that helps to differentiate body self from psychological self (Edgcumbe, 1984). Learning to verbalize one's inner needs and to communicate them symbolically to others promotes a sense of affect and drive regulation that broadens the self-representation. This ability of the mother to raise somatic communication to a symbolic level leads to an internalization of affect and drive regulation and an early sense that one's needs and their regulation are located within the self-representation. Failure at this function leads to affects' and drives' remaining localized in the body self and not being experienced at a symbolic level. Such toddlers remain fixated at the early stage wherein body self is not distinct from psychological self and the self-representation is not well differentiated from the object representation. The predisposition is laid for the later externalization of affect regulation into the object representation (Krystal, 1978).

Differentiation within the body self accompanies its differentiation from psychological self. Id, ego, and superego facets to the body self emerge from the developmental thrust toward intrapsychic differentiation and integration (Lichtenberg, 1978). Drive-related experiences comprise its id aspects; perceptual, motor, and boundary phenomena make up its ego characteristics; and body ideals and prohibitions reflect the integration of the emerging superego with the body self (Lichtenberg, 1978). Early identifications also begin to affect the body self as the concomitant differentiation of self-representations from object representations allows the displacing of traits from object to self-representation that is the mechanism of identification (Sandler, 1960).

Core gender identity coalesces around the sense of having a female body image as body self becomes more differentiated from the more encompassing self-representation and then more integrated with other facets of it (Tyson, 1986). Dawning genital pleasures accompany the formation of a sexually differentiated body self at the separation–individuation stage (Roiphe, 1968). These genital sensations can now be cognitively represented and integrated into the body self. In this way, a self-representation of being female encompasses a body self that includes having female genitals (Silverman, 1981; Person, 1983; Tyson, 1986). (I maintain an emphasis on female body self, given the gender specificity of this syndrome.) Selective identifications with the mother and pleasure at the body self's resemblance to the mother's body occurs when development and mothering proceed normally (Mahler, 1981). But the intense affects that accompany the rapprochement subphase and/or the mother's difficulty in tolerating them can undermine this identification.

The heightened aggression and ambivalence that characterize this subphase can lead to a defensive retreat from autonomy and a fixation at a passive, masochistic posture (Tyson, 1986). Pleasure at being like the mother wanes as idealization of the mother is buffeted. Penis envy is a not unusual result, as having a female body comes to feel worthless (Grossman & Stewart, 1976; Tyson, 1982). The body self becomes narcissistically depleted, and a sense of inadequacy, deprivation, and damage pervades it (Tyson, 1982). A failure to integrate the body self well into the self-representation, which is later exploited unconsciously in bulimia, can occur under these circumstances. The body self can become sexualized and/or aggressivized, leading to the motoric inhibitions and awkwardness that characterize early miscuing between mother and child (Robertson, 1962; Dowling, 1977). An integrated self-representation with a secure sense of self-regulation will, of course, be disrupted, given how integral a component the body self is at such an early stage. And a predisposition to defensive displacement from self to body is formed (Joffe & Sandler, 1967). At this stage there is little defensive value in such a displacement. But later it can help reduce the gap between actual and ideal states of the self-representation to maintain narcissistic equilibrium in bulimic and other psychosomatic symptomatology.

When development proceeds smoothly, the engagement of oedipal issues leads to a re-emphasis on the body self as part of the vertical decalage that accompanies self- and object representation development (Sharpe, 1984). That is, normal development involves changes in both self- and object representations through the interplay of maturation and development, so that they become more complex via a hierarchical organization of systems that allows a repertoire of ever more complex actions, emotions, and thoughts (Rosenblatt & Thickstun, 1977). This hierarchical organization, which promotes ever more differentiated and integrated self-representations, involves a vertical decalage in which all earlier facets of self-representation must be reconstructed again at each new developmental level (Sharpe, 1984). Each more organized level of the self-representation repeats the same structural pattern and sequence, although there are important qualitative differences because of developmental and maturational shifts in id, ego, and superego. Thus, the body self is returned to at each developmental stage in order to promote further expansion and organization of the self-representation. Specifically it must be differentiated and reintegrated with self-as-child, self-as-daughter, and self-as-female (among other self-representational elements) in regard to the developmental antecedents of bulimic symptomatology.

Oedipal-age children demonstrate this recapitulation of earlier emphases on the body self in their prominent preoccupations with genital differences and the integration of these anatomical differences into the gender of their body selves. Successful resolution of a girls' oedipal strivings requires that both parents be sufficiently accepting of her impulses to allow her to identify with the mother, the mother's body, and its functions—most prominently that of procreation. One 6-year-old girl, still struggling toward this resolution, began to become preoccupied with not leaving the house until she was sure that her hair was in place, that her clothes matched, and that her nails were polished. She would even sneak into her mother's room and put makeup on when the opportunity presented itself. Her mother was beside herself about what she felt to be her daughter's excessive vanity until I pointed out how much effort she herself put into her own physical appearance. Explaining the value of this identification made her more accepting of her daughter's behavior. Similar scenarios are seen when little girls at this age place pillows under their shirts in order to mimic a female pregnant body.

Generally this emphasis on the body self around oedipal issues is heralded by the girl's entry into the phallic–narcissistic stage (Edgcumbe & Burgner, 1975). Earlier problems during separation–individuation may lead to a splitting of the girl's ambivalence, so that the mother is maintained as a love object and negative feelings are displaced to the father (Edgcumbe, Lundbert, Markowitz, & Salo, 1976; Rocah, 1984; Tyson, 1986). Such a fixation sets the stage for bisexual conflicts (Ritvo, 1984, 1988; Rocah, 1984; Tyson, 1986). When the earlier relationship with the mother is less fraught with conflict, negative oedipal situations may arise wherein the body self is experienced as active and masculine, while the father becomes a competitor for the mother. Again, such bisexual conflicts lead to a preoccupation with the body and its gender differences that is later expressed in bulimic symptoms.

The transition into latency and the attainment of concrete operational thinking promotes an even more integrated self-representation (Sugarman & Jaffe, 1990). The latency-age child becomes able to transform self- and object representations independently of overt body interactions with the environment as she becomes able to construct inverse and reciprocal relationships between mental constructs (Greenspan, 1979). Phallic–narcissistic and phallic–oedipal conflicts can be modulated by the more ideational defenses promoted by this cognitive shift

(Furman, 1980). A differentiated, hierarchically stratified self-representation emerges as a cohesive structure through the multitude of transformations allowed by cognitive maturation. This structuralization encourages improved competence in coping with drive impulses as well as with reality pressures.

Again, the recapitulation of early stages in the development of the self-representation involved in vertical decalage brings the body self into prominence, as its sexuality must be integrated. Libidinal impulses lead to the masturbation that characterizes latency (Clower, 1977; Kramer & Rudolph, 1980). Such masturbation generally involves clitoral stimulation without vaginal penetration (Clower, 1977). Rhythmic activities such as jumping rope and gymnastics serve to discharge such impulses, as do more directly stimulating activities such as horseback riding or climbing poles. Boys and girls may experience anxiety over masturbatory impulses or fantasies and may regress to other early bodily expressions of drive discharge, such as eating, finger mouthing, hair twirling, mouth stroking, and so on (Clower, 1977; Kramer & Rudolph, 1980).

Both genders also become highly conscious of their bodies as they relate to narcissistic issues during latency. Boys begin to identify with the masculine ideal of being athletic, and their prowess on the baseball or soccer field becomes a significant contributor to their self-esteem. And girls become more aware of feminine ideals, so that prettiness and fashion consciousness become even more accentuated as they progress through this stage. Early conflicts over a feminine body self are fueled by either preoedipal or oedipal conflicts and can be seen in the tomboyishness that characterizes certain latency-age girls. A not uncommon presenting symptom in girls during latency seems to be balking at wearing skirts, dresses, or other apparel that emphasizes a clearly feminine body self.

Adolescence, of course, involves the recapitulation of body emphases, as manifested in the need to integrate major changes in the appearance and sensations of the body into the body representation and then the more encompassing and sexually differentiated self-representation. Pubescence, with its changes in body self that make the adolescent capable of adult sexuality and procreation, leads to intensified drives and affects that strain the developing ego's capacity to integrate the body representation into the self-representation. An initial preoedipal regression develops out of the anxieties posed by the newfound capacity to implement oedipal urges (Rosenthal, 1981). Thus, the body of the early adolescent experiences a sharp increase in libidinal and aggressive urges, which can lead to a longing for a developmentally less mature body (Blos, 1962). Negative oedipal and sadomasochistic impulses continue to buffet the adolescent girl whose preoedipal relationship with her mother has been unusually conflictual (Ritvo, 1988; Rocah, 1984). The bisexual appearance and openly expressed sadism of teenage musical idols may be accounted for by their implications about these girls' ideal self-representations. Through the use of more abstract transitional phenomena, the adolescent girl whose earlier relationship with her mother has been "good enough" is able to develop a hierarchical drive organization where preoedipal drive derivatives are subordinated to oedipal ones and pregenital aims are relegated to foreplay (Blos, 1962; Sugarman & Jaffe, 1989). Such a drive organization, of course, is played out on the body self through the sexual experimentation characteristic of this stage.

Compounding the strain on the adolescent's representational world is the narcissistic vulnerability that strains the self-representation and makes the task of integrating the body representation into the self-representation even more difficult. Both ego ideal and superego prohibitions are reworked and altered during adolescence. Under the developmental thrust toward individuation and psychological emancipation, the ego and superego, as well as the representations that comprise them, are weakened (Blos, 1962). Deidealization of the parental representations occurs leading to a desperate search for new idealizations until more discriminating identifications with the more realistically seen parents can be developed (Tyson & Tyson, 1984). The ideal self-representation is modified and elaborated as part of this process. An emphasis on the ideal body occurs early in the deidentification process, as having an ideal body is used to compensate for the loss of the previously idealized object representations. Only mature shifts in superego and ego ideal can insure autonomous narcissistic regulation and invulnerability to the pathological depression that follows from this search for an ideal body.

> The ideal forms of behavior until adolescence are aimed at assuring the love from the original objects or their equivalence in the superego. In adolescence, the ideal toward which one strives has the added important role of helping the person to free himself from the original source of narcissistic supply and of paving the way to emotional maturity. (Laufer, 1964, p. 210)

But such reworking of the realistic and ideal self-representations, and the need to give up old identifications while developing new ones, mean that the self-representation is in such flux during this stage that the enormous task of differentiating and integrating a new body representation can become only one more drain on the psychic economy.

Complicating the matter even further is the cognitive maturation of this stage. The shift from concrete to formal operational thinking (Inhelder & Piaget, 1958) characteristic at this stage eventually allows for a superordinate self-representation that has greater stability and is able to integrate diverse and separate images of the self into one integrated representation (Sugarman & Jaffe, 1990). It is this added cognitive ability that allows for the predominance of symbolic over somatic expressions of subjective experience, which is necessary for successful integration of preoedipal, negative oedipal, and positive oedipal impulses generated by this developmental stage. But this transition into a new cognitive level carries with it a temporary egocentrism that becomes another source of dynamic pressure and anxiety (Erlich, 1978). Abstract ideals and concepts tend to be treated concretely and vice versa, so that developmentally less mature impulses or conflicts can be treated in both concrete and abstract ways simultaneously. Thus, the search for the new ideals and narcissistic equanimity can be concretized as the ideal body representation substitutes for the more abstract ideals that characterize this stage. When development continues in a progressive manner, however, the more abstract and integrated self-representation emerges to allow a successful transition to early adulthood.

DISRUPTION OF BODY SELF DIFFERENTIATION AND INTEGRATION IN BULIMIA

Development goes awry in those teenage girls who develop bulimia. Overwhelming clinical evidence reports that they have problematic interactions with their mothers (Berlin, Boatman, Sheimu, & Szurek, 1951; Ceasar, 1977; Chediak, 1977; Jessner & Abse, 1960; Krueger, 1988; Lorand, 1943; Rampling, 1978; Ritvo, 1988; Selvini-Palazzoli, 1974; Sours, 1969a, 1969b; Sugarman & Kurash, 1982; Sugarman, Quinlan, & Devennis, 1981; Woodbury, 1966). Many of these mothers tend to be narcissistic women whose relationships with their own mothers were disturbed. Such women tend to be the sort who have trouble being sufficiently attuned to their infant daughters to help them learn to convert somatic communication into verbal, symbolic modes (Edgcumbe, 1984; Krueger, 1988; Krystal, 1988). In other cases, these mothers have been depressed and emotionally unavailable during infancy because of a deteriorating marriage or other life stressors. Regardless of motive, such maternal self-absorption results ultimately either in the daughter's defensive failure to verbalize affect, with affect regulation attributed to the maternal representation (Krystal, 1988), or in a developmental arrest wherein affect regulation is never integrated into the self-representation (Krueger, 1988; McDougall, 1974). The latter difficulties tend to be relative, so that only a small percentage of such women have been truly arrested. More often, a vulnerability and fixation develops that allows for regression when later development proves too difficult.

Not surprisingly, such early misattunement makes separation–individuation a difficult stage for these girls (Chediak, 1977; Masterson, 1977; Sugarman & Jaffe, 1987). A sadomasochistic relationship with the mother and sometimes the father can lead to splitting of ambivalence and a poorly integrated self-representation. Such excessive sadomasochism often results in a sexualization and/or aggressivization of the body self that can lead to motoric inhibition and other constrictions or distortions in the body representation. The early connection between the body self and the object representation from which it first differentiated results in somatic regulation's remaining only tenuously integrated into the expanding self-representation. Anna Freud stressed the vulnerability of such self-regulation when she stated, "The processes of feeding, sleeping, evacuation, body hygiene, and prevention of injury and illness have to undergo complex and lengthy development before they become the growing individual's own concern" (1965, p. 68). Regulation of bodily processes is all too easily ascribed to the maternal introject, given the early interconnectedness between body self and maternal representation.

Such mother–daughter problems make oedipal engagement particularly problematic for such women. Penis envy associated with conflicts over identifying with the mother's body occurs. Consequently, such a girl regresses to a preoedipal position that can masquerade as a triadic, negative oedipal conflict, or she engages a true negative oedipal position (Edgcumbe et al., 1976). Either scenario leads to the maintenance of bisexual conflicts that are displaced onto the body (Ritvo, 1984, 1988). It remains an empirical question whether such girls are then predisposed to more tomboyish behavior and masturbatory conflicts during latency than other girls. The ones I have treated report a tendency to have been chubby during latency, indicating that their intense preoedipal and negative oedipal conflicts were already being displaced onto their bodies. In one way or another, they react to their narcissistic mothers' conception of the ideal body—either by rebelling or by conforming. The latter mode of trying to comply with the mother's image of the ideal body could be seen in one adolescent girl who had spent her latency striving to be an Olympic-caliber gymnast. Yet she also "accidentally" severed a finger while playing with a friend, highlighting the unconscious sadomasochism being displaced into the body self, as well as her unconscious rebellion via masochistic channels. By the time she entered adolescence, she had developed both bulimia and a somatoform pain disorder, wherein soft tissue damage in her back that could not be verified by medical tests inhibited her gymnastic and cheerleading activities.

Such girls are woefully unprepared for adolescence. As their bodily changes make their body selves more clearly approximate their mothers' bodies, it becomes easier to equate (unconsciously) their body represen- tation with the maternal representation. Thus, they easily displace their numerous conflicts with their mothers onto their bodies. Such displace- ment, fueled by the egocentric confusing of concrete and abstract (Erlich, 1978), leads them to experience their bodies as though they were in- dependent objects, like their mothers. This concreteness and displace- ment are probably what lead Selvini-Palazzoli (1974) to conclude that the body becomes experienced as a persecutory object that must be con- trolled totally, lest it devour or smother the patient. Unfortunately, her Kleinian emphasis tends to reify this defensive displacement and con- cretization.

Numerous unconscious conflicts can be expressed via the gorging and purging of the bulimic syndrome. Sadomasochistic conflicts, for example, are expressed, in regard to the torture of the body, which is equated with the maternal representation; the control that is attempted over the body has a sadistic quality (Boris, 1988; Mintz, 1988; Oliner, 1988; Ritvo, 1984, 1988). The misguided attempt to keep the body slim can be an attempt by such a woman to maintain a masculine body self, which can then compete with men for the sexual love of the mother (Ritvo, 1988). Dependent conflicts can be expressed via the bingeing, while hostile repudiation and an attempt to maintain autonomy can be expressed through purging (Sugarman et al., 1981; Sugarman & Kurash, 1982; Krueger, 1988; Reiser, 1988). In those occasional borderline bulim- ics, the alternating between bingeing and purging may even serve to maintain the self–other boundary (Sugarman & Kurash, 1982). Finally, struggles with narcissistic equilibrium can be expressed via the body self. An emphasis on the ideal body self and the bulimic adolescent's struggles to attain it can help her to avoid the more profound sense of despair and inadequacy associated with her defensively distorted, preoedipal idealiza- tion of her mother. Failures to attain this ideal can be circumscribed, so that a more encompassing sense of self-criticism and failure is avoided (Joffe & Sandler, 1967). In this way, the discrepancy between the ideal self-representation and the actual self-representation can be minimized.

CASE EXAMPLE

The psychoanalytic treatment of a young female bulimic, who clearly demonstrated the displacement of the numerous conflicts discussed above into her body, is now presented. Her treatment illustrates not only this defensive displacement, but the way in which these conflicts may become expressed and finally resolved in the transference.

Background

B. was a 18-year-old college sophomore when she sought psychoanalytic treatment for what she termed her "problems," the nature of which she had difficulty articulating without active questioning by me. Such an unusually active stance during the initial consultation led her to clarify hesitantly that she needed help with the emotions that had caused her high school drinking and bulimia. Although not actively bulimic at the time of the consultation, she felt that her long-standing feelings of being lonely, unloved, and lacking in self-confidence left her still vulnerable to the reoccurrence of both symptoms; so did her depression and angry ruminations about her mother.

Her drinking and bulimia were precipitated by a high school boyfriend's terminating their relationship without warning or explanation. At the time of the breakup, she concluded that she must be horrible to have driven him away. Her bulimic symptoms began with a weight gain of 15 pounds and the emergence of intense feelings of loneliness and estrangement after being jilted. Vomiting was used to lose weight, and she rapidly lost 25 pounds. Soon, however, she began to binge and compulsively purge at the same time every day whenever she felt stressed and depressed. She became paradoxically more detached from her friends at this time, despite her conscious hope to gain friends and admiration through being thin and attractive.

B. understood her symptoms as related vaguely to her rage toward her mother at the time of the consultation. She felt that her bingeing and purging relieved her internal tension and all her "horrible feelings" toward her mother. She had always binged and purged when she returned home from school every day. This behavior helped to "numb" her to the mother's increasingly erratic and inappropriate behavior, following her mother's second divorce during B.'s preadolescence. Her own father remained a benign but ephemeral figure during her adolescence despite his weekend custody of her, since the divorce from B.'s mother when B. was young. His own remarriage had been a successful one, and B. reported feeling close to his wife.

The Early Phase of the Analysis

B. began the analysis by asking whether she should put her feet up on the couch; the passivity and dependency implicit in this request were harbingers of things to come. Much of her early content involved bitter recriminations toward her mother, accompanied by intense sobbing. Weeks went by in which she literally spent most of the sessions crying. Both preoedipal dependent longings and negative oedipal wishes seemed to be the impulses that she so desperately had wanted her mother to gratify. Evidence of the latter could be seen in her casual mention of her mother's current husband during the first quarter of the analysis. She seemed surprised when I noted that she had failed to mention this marriage during our evaluation; then she realized that most of her friends also did not know of this marriage. She acknowledged that her dislike and contempt for her stepfather's deference toward her had contributed to her oversight. Soon B. remembered how she used to spend time in front of the mirror, listening to music, and playing out her fantasies "about guys" during her bulimic episodes in high school. Thus, she linked her bulimic symptoms to displaced sexual impulses quite early, although her inability to articulate the fantasy content of these masturbatory equivalents made it impossible to be precise about the nature of her impulses.

B. showed a consistent pattern during the early phase of the analysis to move from sexual to oral content quickly. My effort to bring her complaints about her mother's "bitchiness" into the transference led to these complaints about oral and narcissistic deprivation being expressed toward me. She began to complain about my silence, my failures to reassure her overtly, my ending the sessions on time, and my expectation that she take responsibility for having her parents pay the bill. Simultaneously she took to wearing low-cut sweaters and blouses to sessions while alluding to guilt about her sexuality, with the suggestion that she might be keeping sexual secrets from me. Oral and sexual conflicts remained condensed within the early transference.

Increasingly B. felt disappointment with my passivity and silence, and sought gratification outside the sessions through drinking, smoking marijuana, and taking up cigarette smoking. She liked a brand of cigarettes called Close, seemingly to counteract what she felt to be the lack of closeness between us. Promiscuity began, unabated by her intellectualized insight into how she looked to men to compensate for her many disappointments with her mother. As she began to emphasize more orally and anally demanding content, she began to enact such wishes in the transference. Specifically, she expressed a wish that I actively read her mind and drag her uncomfortable thoughts and feelings out of her. Long silences began to occur as she moved into a stance of feeling victimized and let down by me.

B.'s acting out through bulimic equivalents (Wilson, 1988) increased as marijuana and cocaine began to be used nightly. She began to treat her roommate sadistically after the roommate "betrayed" her by telling mutual friends about B.'s adolescent bulimia. These concerns about others' revealing her secrets led to fantasies about the colleagues and supervisors with whom I might share information about her. But the content of these fantasies were withheld as she cried over her inability to trust me. Sessions took on a repetitive pattern of 15- to 20-minute silences, followed by truncated statements that were punctuated by further silences and conscious withholding. It was not unusual for her never to complete a sentence during this early phase of her treatment. Passive, masochistic pleas that she was unable to talk gave way occasionally to short-lived admissions of active withholding. She acknowledged that revealing herself to me made her feel powerless during these rare moments of insight. I would know more about her than she did herself. Furthermore, she would never know the details of my life, which again unbalanced the power in my favor. Thus she demonstrated early her issues around control and her quickness to defend her own sadism with masochistic victimization. And she also demonstrated her defense avoidance of expressing these impulses and feelings in a verbal, symbolic mode.

But B. was unable to keep her sadomasochistic conflicts within the transference. As her promiscuity intensified, she became attracted repetitively to troubled men who exploited her and failed to gratify her needs. She also began to engage in a pattern of disappointing others' expectations and then feeling misunderstood by their response without realizing her own provocations. Thus, she dropped out of school for a quarter but lied both to her parents and to her roommate about it. More blatant was her provoking an eviction from her apartment by transgressing almost every rule of the building. The childhood antecedents involved her disrespect for authority and regulations. She recalled how she could usually cry her way out of scrapes and was able to manipulate both her mother and father. Early in life, she had learned that manifest suffering could be used to control or to defy.

B.'s acting out reached its zenith when I did not gratify a request for an extra Monday session as we drew close to the summer vacation at the end of her first year of analysis. Her mother and father called (separately) over the weekend to inform me that the patient had spent a large amount of money in the first 8 months of her analysis and had depleted her financial resources. Her father feared that she was addicted to drugs, while her mother fretted about her overdependence on me. Both parents and the patient, during her admission of the predicament, talked as though the analysis accounted for the amount spent; in reality it accounted for 10% of it. She admitted to an illusion that the money would last forever; soon, anger at her parents' refusal to pay for the analysis surfaced. But she still remained unaware of her own provocativeness; consequently, I suggested that spending all the money might be her expression of anger at her father. She then admitted to wanting to rub her father's nose in her financial irresponsibility, and, by extension, his failure as a parent. Because much of the money had been a gift from her maternal grandmother, she could similarly gloat over her mother's discomfort and embarrassed fear of admitting the deed to the grandmother. Finally, she acknowledged her wish to embarrass me in front of both her mother and father.

Separation–individuation and anal conflicts also became clear in the first year of the analysis. My request to be paid by the 10th of the month instead of the 30th led to painful revelations about B.'s contempt and disregard for authority and rules. Rules were felt as assaults to her autonomy, and so she rebelled against them. At the same time she struggled with conscious wishes for an idealized object, usually a man, to meet her needs. Thus, she complained that her own sense of self was ephemeral and largely unknown to her because she had so long tried to maintain the facade of happiness, gaiety, academic achievement, and compliance that she felt was necessary to be loved by her father.

The Emergence of a Transference Neurosis

B. began to admit her dependency on me as she approached midphase and the emergence of a transference neurosis. In direct and indirect ways, she let me know that I and the analysis were the most important relationship in her life. Her grudging and helpless description of a typical week poignantly captured her plight: "During the week I find myself not doing much during the day, like I'm waiting for the next session. After Friday I can get things done." Such dependence was terrifying to her because of both her fear of rejection and her fear of relinquishing her efforts to separate and individuate. Anger, retentiveness, and devaluation were all used to keep me at a safe distance.

The early transference neurosis coalesced around a paternal transference as I became the idealized academic whom B. could not please. She hated for me to see any "weakness" or "failure" in her because she would feel humiliated. Turning her passive experience of being scrutinized by me into active scrutinizing led her to begin to search through library abstracts to find out information about me. Finding some of my publications and previous academic affiliations led her to feel that she was being "analyzed by Superman" and only added to the pressure that she felt to meet my standards. Her wishes to be regarded so highly made it difficult to find ways of phrasing interventions that would not feel critical. To focus on a "problem" felt to her like an attack for not being perfect. When she began shamefully to reveal the details of her high school bulimia, she felt particularly embarrassed admitting how she would "mark" where she had started bingeing with some clearly discernible food so that she would know when to stop vomiting. Out of a misguided attempt at support, I reassured her that such "marking" was not uncommon. Not surprisingly, she became enraged at my treating her "like a statistic and categorizing" her. I was all too aware of feeling provoked and angry with her during this period, as it seemed that whatever I said only incited her.

Some progress was made toward clarifying the defensive nature of B.'s sadomasochistic interactions after I took a 2-week vacation that "spoiled" our first anniversary. Adding insult to injury was her suspicion, a correct one, that I was gone because my wife had delivered a baby. She was reading Judith Rossner's novel *August* when I returned, and soon brought me a photo album in the way that the patient in the book brought sketches to her analyst. This album had been put together by her mother and marked a shift to a maternal transference neurosis. She berated me for not caring, and complained that I only cared about my training, not her, when I took longer to look through it than she desired. I interpreted that she wished I would be like the mother she had always wanted and say that I loved her. Her confused associations to this interpretation revolved around the statement that it hurt too much to be so involved. I then suggested that she used sex, silence, and drinking to distance herself and not feel the pain of these wishes. In response, she "remembered" how she would fantasize saying "I love you" during her bulimic binges and would hear the words "Marry me" at those times.

Wishes that I become active and teach her soon followed, amidst complaints that her mother had never taken time to do so. She began to complain more openly of my lack of magical powers as her maternal transference neurosis deepened. She felt hurt that I failed to foresee the future and warn her about the consequences of her actions. Sadomasochism flared up around another vacation of mine as she missed sessions, requested schedule changes at the last moment, and began having intercourse without birth control. Her fantasy of being overwhelmed by finding that she was pregnant while I was on vacation spoke to her self-destructive expressions of rage. The competition over my wife's presumed pregnancy was inaccessible at this time.

B. developed another somatic symptom within the transference as a full-fledged maternal transference evolved, illustrating her vulnerability to regress to somatic pathways of communication. Thus, she began to worry frequently about losing control of her bladder and/or needing to use the bathroom during our sessions; in fact, several sessions were interrupted by trips to the bathroom. Her shame made it impossible to clarify the nature of these bathroom impulses, but the speed of her return suggested that she was urinating. This symptom appeared to be another bulimic equivalent. She feared discussing the matter in our sessions, as she anticipated that talking about it would only stimulate her urgency, just as interpretation of impulse in young children is likely to lead to its expression.

At first the symptom seemed a symbol of B.'s fear of losing control of her anger, because it initially emerged in a discussion of her hatred toward her mother. My interpretation that she was displacing her anger from me onto her mother led her to interrupt that session to go to the bathroom, confirming the interpretation somatically. But the symptom was multiply determined and so did not abate with this interpretation. Soon she interrupted another session for the bathroom in the midst of repeating my words to her during a frankly sexual transference dream. In that dream she stated her plans to leave town and I begged her to stay, saying that I had the same feelings that she did. Interpretation of her fear of letting go of her sexual impulses led to the symptom's temporarily disappearing, but failed to allow her to discuss her sexual fantasies openly.

The layering of meanings in this bulimic equivalent highlighted how B.'s anger was used as a defense against her sexuality. But remaining immersed in a sadomasochistic maternal transference neurosis continued to be more comfortable for her than the homosexual impulses associated with her negative oedipal feelings, just as she preferred anger to acknowledging her sexual tie to her mother. The ego syntonicity of her sadomasochism in the transference posed a troublesome technical problem, however. She could easily acknowledge her hurt, anger, and retaliation for my vacations, silences, and interpretations; however, she would then tearfully demand to know why I continued to act in such a manner, since I knew that it was hurtful to her. It particularly hurt her that I did not seem to care as much about her as she did about me. Frequently she would bemoan her single-minded preoccupation with me and the analysis. She demanded stubbornly that I demonstrate my caring in just the manner that she wished. Just to listen and analyze meant that she was only a specimen whom I managed according to the rules of analytic technique. Her forays into the literature of psychoanalytic technique only documented both my technical appropriateness and the expectability of her responses; consequently, she felt further manipulated. She angrily berated me for making a mockery of our relationship by pretending to feel for her in order to facilitate the transference. Out of desperation, I began to make genetic links to her childhood feelings about her mother earlier than I usually do; these links allowed her to take some distance and to consider the intensity of her reactions.

Erotic feelings began to emerge in several dreams as we worked through some of B.'s rage and her fear of losing control of it. One dream involved her taking off her shirt in a class taught by a professor who claimed to be a lay analyst. Another one involved an obese child with an adult chest. Her associations always came back to fears of being exposed and having her "craziness" seen by me. Her exhibitionistic sexual impulses were seen as crazy, and so had to be defended through anger and/or withdrawal. Defensive flights back into sadomasochism, as well as her underlying dependency, were repeatedly worked through; this eventually allowed clear-cut homosexual material associated with negative oedipal conflicts to emerge.

Overt homosexual content was introduced through a series of dreams, none of which could be worked with consistently because of B.'s anxiety about their content. The first of them involved being in bed with her sister, who had male genitalia attached to her in some fashion. Soon afterward, she had another dream in which her sister "touched" her and brought her to orgasm. She stressed how uninterested in "touching" her sister she had been in the dream. Another dream in which she was kissing a female friend followed. Associations led to wanting to hit her sister in the face just as her stepbrother used to hit her. She then admitted a fantasy of seeing her female friend in conversation with me. Thus, sexuality remained a melange of sadomasochistic, negative oedipal, and positive oedipal impulses.

This series of dreams peaked with one wherein her mother and former stepfather excluded her while her own father made a sexual innuendo to her. Her sister than spilled coffee over her mother's rug in order to be mean. She associated to needing to protect her mother from her sister, which I interpreted as a defense against feeling excluded. She heard this interpretation as siding with her mother and refusing to believe her earlier accusations about her mother's actual malevolence. Realization of how much she wanted me to side with her led to remembering how much her mother's overt sexual interest in men had bothered her as a child. She recalled being told that she had disliked her former stepfather early in their relationship. Her wishes to be exclusively close to her mother had intensified in adolescence after the second divorce.

In part, B.'s passive dependency began to appear as a defensive regression from a negative oedipal constellation. She began to realize her positive feelings toward her mother as she hesitantly faced her jealousy that her mother had not rushed to her for comfort after the divorce. But her mother always seemed to withdraw in response to her advances, leaving her feeling that she must be passive and await the mother's overtures. Soon she lamented her need to be sexually attractive in order to have people like her; she felt that she had become popular only when her body matured. In addition, her mother had always been preoccupied with being sexually attractive.

B.'s anxiety about needing to go to the bathroom during the session resurfaced at this time, and more clearly had to do with her fear of losing control of her sexual impulses toward me as mother. She talked about passionately kissing her boyfriend during intercourse and thinking that even if she lost control of her bladder at that moment, he would understand. Her earlier problems of being unable to achieve orgasm with him became comprehensible as she realized how her sexuality had become inbued with urethral and anal connotations.

The next elaboration of her negative oedipal theme occurred via her idealization of a female professor who had everything—a career, a husband, and a baby boy. Her fantasies of having her own baby and an idyllic life felt so powerful that they made her cry in the session. Further associations to needing to lie in order to impress her professors and a fantasy about a little boy led me to reconstruct her fantasy that her mother would have loved her more if she were a boy. She remembered having thought this consciously and being mistaken for a boy during latency. A dream of her mother breastfeeding ensued and was followed by one in which her high school boyfriend was sucking her nipples after the death of his grandmother. She awoke from the dream wondering how she could ever breastfeed, since it was so erotic. Further associations indicated an unconscious assumption that being a male child would allow her to have her mother to herself.

Masturbatory anxieties from latency were alluded to when B. next remembered fearing that she had cancer from the fifth to seventh grades, because it hurt whenever she leaned against a table. For the first time, she acknowledged that her fear of going to the bathroom during sessions had begun when she bought a vibrator. At that point she had been feeling "not sure" whether she was having orgasms with her boyfriend, even though just kissing her high school boyfriend had always led to orgasm. She became obsessed with the vibrator and consciously equated it with her high school bingeing. Being able to bring herself to orgasm whenever and with whatever fantasies she wanted made it compelling, just as being in control of her weight had made her bingeing and purging so compelling. Thus, she could enjoy sex once she had her own penis. Her linking the vibrator with bingeing also suggested that the bulimia had, in part, expressed her unconscious wish to have a penis in order to actualize her homosexual impulses toward her mother.

These impulses toward her mother soon became more articulated within the transference, when it became easier for me to interpret her sadomasochistic demands as a defense against her fear of becoming sexually excited. She responded that she was not uncomfortable thinking about sex, just with telling me about her fantasies. A dream about her mother led to memories of masturbating on the bathroom floor as a child while she listened through the vent to her mother and stepfather having intercourse. Then she wondered whether she had sexual feelings for her mother. A sadomacochistic regression within the transference followed as a temporary defense against her sexualized maternal transference. Finally, her refusal to tell me the details of a dream in which she was tortured allowed me to interpret her wish that I sadistically force the details out of her. She responded with a dream in which she was babysitting my babies. I interpreted her wish to have my baby, to which she responded, "I knew you'd say that."

Looking in the phone book to see whether my wife's name was the same as a female psychologist listed in the *Psychological Abstracts* led B. to admit that she constantly fantasized about me and felt attracted sexually. Anger over being narcissistically deprived by me alternated with such material as did her crying that I did not care about her when I ended sessions on time. Cancellations, tardiness, and silence again were used to retaliate. Only when I interpreted that her acting out seemed a re-enactment of her adolescent feelings toward her mother did she regain control. She admitted that she had behaved the same way during adolescence. Anxiously, she realized that she felt out of control about her sexual feelings toward me. An immediate association to both her mother's uncleanliness and her mother's masculinity clarified the homosexual nature of the seemingly heterosexual transference. She found herself wanting to eat a great deal and began bingeing and purging, which she felt allowed her not to have to control her eating. I maintained analytic neutrality and chose only to analyze the symptoms rather than to focus on attenuating them. She explained that her excessive drinking aroused her sexually but that eating did not do so. At that point I prematurely interpreted her binge-eating as a defense against homosexual impulses. She puzzled over why I thought so, while emphasizing that her homosexual dreams did not seem so strange to her. Soon she recalled that she and a girlfriend used to kiss and hug each other in the fifth grade while pretending to be a male and female teacher. Then she began to worry that I would take away these fantasies, which felt crucial for maintaining narcissistic equilibrium.

Not surprisingly, B. regressed back to her preferred sadomasochistic stance and withheld associations, feelings, and insights from me because she felt so hurt and enraged that I would not encourage her, reward her, or say that I cared about her. But glimpses of insight into her depressive masochism did occur. At one point she recognized that being depressed meant that she was like her sister, mother, and maternal grandmother. Then she recalled a high school fantasy wherein she would be almost raped by her boyfriend's uncle and then enjoy the sympathy she gained. This adolescent beating fantasy (Novick & Novick, 1987) highlighted how suffering was a way to be dependent and narcissistically gratified. She then associated to wishing to be dependent and then to being angry at her mother for not taking her childhood anger seriously. Thus, her masochism reflected both an attempt to remain attached to a sadistic maternal introject and a defense against her guilt over her own considerable sadism.

Progress in the Analysis

A gradual and fluctuating increase in B.'s self-reflectiveness occurred after 3 years of working through these various conflicts. Prolonged silences, cancelled sessions, phone calls, and angry recriminations were punctuated more often by her attempts to understand her labile reactions in and out of the analysis, rather than to see them as justified. The prominent role of her own feelings in her conflicts began to become apparent. In particular, she realized her lifelong competition with her sister, as well as her identification with her sister's sadomasochism. Such insights led to greater acknowledgment of her passive, dependent longings. She even acknowledged her wish to remain dependent but complained that others would not support it. Then she talked about being so bad that nobody could like her. I interpreted that feeling so bad was an attempt to remain unique in order to be allowed to stay dependent. She responded by admitting that she was doing much better outside of the analysis than she was admitting to me.

Guilt over her sadism was expressed in a dream where B. killed somebody. Her associations led to how much she felt guilty in her life. Two weeks before another of my vacations, she underlined the defensive use of her anger with a dream to which she associated for an entire week. It was a lengthy, multisegmented dream starting with three people lying on beds, moving to dangerous sharks circling the beds, and ending with seeing a daughter beheaded by the father. She began her associations by negating the dream's sexual overtones and then associated to castration, menstruation, and me as the father in the dream. Toward the end of the week, she realized that she had become aware of the sexual implications of the dream while she was actually dreaming it and had negated them during the dream itself by intentionally moving the plot into violence. I interpreted the obvious defense of anger and violence to avoid her sexual impulses. She distinguished these sexual feelings from her manifestly sexual dreams about me early in the analysis. This time I seemed stilted in the dream, like her father, whereas she tended to be attracted more to men like her former stepfather. Then she recalled that this stepfather used to flirt with her when she would see him after he divorced her mother. Thus, more oedipal determinants to both her character pathology and her bulimia began to be more evident.

But B. remained more comfortable with a preoedipal stance. Her realization that her shyness was an attempt to seduce men led me to suggest an unconscious sexual motive to her continued insistence that I draw her out. She started crying and admitted that this motive was "not all that unconscious." When I then interpreted her subsequent anxiety as related to sexual feelings toward me, she talked about "needing so much."

Then she wondered whether she got more by not talking. She preferred to emphasize sex as a means to gratify oral needs. In this context, she became increasingly aware of how she used her anger to control her dependency, as she lamented caring so much. She actually quit the analysis for half a day in retaliation for my not caring enough at this point. But she returned, acknowledging her continued attempts to get the love and attention that she felt her mother had not provided her with as a child.

This acknowledgment led B. to realize that her sadomasochistic transference was also to avoid leaving the analysis. So long as her problems continued, she was obviously not ready to terminate. Soon she raised the question of termination as she considered a foreign fellowship. Her self-destructive failure at her interviews, however, insured that she would not need to terminate before she felt ready. Even her anxious checking of my publications in the library's abstracts every few months became a manifestation of her wish to remain dependent. Finally, I interpreted her wish to be uniquely pathological, so that I would keep our relationship alive forever by writing about it. Grudgingly, she admitted the possibility of this interpretation and went on to admit sexual fantasies toward a professor.

The magical thinking associated with B.'s anal sadism soon became highlighted as a source of resistance. It became clear that one of her motives for telling me so little about her external life had to do with her assumption that I magically could know what transpired without her telling me. A rather gross example occurred when she withheld the fact that she graduated from college. Her college career had been so erratic throughout the course of the analysis that I did not know how far along she was, even though I did realize she must be approaching the point of graduation. Thus, she graduated without ever telling me and then wondered why I failed to congratulate her. Little perspective was available into how unrealistic her expectation that I knew about it was.

But the contamination of B.'s sexuality by her anger did receive greater scrutiny. She realized that she was obsessed with being sexually attractive to men in order to make them uncomfortable over feeling so attracted to her. I interpreted how she used her sexuality both to express and to defend against her anger. She responded that she found trying to attract me a challenge, which she realized was motivated by her hostility. Then she wondered whether her anger at men had to do with her father and her first stepfather leaving her. Memories of being angry at this stepfather were mentioned. Soon she recalled how she would always accentuate her own happiness when visiting her own father, in order to sadistically highlight his own depressive personality.

Further work on her sadism led B. to wonder about her need to sabotage things in order to avoid the excitement she felt when they went well. She acknowledged keeping herself from obtaining things she wanted for reasons beyond her understanding. Then she realized how strange she felt during those rare moments when she did not feel guilty or bad. Memories of her victimizations during high school began to be recast as having been caused by her own need to suffer. For the first time, she revealed how she had rejected the boy who had sexually exploited her during high school whenever he tried to introduce emotional closeness into the relationship. She allowed herself only to have sex with him because that made her feel cheap and guilty. Plaintive questioning emerged about why she could not allow herself to enjoy anything. She realized that, in part, she feared doing things she would regret, were she to get overly excited by a sense of success; she would not expand on these fears, however. In addition, she feared that if she "got things together" her parents would abandon her, go off on their own, and feel good about their parenting.

This fear reverberated within the transference at the time B. graduated from college. For the first time, she assessed what she needed to do in order to finish the analysis. She realized that her goals for analysis had always been vague and had to do with improving her self-esteem and stopping drinking. A fear was voiced that at some point I would declare her problems to be solved and unilaterally terminate, just as her therapist during high school had written a paper claiming that his treatment had helped her a great deal. She realized, moreover, that part of her would like to stay forever in analysis.

Her realization of the connection between her masochism and dependent longings allowed me to connect them to her relationship with her mother. A dream about her mother led to associations about how her mother always ruined everything. But this externalization soon gave way to embarrassed acknowledgment that I was correct with my earlier interpretations about how much she still tried to please her mother. She realized that she always called her mother to keep her abreast of her life and then felt angry because her mother seemed to take over her successes. Therefore, she failed at life in order to rebel against what felt to be her mother's unfair demands. But she felt conflicted, since many of the things she wanted were the same as what her mother valued.

Soon there were enough negative oedipal and homosexual themes in B.'s associations to allow me to interpret that her sexual feelings kept her so tied to her mother. She remembered that one time her mother had offhandedly commented that her family was "bright and gay." Shamefully, she admitted knowing that these feelings were important and that she had been aware of sexual feelings toward her mother and other women growing up. But she wished that I would reassure her that such feelings were normal and acceptable to discuss. Negative oedipal material continued to build until she had a dream 2 months later wherein she occupied the pinnacle of a hierarchy of women. In the dream she wore no shirt and a girl from high school kissed her breasts. She felt very excited, but refused to let the girl know how excited it made her. Associations led to her wish to be important and that being important was highly valued by her mother. Thus, her negative oedipal wishes expressed her wishes to be as phallic and powerful as her mother.

The relationship between these wishes and B.'s bulimia were alluded to in a dream in which she was riding up in an elevator with Nancy Reagan. She saw an old boyfriend from high school and felt very important because she was accompanied by a famous person. After seeing him, she went to the bathroom and defecated food that came out in undigested sections. Snakes that were covered with a film also emerged. They moved rapidly; she slammed the toilet lid shut and went to tell her mother because she was so frightened by their fangs. Her first association was that something bad, like shit, was inside her. She went on to expound how different and important she felt being with somebody famous; this was linked to her mother's values. At that point she admitted suspecting that I would think the snakes represented something phallic. It seemed that the dream represented her unconscious wish to incorporate a maternal penis, which then led to her need to vomit it out.

Greater self-observation and awareness into her defensive externalization and displacing of her aggressive, dependent, and sexual impulses occurred. B. talked about how it had never been clear to her, in the analysis or outside it, that she had any effect on the other person or situation. I interpreted that she preferred to feel powerless because it made her uncomfortable to think that she could have power. She was struck by this possibility, but wondered why it would be. I suggested that being powerful felt like being her mother and that she did not want to be like her. She recalled how she had always wanted to be like her mother as a child. Now she always wanted a situation in which somebody would be like her mother and take care of her. I suggested that feeling powerful would preclude the option of somebody taking care of her. She hesitated and said that she did not know. Then she said, yes, that was the problem. She did not want to take care of herself because she wanted somebody else to do so. In retrospect, she had come to analysis to be taken care of 5 years earlier.

Termination

With this awarenes, she struggled between her wishes to remain in analysis and achieve the perfect state of self that she had fantasied, and her wish to apply to graduate school and get on with her life. An offer of a desirable fellowship to a prestigious graduate program proved too enticing, and she accepted that she could live with her analytic accomplishments, even though they were less than her idealized ones. Her choice of this program (which made her financially independent of her parents and put her 3,000 miles away from her mother) over one on the West Coast (which would have left her financially dependent) spoke to the resolution of many of her dependent and negative oedipal longings.

Not surprisingly, the termination phase was difficult for her. All the conflicts that underlay her bulimic symptomatology resurfaced and were worked through once more. Brief upsurges of drinking and bulimia occurred in this context, but were quickly mastered by her ability to use her insight, so that no extra analytic parameters were necessary. Finally, positive oedipal issues began to emerge, and for the first time she revealed how sexually stimulating her father and his second wife had been during her late latency and early adolescence. Some of the displacement of her oedipal longings from her father to her former stepfather were worked through. But these issues failed to achieve the prominence or intensity that her preoedipal and negative oedipal ones had occupied in the analysis. It remained unclear whether they were less important or better defended. Nonetheless, she achieved significant symptomatic and characterological improvement. After 5½ years, she left the analysis still mourning her failure to achieve her idealized self-aspirations, but with a far greater self-confidence and a sense of being in control of her own life than she had had when she began.

CONCLUSION

This patient's material reveals that her bulimic symptomatology was a compromise formation born of intrapsychic conflict. Her mother's emotional unavilability during her earliest years had undermined her ability to communicate in a verbal, symbolic manner. Instead, her communication of her dependent and narcissistic needs remained fixated at a somatic level and left her body representations insufficiently differentiated from her psychological self (Edgcumbe, 1984). In particular, she learned to externalize the regulation of these needs and saw first her mother, and then me in the transference, as responsible for regulating them. Conflict over gender identity developed from her ambivalent identification with her mother, her mother's body, and her mother's femininity. The defensive retreat from autonomy and fixation to a passive, masochistic posture characteristic of rapprochement difficulties ensued and was repeatedly enacted in the transference. Over time it became obvious that this defensive retreat also served to avoid the negative oedipal and positive oedipal conflicts that only emerged in the second half of the analysis. At each stage of development, this patient had difficulty integrating her body self with other key facets of her self-representation (self-as-child, self-as-daughter, and self-as-female). By latency she had concluded that her mother would have loved her more if she had been a male child with a male body. Thus, she displaced her conflicts into her body self. And adolescence was interpreted to bring happiness only when she had developed a mature and attractive body.

Her analysis bears out Ritvo's (1984, 1988) contention that bulimic patients displace their sadomasochistic and bisexual conflicts onto their bodies. Only as these conflicts could be displaced and externalized in the transference was the patient able to work them through and realize that her own self-representation as masochistic victim, and her complementary representation of her mother as powerful sadist, were not the veridical images of her childhood that she claimed. As she could acknowledge and resolve her dependent, sadistic, masochistic, and negative oedipal wishes, she could admit how her representations had been distorted by these wishes and her defenses and superego injunctions against them. Eventually such acknowledgment alleviated the need to defensively displace these conflicts into her body self. Her self-representation expanded as it came to include a sense of mastery and ability to regulate a variety of emotions and impulses that had previously been outside its aegis.

Throughout the analysis she demonstrated her tendency to regulate and express these various conflicts through somatic channels and bodily action. Bodily communication felt more safe than symbolic, verbal channels, because it allowed her to feel that she was not responsible for her impulses. She could avoid the guilt and anxiety she felt about trying to control them. It would be tempting to say that this woman used her body as a transitional phenomenon to regulate the immature conflicts over separation–individuation that she initially presented as her problems. But such a conclusion would be fallacious in her case; its acceptance would only lead to treatment stalemate if one accepted her distorted view of her mother and her childhood as all bad and colluded with her image of herself as helpless victim of her sadistic mother. Instead, it is crucial with such a patient to realize the defensive displacement from psychological self to body self that reduces the distance between her idealized self-representation and actual self-representation (Joffe & Sandler, 1967). This means of maintaining narcissistic equilibrium is an inherently fragile one, because it fails to address the discrepancy that is at the core of the low self-esteem. Essentially the patient says that the problem is not hers, it is her body's. The rigidity with which neurotically organized bulimics cling to their insistence that their problem is that their bodies are not perfect enough or that their symptom is their only problem highlights the brittleness of such a defense. Only when such a patient is helped to understand and accept her own feelings, impulses, and wishes rather than focusing on symptomatic relief can she revise her ideal self-representation and bring it in line with her actual self-representation. A better ability to tolerate the mother's imperfections and not exaggerate them for defensive purposes is a key step in this process. As this modification of ideal object representations occurred in this patient, she could regulate her nacrissistic equilibrium much better. She no longer had to maintain that she was a helpless infant, controlled by her body, and unable to enlist maternal help in regulating her impulses.

Such a case illustrates the need to distinguish diagnostically between the bulimic whose personality is so arrested that her body literally serves as a transitional phenomenon (Sugarman & Kurash, 1982; Sugarman & Jaffe, 1987), and the bulimic who defensively adopts such a stance because of intrapsychic conflict. This distinction parallels that between narcissistic and pseudonarcissistic personality disorders (Tyson & Tyson, 1982). Those patients whose problems arise from intrapsychic conflict should be treated with psychoanalysis, provided that their impulse control and psychological-mindedness make them suitable for such a treatment. Only the controlled regression offered by this treatment will allow their conflicts to emerge enough in the transference neurosis to allow the various defended impulses to be symbolically communicated and integrated into the psychological self. In this way the self-representation is expanded, and the body self becomes both more circumscribed and better integrated within the self-representation.

REFERENCES

Berlin, I., Boatman, M., Sheimu, S., & Szurek, S. (1951). Adolescent alteration of anorexia and obesity. *American Journal of Orthopsychiatry, 21,* 387–419.

Blos, P. (1962). *On adolescence—A psychoanalytic interpretation.* New York: Free Press.

Boris, H. N. (1988). Torment of the object: A contribution to the study of bulimia. In H. Schwartz (Ed.), *Bulimia: Psychoanalytic treatment and theory* (pp. 89–110). Madison, CT: International Universities Press.

Ceasar, M. (1977). The role of maternal indentification in four cases of anorexia nervosa. *Bulletin of the Menninger Clinic, 41,* 475–486.

Chediak, C. (1977). The so-called anorexia nervosa: Diagnostic and treatment implications. *Bulletin of the Menninger Clinic, 41,* 453–474.

Clower, V. (1977). Theoretical implications in current view of masturbation in latency girls. In H. Blum (Ed.), *Female psychology: Contemporary psychoanalytic views* (pp. 109–125). New York: International Universities Press.

Dowling, S. (1977). Seven infants with esophageal atresia. *Psychoanalytic Study of the Child, 32,* 215–256.

Edgcumbe, R. (1984). Modes of communication: The differentiation of somatic and verbal expression. *Psychoanalytic Study of the Child, 39,* 137–154.

Edgcumbe, R., & Burgner, M. (1975). The phallic–narcissistic phase: A differentiation between preoedipal and oedipal aspects of phallic development. *Psychoanalytic Study of the Child, 30,* 161–180.

Edgecumbe, R., Lundbert, S., Markowitz, R., & Salo, F. (1976). Some comments on the negative oedipal phase in girls. *Psychoanalytic Study of the Child, 31,* 35–60.

Erlich, H. S. (1978). Adolescent suicide, maternal longing and cognitive development. *Psychoanalytic Study of the Child, 33,* 261–277.

Freud, A. (1965). *Normality and pathology in childhood.* New York: International Universities Press.

Freud, S. (1961). The ego and the id. In J. Strachey (Ed. and Trans.), *The standard edition of the complete psychological works of Sigmund Freud* (Vol. 19, pp. 3–66). London: Hogarth Press. (Original work published 1923)

Frosch, J. (1964). The psychotic character: Clinical psychiatric considerations. *Psychiatric Quarterly, 38,* 81–96.

Furman, R. A. (1980). Some vicissitudes of the transition into latency. In S. I. Greenspan & G. H. Pollack (Eds.), *The course of life: Psychoanalytic contributions toward understanding personality development, V. II* (pp. 33–43). Adelphi, MD: National Institute of Mental Health.

Garfinkel, P., Moldofsky, H., & Garner, D. (1977). Prognosis in anorexia nervosa as influenced by clinical features, treatment, and self-perception. *Canadian Medical Association Journal, 117,* 1041–1045.

Goodsitt, A. (1983). Self-regulatory disturbances in eating disorders. *International Journal of Eating Disorders, 2,* 51–60.

Greenspan, S. I. (1979). *Intelligence and adaptation.* New York: International Universities Press.

Grossman, W., & Stewart, W. (1976). Penis envy: From childhood wish to the developmental metaphor. *Journal of the American Psychoanalytic Association, 24,* 193–212.

Hartmann, H. (1939). *Ego psychology and the problem of adaptation.* New York: International Universities Press.

Hoffer, W. (1950). Development of the body ego. *Psychoanlytic Study of the Child, 5,* 18–23.

Inhelder, B., & Piaget, J. (1958). *The growth of logical thinking from childhood to adolescence.* New York: Basic Books.

Jacobson, E. (1964). *The self and the object world.* New York: International Universities Press.

Jessner, L., & Abse, D. (1960). Regressive forces in anorexia nervosa. *British Journal of Medical Psychology, 33,* 301–312.

Joffe, W. G., & Sandler, J. (1967). On the concept of pain, with special reference to depression and psychogenic pain. *Journal of Psychosomatic Research, 11,* 69–75.

Kramer,. S., & Rudolph, J. (1980). The latency stage. In S. I. Greenspan & G. H.

Pollack (Eds.), *The course of life: Psychoanalytic contributions toward understanding personality development, V. II* (pp. 109–119). Adelphi, MD: National Institute of Mental Health.

Krueger, D. (1988). Body self, psychological self, and bulimia: Developmental and clinical considerations. In H. Schwartz (Ed.), *Bulimia: Psychoanalytic treatment and theory* (pp. 55–72). Madison, CT: International Universities Press.

Krystal, H. (1978). Self representation and the capacity for self care. *Annual of Psychoanalysis, 6,* 209–246.

Krystal, H. (1988). *Integration and self-healing: Affect, trauma, alexithymia.* Hillside, NJ: Analytic Press.

Laufer, M. (1964). Ego ideal and pseudo ego ideal in adolescence. *Psychoanalytic Study of the Child, 19,* 196–218.

Lichtenberg, J. (1978). The testing of reality from the standpoint of the body self. *Journal of the American Psychoanalytic Association, 26,* 357–386.

Lorand, S. (1943). Anorexia nervosa: Report of a case. *Psychosomatic Medicine, 5,* 188–292.

Mahler, M. S. (1981). Aggression in the service of separation–individuation: A case study of a mother–daughter relationship. *Psychoanalytic Quarterly, 50,* 625–638.

Mahler, M. S., & McDevitt, J. B. (1982). Thoughts on the emergence of the sense of self, with particular emphasis on the body self. *Journal of the American Psychoanalytic Association, 30,* 827–848.

Mahler, M. S., Pine, F., & Bergman, A. (1975). *The psychological birth of the human infant.* New York: Basic Books.

Masterson, J. (1977). Primary anorexia nervosa in the borderline adolescent. In P. Hartocollis (Ed.), *Borderline personality disorders* (pp. 475–494). New York: International Universities Press.

McDougall, J. (1974). The psychosoma and psychoanalytic process. *International Review of Psychoanalysis, 1,* 437–454.

Merleau-Ponty, M. (1962). *Phenomenology of perception.* Atlantic Highlands, NJ: Humanities Press.

Mintz, I. (1988). Self-destructive behavior in anorexia and bulimia. In H. Schwartz (Ed.), *Bulimia: Psychoanalytic treatment and theory* (pp. 89–110). Madison, CT: International Universities Press.

Novick, K. K., & Novick, J. (1987). The essence of masochism. *Psychoanalytic Study of the Child, 42,* 353–384.

Oliner, M. D. (1988). Anal components in overeating. In H. Schwartz (Ed.), *Bulimia: Psychoanalytic treatment and theory* (pp. 227–254). Madison, CT: International Universities Press.

Person, E. S. (1983). The influence of values in psychoanalysis: The case of female psychology. In L. Grinspoon (Ed.), *Psychiatry update: The American Psychiatric Association annual review* (Vol. 2, pp. 36–50).

Piaget, J. (1937). *The construction of reality in the child.* New York: Basic Books. Washington, DC: American Psychiatric Press.

Rampling, D. (1978). Anorexia nervosa: Reflections on theory and practice. *Psychiatry, 41,* 296–301.

Reiser, L. W. (1988). Love, work, and bulimia. In H. Schwartz (Ed.), *Bulimia:*

Psychoanalytic treatment and theory (pp. 373–398). Madison, CT: International Universities Press.

Ritvo, S. (1984). The image and uses of the body in psychic conflict: With special reference to eating disorders in adolescence. *Psychoanalytic Study of the Child, 39,* 449–469.

Ritvo, S. (1988). Mothers, daughters, and eating disorders. In H. Blum, Y. Kramer, A. K. Richards, & A. D. Richards (Eds.), *Fantasy, myth, and reality: Essays in honor of Jacob A. Arlow, M.D.* (pp. 423–434). Madison, CT: International Universities Press.

Robertson, J. (1962). Mothering as an influence on early development. *Psychoanalytic Study of the Child, 17,* 245–464.

Rocah, B. S. (1984). Fixation in late adolescent women: Negative oedipus complex, fear of being influenced, and resistance to change. In D. D. Brockman (Ed.), *Late adolescence: Psychoanalytic studies* (pp. 53–90). New York: International Universities Press.

Roiphe, H. (1968). On an early genital phase. *Psychoanalytic Study of the Child, 23,* 348–365.

Rosenblatt, A., & Thickstun, J. (1977). *Modern psychoanalytic concepts in a general psychology.* New York: International Universities Press.

Rosenthal, P. A. (1981). Changes in transitional objects: Girls in mid-adolescence. *Adolescent Psychiatry, 20,* 395–416.

Sandler, J. (1960). The concept of superego. *Psychoanalytic Study of the Child, 15,* 128–163.

Sandler, J., & Rosenblatt, H. B. (1962). The concept of the representational world. *Psychoanalytic Study of the Child, 17,* 128–145.

Schwartz, H. J. (1988). Bulimia: Psychoanalytic perspectives. In H. J. Schwartz (Ed.), *Bulimia: Psychoanalytic treatment and theory* (pp. 31–53). Madison, CT: International Universities Press.

Selvini-Palazzoli, M. (1974). *Self starvation: From the intrapsychic to the transpersonal approach in anorexia nervosa.* London: Human Context Books.

Sharpe, S. (1984). *Self and object representations: An integration of psychoanalytic and Piagetian developmental theories.* Unpublished doctoral dissertation, The Fielding Institute, Santa Barbara, CA.

Silverman, M. A. (1981). Cognitive development and female psychology. *Journal of the American Psychoanalytic Association, 29,* 581–605.

Sours, J. (1969a). Anorexia nervosa: Nosology, diagnosis, developmental patterns and power-control dynamics. In G. Caplan & S. Lebovici (Eds.), *Adolescence: Psychosocial perspectives* (pp. 185–212). New York: Basic Books.

Sours, J. (1969b). The anorexia nervosa syndrome: Phenomenologic and psychodynamic components. *Psychiatric Quarterly, 43,* 240–256.

Sugarman, A., & Jaffe, L. (1987). Transitional phenomena and psychological separateness in schizophrenia, borderline, and bulimic patients. In J. Bloom-Feshbach & S. Bloom-Feshbach (Eds.), *The psychology of separation and loss* (pp. 416–458). San Francisco: Jossey-Bass.

Sugarman, A., & Jaffe, L. (1988). Body representation in paranoid and undifferentiated schizophrenics. In H. Lerner & P. Lerner (Eds.), *Primitive mental states and the Rorschach* (pp. 229–254). Madison, CT: International Universities Press.

Sugarman, A., & Jaffe, L. (1989). A developmental line of transitional phenomena. In M. G. Fromm & B. L. Smith (Eds.), *The facilitating environment: Clinical applications of Winnicott's theories* (pp. 88–129). Madison, CT: International Universities Press.

Sugarman, A., & Jaffe, L. (1990). Toward a developmental understanding of the self schema. *Psychoanalysis and Contemporary Thought, 13*.

Sugarman, A., & Kurash, C. (1982). The body as a transitional object in bulimia. *International Journal of Eating Disorders, 1*(4), 57–67.

Sugarman, A., Quinlan, D., & Devennis, I. (1981). Anorexia nervosa as a defense against anaclitic depression. *International Journal of Eating Disorders, 1*(1), 44–61.

Taylor, G. J. (1987). *Psychosomatic medicine and contemporary psyschoanalysis*. Madison, CT: International Unversities Press.

Tyson, P. (1982). A developmental line of gender identity, gender role, and choice of love object. *Journal of the American Psychoanalytic Association, 30*, 61–68.

Tyson, P. (1986). Female psychosocial development. *Annual of Psychoanalysis, 14*, 357–373.

Tyson, P., & Tyson, R. L. (1984). Narcissism and superego development. *Journal of the American Psychoanalytic Association, 32*, 75–98.

Tyson, R. L., & Tyson, P. (1982). A case of "pseudonarcissistic" psychopathology: A reexamination of the developmental role of the superego. *International Journal of Psycho-Analysis, 63*, 283–293.

Wilson, C. P. (1988). Bulimic equivalents. In H. Schwartz (Ed.), *Bulimia: Psychoanalytic treatment and theory* (pp. 489–522). Madison, CT: International Universities Press.

Winnicott, D. (1953). Transitional objects and transitional phenomena. *International Journal of Psycho-Analysis, 34*, 89–97.

Wolff, P. (1960). The *developmental psychologies of Jean Piaget and psychoanalysis* (Psychological Issues, Monograph No. 5). New York: International Universities Press.

Woodall, C. (1987). The body as a transitional object in bulimia: A critique of the concept. *Adolescent Psychiatry, 14*, 179–184.

Woodbury, M. (1966). Altered body-ego experiences: A contribution to the study of regression, perception, and early development. *Journal of the American Psychoanalytic Association, 14*, 273–303.

∴ *2* ∴

Bulimia, Dissociation, and Empathy: A Self-Psychological View

SUSAN SANDS
*Stanford University
and The Wright Institute, Berkeley*

In this chapter I use a self-psychological perspective to challenge a central self-psychological belief: Namely, that if one provides an empathic environment and analyzes the patient's fears of retraumatization, the archaic narcissistic needs will be spontaneously mobilized within a self-object transference. I suggest that the situation is more complicated in the case of eating disorders (or other addictive disorders) in which the archaic needs have been dissociated and then detoured into eating-disordered pathology, and, as a consequence, are not as available to fuel a self-object transference.

I propose first that it is not enough to see bulimia as a symptom; rather, the bulimic symptomatology must be viewed as the behavioral component of a split-off bulimic *self*, with needs, feelings, and perceptions quite different from the patient's ordinary self-experience. Second, I suggest that one must actively seek out and empathize directly with the bulimic self in order to uncover the archaic needs embedded within it. Finally, I argue that it is particularly important to empathize with the *healthy*, albeit distorted, attempts of the bulimic self to express the archaic nuclear needs.

The task of approaching this hidden self is an intricate one, for it is by nature paradoxical and secretive. In this chapter I use clinical examples to address various technical questions that arise in working with the bulimic self or, more generally, with any such subjectively experienced "splits" in the personality. First, however, I present a brief conceptualization, from a self-psychological perspective, of the development of eating disorders.

THE DEVELOPMENT OF EATING DISORDERS

Eating disorders are disorders of the self—that is, they are disorders that develop due to chronic disturbance in the empathic interplay between the growing child and the caregiving environment. The child's genuine narcissistic needs, as well as the affects that surround them (Stolorow, Brandchaft & Atwood, 1987), are not empathically responded to, because they somehow threaten the caregivers' narcissistic equilibrium. As a result, these needs and affects are disavowed, repressed, or split off from the total self-structure. The child's developing self thus incurs structural deficits in its capacities for self-cohesion, temporal stability, and self-esteem regulation (Stolorow et al., 1987), which render it susceptible to fragmentation and depletion.

At some crucial point in development, the individual invents a new, restitutive system by which disordered eating patterns rather than people are used to meet self-object needs, because previous attempts with caregivers have brought disappointment, frustration, or even abuse. Kohut (1977, 1978, 1984) and others writing from a self-psychological perspective (Brenner, 1983; Goodsitt, 1984; Geist, 1985; Gehrie, 1990; Zadylak & St. Pierre, 1987) have consistently viewed eating disorders as attempts to supply missing self-object functions, as have object relations theorists like Sugarman and Kurash (1982), Krueger (1989), or McDougall (1980), the latter of whom conceptualizes addictive processes as attempts to "make an external agent do duty for a missing symbolic function" (p. 385). Food is, of course, a particularly compelling self-object substitute, since it is developmentally a first bridge between self and self-object—a first medium for the transmission of soothing and comfort.

By turning to food, the eating-disordered individual tries to circumvent the need for human self-object responsiveness and to avoid further disappointment and shame. Food is seen as trustworthy, while people are not. The new system also allows the individual to maintain some sort of connection with his or her (most often her; see below) caregivers by relieving the relationship of the burden of having to meet the individual's self-object needs. Because the food and eating rituals are seen as the only reliable self-objects, they are defended with as much ardor as the self-object connection to a human being.

It has been my experience that the disordered eating behavior most often substitutes for *idealized* self-object functions (Sands, 1989). It provides soothing and comfort, helps regulate painful affect states, like anger, depression, or shame, and it is also seen as omnipotent—that is, capable of curing any and all ills. Indeed, many patients describe their relationship with particular foods as one might talk about a passionate love affair. One time when I naively asked a patient what would happen if she let herself eat just a little of her favorite binge food, she hesitated, looked worried, and said, "If I could just eat it like that, any time I wanted to, it wouldn't be so wonderful . . . you have to have something to love." For a smaller subset of patients, the bulimia activates unconscious fantasies of grandiose omnipotence. Indeed, the act of vomiting itself can be regarded by the patient as a highly developed and refined athletic skill, as will be illustrated later in this chapter.

Previously, I have suggested how an understanding of three problem areas specific to female development can help explain women's greater susceptibility to eating disorder pathology (Sands, 1989). First, the culturally determined, distorted mirroring of little girls' exhibitionism, particularly the selective and ambivalent focus on physical appearance, encourages the use of the body as a pathway for expressing exhibitionistic concerns later on. Second, the relative paucity of idealizable female figures interferes with the internalization of self-regulatory functions, later necessitating external self-soothing mechanisms such as eating disorders. Third, the fact that little girls are usually the same sex as their primary caretakers can lead to their misuse as narcissistic extensions of their mothers and, consequently, to the need to create self-definition through behaviors such as eating disorders.

The problem with the new restitutive system organized around food or other substances is that it does not "work," because the self-regulatory functions it provides, while often seductively powerful in the moment, are only temporary. These self-object functions cannot be taken in and transformed into self-structure through the gradual transmuting internalization process. The individual remains dependent on using an external agent or action to fill in for missing internal structure. Kohut (1978) writes of addictive processes in general:

> It is the tragedy of all these attempts at self-cure that the solutions they provide are impermanent, that in essence they cannot succeed. . . . They are repeated again and again without producing the cure of the basic psychological malady. . . . no psychic structure is built; the defect in the self remains. It is as if a person with a wide-open gastric fistula were trying to still his hunger through eating. He may obtain pleasurable taste sensations by his frantic ingestion of food, but, since the food does not enter the part of the digestive system that absorbs it into the organism, he continues to starve. (pp. 846–847)

Moreover, once this new restitutive system based on disordered eating patterns is employed, the individual's development is derailed.

The structure-building process is severely disrupted as eating rituals are substituted for self-object responsiveness. The early needs remain split off and cannot be integrated into the adult personality. If the eating-disordered individual is fortunate enough to find her way into psychoanalytic treatment, she will find it a long and arduous journey back to the primary route—the route by which the individual dares to seek *human* responsiveness in order to complete her self-development.

With the majority of self-disordered patients, the early self-object needs will be mobilized spontaneously within a self-object transference if one provides an empathic environment and analyzes the resistances to developing such a transference. In the case of eating-disordered patients or patients with other addictive disorders, however, the situation is slightly more complicated. As described above, the archaic self-object needs in the eating-disordered individual are not only repressed or split off; they have been detoured into eating-disordered pathology and thus are less available to fuel a self-object transference. Thus, waiting for the needs to emerge as the self-object transference unfolds is often not enough—a fact that I do not think has been sufficiently acknowledged by self psychologists working with eating disorders. I believe that we must more actively search for and rekindle the needs by empathizing directly with the bulimic self. Only then can a self-object transference develop.

THE BULIMIC SELF

The archaic self-object needs that have been repressed and detoured into eating-disordered pathology have, more precisely, been split off into what is subjectively experienced as a bulimic *self*. The bulimic symptoms are but the behavioral component of a sector of the self with a set of needs, feelings, perceptions, and behavior that has been dissociated from the patient's total self-experience. Thus the patient will feel more understood if the therapist talks with her about "the part of you that needs to binge and vomit" rather than referring to "the bingeing and vomiting." When the therapist talks more directly to the "bulimic self," he or she will often find that the patient has already given it her own personal label—for example, "the body," "the monster," "the little girl," the "dark side"—all of which are discussed further shortly.

Of course, the presence of various "splits" in the bulimic psyche has long been recognized, particularly by object relations theorists writing on the subject of bulimia who have described the conflicts between "good" and "bad" maternal introjects (e.g., Selvini-Palazzoli, 1978; Masterson, 1977), or, following Winnicott, between "false self" and "true self" (e.g., Jones, 1985; Johnson & Connors, 1987), or between "body self" and "psychological self" (e.g., Goodsitt, 1984; Sugarman & Kurash, 1982; Krueger, 1989). Those formulations that dichotomize "good" and "bad" internal objects can be dangerous. They can tempt the therapist to view these parts as all-healthy or all-pathological, or even to form an alliance with the patient against the "bad" bulimic self by, for example, trying to ignore it, eradicate it, or convince it to go away. In particular, those theories that conceptualize the purging or fasting as an attempt to destroy the "bad" object (e.g., Selvini-Palazzoli, 1978) can be misused by the therapist to overlook the healthy, self-defining functions of the bulimic's behavior.

Moreover, the patient herself asks the therapist to see her bulimia in a negative light. She comes into treatment complaining of her bingeing or her vomiting or her laxative abuse, and tries to enlist the therapist's help in eradicating the symptom. However, if the therapist were to undertake this charge literally, he or she would be making a serious error, for the patient's deepest and most archaic self-object needs are interwoven with the symptom. The patient, moreover, unconsciously recognizes the value of the bulimic self and holds it sacred. Nor is it enough simply to explore the "function" of the eating-disordered symptom. As shall be seen shortly, talking with the patient *about* the symptom yields dramatically different material than does directly addressing the bulimic self.

The bulimic symptomatology expresses and temporarily fulfills the needs of a sector of the self that is at odds with the patient's ordinary self-experience. In most cases of bulimia, the patient is more closely identified with the false, pleasing, perfectionistic self that has grown up in compliance with the narcissistic needs of the parent—the result of what Kohut (1971) calls a "vertical split" in the psyche. (See also Jones, 1985, or Johnson & Connors, 1987, for a discussion of "false self" in bulimia.) However, in a bulimic patient there can always be found this other more secret self, the bulimic self, which both symbolizes and expresses the more genuine, nuclear needs for emotional connection as well as for autonomy. I do not agree with Jones (1985) that the needs of the true self are expressed only through the binges and not through the purges. I think the true needs are communicated through both: The binges reveal the needs for nurturance and connection with the self-object; the purges express the needs for self-definition and separation for the self-object.

It is the highly paradoxical nature of the bulimic self that makes it so complicated both to approach and to engage. On the one hand, the patient experiences the bulimic self as negative and "not me" because it is self-destructive and out-of-control, almost involuntary. It expresses the rage that usually follows when needs are unmet. Moreover, this punitive aspect of the bulimic self often involves experiencing the self as the unempathic parent—an identification with the aggressor. The lack of empathy for the body shown through the punitive bulimic behavior recapitulates the lack of empathy the patient experienced as a child. On the other hand, the bulimic self is unconsciously regarded by the patient as intensely positive, the only "true" part of her, because its actions are *for her*, not for her parents or anyone else. Because the bulimic self represents her urgent demand for selfhood, it is unspeakably precious to her. The bulimic behavior is thus both an assertion of self *and* a punishment for it. The patient will not begin to reveal her hidden self until its paradoxical and multidimensional nature is fully acknowledged and accepted. The therapist must let the patient know that he or she can appreciate the self-affirming as well as the self-destructive intentions of the bulimic self, and must also communicate a kind of reverence for this secret, sacred part.

The bulimic self is also paradoxical in that it is both an expression of and a defense against the archaic needs and feelings. It expresses and temporarily meets the needs, in that it *does* in fact provide temporary tension relief, euphoria, and so forth, as well as a sense of separateness. It operates as a defense in that it "numbs" the painful affects, like rage, surrounding the unmet nuclear needs. Thus, while the bulimic state protects the patient from fears of disintegration and depletion, it also prevents the needs and feelings hidden in this bulimic state from being mobilized, worked through, and integrated within the total self-structure. Moreover, the bulimic behavior numbs the patient's feelings to such an extent that it prevents her from processing current traumas in her life.

We can learn from those who study multiple personality disorder (e.g., Watkins & Watkins, 1988) who caution us never to make an enemy of any of the split-off parts of the patient's psyche. Since the bulimic self came into existence to protect the survival of the patient, its greatest fear (and hence source of resistance) lies in the conviction that the therapist is out to eliminate it. If the bulimic self is threatened with extinction, therefore, it will fight for its life—if need be, sacrificing other parts of the patient.

The Bulimic Self and Dissociation

The connection between bulimia and dissociation—a defense that serves to "compartmentalize and separate aspects of experience" (Spiegel & Cardeña, 1990)—needs further clarification. My own (incomplete) understanding of the role of dissociation in bulimia is as follows. When the nuclear needs (and the affects surrounding them) are not responded to empathically because they somehow threaten the caregivers' narcissistic equilibrium, they are split off from the total self-structure and may then be organized into a separate sector of the personality. Then, I propose, when the individual later begins to experiment with bulimia, the biochemical effects of the binge–purge cycle create an altered state that serves to reinforce the already existing split in the psyche and further organize the dissociated needs into a "bulimic self." The split-off state becomes associated with the bulimia, and the bulimic behavior becomes a way of voluntarily accessing this hidden self.

From those who use hypnosis to study multiple personality (e.g., Watkins & Watkins, 1988) comes increasing evidence that divisions within a personality are quite common and range along a continuum from normal adaptive differentiation at one end to multiple personality disorders at the other. My experience suggests that most bulimic patients subjectively experience internal splits to a lesser or greater degree. The extent of the organization of their early, dissociated needs into a distinct self-state varies, with those who have suffered the most traumatic breaches of empathy having the most distinct self-states. This observation is in line with mounting research evidence of a clear relationship between dissociative symptoms and childhood trauma.

That many bulimic patients are expert at dissociation is well-known to clinicians; in fact, there is research evidence (e.g., Pettinatti et al., 1985) in support of the dissociative abilities of bulimics.[1] Many portray their bingeing episodes as one might describe a trance state, drug trip, or delirium. Most become wholly identified with—"taken over" by—the bulimic self-state. No amount of cognitive persuasion or exhortation can stop them, because the bulimic self has been dissociated from the more reflective, observing self. The early needs *must* be expressed. To try to talk the bulimic self out of bingeing or purging is like telling a cat stalking a bird to stop its carnivorous pursuit. What the bulimic self *is* able to hear is, first, an acknowledgment of its deeper needs in the present, and then, later on, an explanation of its genetic roots.

I have found that many eating-disordered patients will report a history of dissociative abilities, particularly those, of course, who are in the "borderline" range of psychopathology and/or who have experienced the trauma of physical or sexual abuse. In fact, several of my bulimic patients have reported being "better" at dissociating spontaneously as children than they are now. One patient described how as a child she used to be able to "go numb" at will to find relief from her emotional pain, and how as she got older she began to lose this ability. During one session, she realized with a jolt that she was now using her bulimia and her drug use as external techniques to reach the same dissociative state she had been able to reach internally as a child.

The Bulimic Self and the Body

The bulimic self is at bottom a body self. It "speaks" through the body. The body, however, does not have language, so the archaic needs must be enacted. Self-object failure during the earliest years has undermined the patient's ability to communicate in a verbal, symbolic manner, and her deepest needs are still expressed at a somatic level. According to Sugarman et al. (1981, p. 46), she is "cognitively fixated at a level of sensorimotor self- and object-representations," wherein "the object can be internalized only as part of an action sequence." McDougall (1974) also believes that psychosomatic transformations (among which she includes eating disorders) represent a failure of symbolization, and she adds that they derail the capacity for psychic defense work, such as the creation of protective neurotic symptoms.

The bulimic self, therefore, is usually mute when treatment begins and will remain mute until, with the aid of the therapist's empathy, it is finally helped to verbalize its needs and feelings. Indeed, eating-disordered patients themselves indicate their lack of belief in verbal communication when, for example, they express the conviction that asking for what they want won't work. And it is precisely because they do not believe in the effectiveness of words that, when they *do* begin to assert their needs, they often either act them out or verbalize them in such a way as to insure that they do not get what they are asking for.

The child's early recruitment of the body to enact the deepest needs and conflicts is reinforced by her later experience in society and in her family (Sands, 1989). First, there is the general societal preoccupation with the female body and encouragement for females to display their exhibitionistic strivings through their physical appearance. Second, all evidence suggests that in families of eating-disordered patients there is a particular emphasis on physical appearance, and, more precisely, a pathological focus on body *fragments*. The child looks into the mirror of her parent and sees what Geist (1985) has called "a prismatic image of isolated parts," the impact of which is psychological fragmentation, loss of self-cohesion, and fixation on parts of the body (Kohut, 1971, 1977). I have argued that it is precisely because these children have been encouraged to offer the fragmented body for mirroring that they later in life tend to reveal their psychopathology through *bodily* symptoms, such as eating disorders. These patients use the body to express their deepest needs because this has been one of the few avenues of expression reliably open to them. This focus on bodily appearance and body fragments, to the exclusion of other parts of the self, leads both to the loss of cohesion of the body-self and to its lack of integration into the total self structure. Body exhibitionism becomes a continuing source of shame. In adolescence, when bodily concerns take central stage in development, the girl whose body-self-esteem is less intact because of early failures in attunement will have greater difficulty accepting her body's developing imperfections. She will experience her limitations as cruel narcissistic injuries, and she may develop an eating disorder to aid in self-restoration. It is because the body-self has not been integrated into the total self structure that our patients so often experience their bodies as somehow foreign and almost extraneous to the rest of their self experience, and why they are strangely indifferent to the needs of the body and to the damage inflicted by behaviors like binge eating and purging.

Approaching the Bulimic Self

It is the therapist's empathic stance that allows the needs and feelings hidden beneath the bulimic symptoms to be articulated, welcomed into the total self-structure, and experienced at last as part of "me." If the bulimic self is not empathized with, it will continue to clamor for attention, or it will go underground for a while, only to sprout up in unpredictable and often self-destructive manifestations. The reach of empathy—which can be defined as understanding the patient's expressions from *within* her subjective frame of reference (Stolorow et al., 1987)—extends beyond the patient's *conscious* productions. The accurate use of empathy requires that the therapist be able to respond to the patient in her totality—to acknowledge and simultaneously hold in mind as many different parts of the patient as possible, whether conscious or unconscious. This ability to hold all of the patient at one time is particularly important when the bulimic patient becomes wholly identified with the bulimic self-state and feels as if it were fully in charge of her personality.

Some patients may feel comfortable with our initially referring to the bulimic self as "you," but many do not, because this secret part has been split off from the main sector of the personality for as long as they can remember. In my experience, the process of approaching the bulimic self for the very first time often goes something like this: I sense the electricity in the room of a new, vulnerable presence; when I gently and empathically ask *about* her, the patient is then able to simultaneously feel her way into the bulimic part and use her observing self to communicate what the bulimic part is feeling. As the bulimic self becomes more integrated into the total self-structure, of course, it no longer has to be talked *about* and can more and more be addressed directly.

I must emphasize that in discussing the technical aspects of working with the bulimic self, I am *not* suggesting that we stray from the empathic openness of the psychoanalytic approach. I am not advocating the imposition of a particular systematic technique upon the patient. The therapist should not, for example, suggest to the patient that she has a hidden self, or, for that matter, suggest to the patient that she behave in *any* predetermined way. Rather, the patient's shy revelation of the bulimic self will usually be painstakingly slow, and will only come about after the therapist has interpreted again and again her fears of retraumatization and the patient has been assured of the safety of the therapeutic container. The purpose of this chapter is to alert therapists to the fact that many bulimic patients have dissociated self-states, so that therapists can better know what to look for and what to empathically pursue.

TECHNICAL ISSUES IN TREATMENT: CLINICAL ILLUSTRATIONS

The crucial turning point in case after case has come when the patient realized that I could empathize with—even appreciate—her bulimic self. In the clinical vignettes that follow, I address some of the technical questions that arise in working with the bulimic self.

The first case example illustrates how a patient will invariably present her bulimic self in the worst possible light to see whether the therapist will reject it as other important figures have denied her true needs and feelings. Marilyn, a 24-year-old bulimic patient, alternated between two distinct modes of being during the first 6 months of therapy. In the first mode, she would stringently "manage" her behavior and socially isolate herself to keep from getting into trouble. During these times she would present herself to me as righteously proud of her accomplishments, but anxiously "holding on" and fearful of "losing it." In the second mode, she would abandon herself to promiscuity and drug abuse, precipitating one emotional crisis after another, around which she would become intensely bulimic and suicidal. During these crisis periods she would make numerous emergency phone calls to me, presenting herself as an emotional "wreck" who was hopelessly out of control and unable to work or care for herself. Although she presented the "controlled" periods as desirable, it was clear that this "false self" was no fun at all and was maintained at a tremendous emotional cost. The bulimic, acting-out self, on the other hand, which was presented as completely unacceptable, was also clearly cathartic and stimulating. It was not until 6 months into treatment that she first alluded to the inner bulimic part of her. An excerpt from this session follows, in which she tested me to see whether I too would view this part as unhealthy:

> PATIENT: There's this monster in me that always has to "fuck up." She's bulimic. She takes drugs. She's mean to people. . . . I've got to get rid of her.
> THERAPIST: Wait a minute. I'd like to hear from her.
> PATIENT: *(Stares at me silently, questioningly.)*
> THERAPIST: She needs to be heard too.

PATIENT: Yes, she does. *(She suddenly looks like a little girl.)*

THERAPIST: I think she's pretty young.

PATIENT: *(Misunderstanding, feeling judged)* Oh, yeah. She's pretty immature sometimes.

THERAPIST: When I said "young," I was thinking about her feelings.

PATIENT: *(Long pause, then in a tiny voice)* That's because she's never been out.

THERAPIST: She hasn't had a chance to develop.

PATIENT: She's never talked with anybody. But you know what? She's the only part I love. . . . *(Sobbing for some time)* I think you can really help me.

I believe this was the very first time that the patient felt I *would* be able to help her. She was testing me by presenting her "bulimic self" in the terms her mother had used to determine whether I too would see her as a monster, while at the same time secretly continuing to treasure this hidden part of herself. She needed to know whether I really could accept all of her. If not, the most important part of her would again have to go underground and express itself through self-destructive acting out, in the hope that sometime someone would "hear" her.

I would now like to present another clinical vignette in order to clarify the distinction between talking with the patient *about* the bulimic symptoms versus addressing the bulimic self directly. Dorothy, a 46-year-old business executive, and I had explored the function of her bulimic symptoms and her relationship to her body many times over the course of treatment. During these discussions, she had many insights: that she ate when she was lonely; that she ate because she felt empty and wanted to fill herself up; that she ate to give herself comfort; that she remained overweight as an excuse to remain socially isolated; that she ate because she was afraid of sexuality. It became more and more clear to me—in the way that Dorothy talked about her body as betrayer and enemy—that her bulimic self was completely mute and communicating *only* through her body. When I finally asked to hear from her *body*, we were both surprised by what happened. The exchange that follows occurred during a session in the third year of treatment, after Dorothy had once again declared that there was nothing she could do to stop her bingeing and vomiting:

THERAPIST: What would your body say about this?

PATIENT: *(Startled, then a quick switch to anger)* I don't care!

THERAPIST: You don't care to hear what your body has to say?

PATIENT: No! Absolutely not! It's had plenty to say, and everything it has to say is negative!

THERAPIST: Negative, how?

PATIENT: It demands! It always wants more than it needs! It never gets enough.

THERAPIST: *(Choosing to shift from the estranged body self to the self the patient is identified with.)* Well, you haven't gotten enough.

PATIENT: *(Quick tears)* I know. *(Softens for a minute, then stiffens again.)* But the body demands priority!

THERAPIST: So this body doesn't give up its own needs for other people's. It demands priority.

PATIENT: I see what you're getting at. *(Begins crying quietly and continues tearfully for the remainder of the session.)* I was always hungry as a child. They told me I had a *huge* appetite. I never got enough. They told me there was something wrong with my body.

THERAPIST: So you learned you'd better not listen to your body.

Because Dorothy's needs had been split off into the mute bulimic body self, my asking her to talk *about* her bodily symptoms brought only cognitive approximations of what she thought her body might be feeling. In the example above, my asking to hear directly from the body provoked a spontaneous response, which surprised the patient's cognitive mind and which gave her an experience of her body's needs—more exactly, her excruciating fear of her body's needs and her conviction that these needs must be squashed at any cost. This powerful experience then led immediately back to memories that vividly revealed the painful genetic roots of her contempt for her body.

When patients find themselves confonted with a therapist who seeks to learn more about the healthy intentions of the bulimic self, they are uniformly dubious, and they will need to test the therapist repeatedly to assure themselves of his or her trustworthiness. Tanya, 30, disclosed with a good deal of shame after 6 months of treatment that when she was 18 years old and undergoing overwhelming family stress, she had been violently bulimic, using ipecac to make herself vomit 12 to 15 times a day. After asking to hear more about her behavior, I suggested simply that she was trying to make herself feel better in the only way she knew how. She first looked very pleased, then became pensive. In the next session, she told me that she had been doing a lot of thinking about what I had said and that she had decided that perhaps I was too "far out," too "off the wall" for her. Her previous therapist, she said, had interpreted her behavior at age 18 as being "suicidal." She then tested me even further. She said, "You mean to tell me if an 18-year-old walked in here and said she was taking poison to make herself throw up 15 times a day, you'd say, 'How wonderful, you're trying to make yourself feel better?' " I stuck to my guns. While I assured her that I would take any and all steps necessary to protect the 18-year-old's health and safety, I also said that, yes, I would definitely then talk with her about how she was trying to make herself feel better. At this point the patient, having assured herself of my sincerity, visibly softened; she then pulled out a journal she had written at age 18 and read to me passages in which she herself had described her bulimic self in terms surprisingly similar to those I had used.

Of course, Tanya would also have felt misunderstood if the self-destructiveness and rage inherent in her bulimia were not also recognized at the same time that we acknowledged the healthy needs. She came to understand that her "bulimic self" was in many ways identified with her destructive and unpredictable mother. But we also came to see how, on an even more significant level, this fierce "bulimic self" had developed in order to *protect* her from this mother. And we understood how her violent bulimic behavior was an attempt to "control the pain"—first, by inflicting it *on herself*, rather than dreading the mother's inflicting it on her (turning passive into active), and, second, by making the emotional pain physical by moving it from her "heart" to her stomach.

When a patient senses that the therapy process is threatening a part of her personality, she will fight for its life. A good example of this again involves Marilyn—but in this instance, it was her cocaine use that was at issue. Although I knew better than to try to banish this patient's bulimic behavior, I temporarily "lost the concept" when she used cocaine for the first time. My knowledge of the extreme addictive potential of this dangerous drug made me hope naively that a short, firm lecture from me on the subject could nip this new behavior in the bud. Of course, a few days after my lecture Marilyn used cocaine again, calling me at 6:30 A.M. to tell me she had been up all night freebasing. In the next session, just in case I had missed the point, she educated me on what not to do by telling me about her mother's reaction: "My mom was really disapproving of me for using cocaine. I didn't say anything, but I felt like telling her, 'You don't know what you're saying. You're disapproving of the best part of me.'" Marilyn was using cocaine (as she used bulimia) to define her independent selfhood. My telling her to give *that* up immediately cast me in the role of the impinging mother whom she needed to defy at any cost.

Sandy, a 19-year-old student, literally fought for her bulimic self. She reported an incident in which she was at a party vomiting in the bathroom when a male friend accidentally walked in on her. Without thinking, she wheeled around and punched him in the face. "My purging is the one thing I won't let anyone mess with," she said, clenching her fist. She defended the purging ritual so desperately, because she unconsciously knew that if she were deprived of the ritual before genuine self-object functions could be internalized, she would be seriously endangering her self-cohesion. For this shame-prone, apologetic patient, the purging ritual served not only a tension-regulating and a self-defining function, but was also virtually the only expression of her grandiose exhibitionistic needs. In her own words:

> I was the Miss America of purging. I was the best. Friends of mine got exhausted after two times. I could do it 9 or 10. I could *always* make the food come up. If it wouldn't I would reach down in my throat, open the flap, and bring it up! It was amazing what I could do. . . . Some girls felt really good about being a cheerleader. I never felt proud of that like I did about purging. Purging was mine. No one knew about it, so they couldn't criticize me for it.

If the needs hidden in the bulimia are not analyzed before the bulimic symptoms are given up, the needs will remain split off and will eventually demand discharge. This happened in the case of Gina, who at first could only present either her falsely exuberant self or her bulimic symptoms. As a child, when Gina was depressed, her mother had told her to "snap out of it" and "be strong"; as a consequence, her depressive affect was split off, and she developed a falsely cheerful face to present to the outside world. During the first 2 years of treatment, the "needy self" showed itself only through bulimic symptoms.

The first direct allusion to a hidden self came 2 years into treatment, during the session marking the 1-year anniversary of her last purge. Gina came in wanting to celebrate. She thanked me for my help, then added tearfully, "Sometimes I came in here wanting to die and saying, 'Everything's fine,' but *I knew you saw through me,* and you seemed to believe that I could do it." Clearly, she wanted me to continue to see through her. Following this session, during which she "officially" gave up her bulimia, she entered a period of extreme ambition at her workplace. She discovered her intelligence, worked long hours, became politically adept at flattering the right people, and reveled in her independence. She presented everything as wildly exciting and gratifying; try as I might to explore the other, more vulnerable parts of her, she persisted for months in presenting this rather brittle, hypomanic self to me.

Then, unexpectedly, following a 1-month separation due to our sequential vacations, she called me in a panic on a Sunday. It was her first emergency phone call in almost 3 years of treatment. She reported that she had discovered that her husband had been dishonest with her, felt as if "the floor had fallen out from under her," and had begun bingeing and vomiting again. The next session was filled with long, amusing, irrelevant stories, which I had to interrupt to ask about her feelings. Then came another phone call on a Friday night to tell me that she had been fasting and that her weight loss was beginning to alarm the people around her. I insisted on her coming in sooner than scheduled. She again began that next session with entertaining stories, until I interrupted her, and the following exchange ensued:

> THERAPIST: How are you feeling underneath?
> PATIENT: I feel like two people. Do you know how hard it is to say this? Beginning before the holidays—I didn't tell you this—I started to have dark days, high highs and low lows. . . . I was afraid that if I showed the "dark side," the light side would get lost. It used to be 100% dark, when I wanted to kill myself. Then it became 80% light. Now it's about 50–50.
> THERAPIST: I think by calling me those two times, you really grabbed hold of me and made me see the dark side when I had been ignoring it.
> PATIENT: (Suddenly, with great feeling) Don't let go! My husband's let go. Even my mother's let go. If you let go, it's the end.
> THERAPIST: I guess it felt like I was letting go when I kept failing to see the dark side, failing to see all of you.

Following this session, Gina's bulimic symptoms abated. Shortly afterwards, she hurt her knee in a skiing accident and for several weeks had to miss her sessions. When she did come in, she was for the very first time not wearing makeup, and she tearfully complained about how awful she felt:

> PATIENT: Well, here *I am*. Maybe it took all this for me to show you this part . . . this dark side. I have really looked at myself and seen things I don't like. I'm vulnerable inside. I can be hurt. I'm gushy inside, the opposite of the way I've been this past year. . . . I feel like a different person, so needy, so vulnerable.
> THERAPIST: I think you're the you today that used to be bulimic.
> PATIENT: Yes! Yes, that's right. . . . Do you think that if I let her be, then she would let me be? That she would let me get on with my life and not get in the way of my work and my relationships?
> THERAPIST: A very good chance.
> PATIENT: A few months ago she got lost and I got in trouble.
> THERAPIST: She wasn't being seen by you or by me.

CONCLUSION

I have suggested that the bulimia be viewed not merely as a symptom but as the behavioral component of a dissociated self-state, with its own feelings and perceptions and behaviors. I have argued for the importance of actively seeking out and empathizing with the bulimic self, for it is within this self that the archaic nuclear needs have been hidden. The task of empathizing is made difficult, however, by the fact that the bulimic self is by nature paradoxical. It is both self-destructive and self-affirming, and the patient will not begin to reveal her bulimic self until the therapist fully accepts both sides and communicates a kind of reverence for this secret, sacred part. Clinical material has been presented that addresses technical questions of how to recognize and encourage the hidden self to reveal itself, how to respond to its healthy needs and intentions, how to recognize and pass its tests of the therapist's sincerity, and how to assuage its fears of annihilation. It is my hope that these reflections on the bulimic self may serve as an example of how, more generally, to work with the various splits in the personality that may occur when parts of the nascent self are not responded to empathically.

Acknowledgments. I would like to thank Abby Golomb Cole, PhD, Karen Peoples, PhD, John Schneider, PhD, and Deborah Weinstein, MFCC, for their helpful critiques of this chapter. Earlier versions of the chapter were presented at the 12th Annual Conference on the Psychology of the Self, San Francisco, October 12–15, 1989, and the Division 39 (psychoanalysis) American Psychological Association meeting, New York, April 5–8, 1990.

NOTE

1. Pettinati et al. (1985) measured hypnotizability—one measure of dissociative ability—in 86 female bulimic and anorexic patients and found that the bulimic patients were highly hypnotizable, significantly more so than the anorexic or normal patients.

REFERENCES

Brenner, D. (1983). Self-regulatory functions in bulimia. *Contemporary Psychotherapy Review, 1,* 79–96.

Gehrie, M. (1990). Eating disorders and adaptation in crisis: An hypothesis. *American Psychiatric Press Annual Review of Psychiatry, 9, 369–383.*

Geist, R. (1985). Therapeutic dilemmas in the treatment of anorexia nervosa: A self-psychological perspective. *Contemporary Psychotherapy Review, 2,* 115–142.

Goodsitt, A. (1984). Self psychology and the treatment of anorexia nervosa. In D. M. Garner & P. E. Garfinkel (Eds.), *Handbook of psychotherapy for anorexia nervosa and bulimia* (pp. 55–82). New York: Guilford Press.

Johnson, C., & Connors, M. (1987). *The etiology and treatment of bulimia nervosa: A biopsychosocial perspective*. New York: Basic Books.

Jones, D. (1985). Bulimia: A false self identity. *Clinical Social Work Journal, 13*(4), 305–316.

Kohut, H. (1971). *The analysis of the self*. New York: International Universities Press.

Kohut, H. (1977). *The restoration of the self*. New York: International Universities Press.

Kohut, H. (1978). Preface to *Der Falsche weg sum selbst, studien zur drogenkarriere* by Jurgen vom Scheidt. In P. Ornstein (Ed.), *The search for the self* (Vol. 2, pp. 845–849). New York: International Universities Press.

Kohut, H. (1984). *How does analysis cure?* Chicago: University of Chicago Press.

Krueger, D. (1989). *Body self & psychological self*. New York: Brunner/Mazel.

Masterton, J. F. (1977). Primary anorexia nervosa in the borderline adolescent: An object relations view. In P, Hartocollis (Ed.), *Borderline personality disorders* (pp. 475–494). New York: International Universities Press.

McDougall, J. (1974). The psychosoma and psychoanalytic process. *International Review of Psychoanalysis, 1*, 437–454.

McDougall, J. (1980). *A plea for a measure of abnormality*. New York: International Universities Press.

Pettinati, H., Horne, R., & Staats, J. (1985). Hypnotizability in patients with anorexia and bulimia. *Archives of General Psychiatry, 42*, 1014–1016.

Sands, S. (1989). Female development and eating disorders: A self psychological perspective. In A. Goldberg (Ed.), *Progress in self psychology* (Vol. 5, pp. 75–103). Hillsdale, NJ: Analytic Press.

Selvini-Palazzoli, M. (1978). *Self-starvation: From individual to family therapy in the treatment of anorexia nervosa*. New York: Jason Aronson.

Spiegel, D., & Cardreña, E. (1990). Dissociative mechanisms in post traumatic stress disorder. In M. Wolf & A. Mosnim (Eds.), *Post traumatic stress disorder: Etiology, phenomenology, and treatment*. Washington, DC: American Psychiatric Press.

Stolorow, R., Brandchaft, B., & Atwood, G. (1987). *Psychoanalytic treatment: An intersubjective approach*. Hillsdale, NJ: Analytic Press.

Sugarman, A., Quinlan, D., & Devennis, L. (1981). Anorexia nervosa as a defense against anaclitic depression. *International Journal of Eating Disorders, 1*(4), 57–67.

Sugarman, A., & Kurash, C. (1982). The body as a transitional object in bulimia. *International Journal of Eating Disorders, 1*(4), 57–67.

Watkins, J., & Watkins, H. (1988). The management of malevolent ego states. *Dissociation, 1*(1), 67–72.

Zadylak, R., & St. Pierre, A. (1987, October 23–35). *A self psychological approach to the treatment of eating disorders*. Paper presented at the 10th Annual Conference on the Psychology of the Self, Chicago.

∴ *3* ∴

Bruch Revisited: The Role of Interpretation of Transference and Resistance in the Psychotherapy of Eating Disorders

WILLIAM JAMES SWIFT
University of Wisconsin Medical School

BRUCH'S CONTRIBUTIONS

I believe that most authorities would agree that Hilde Bruch (1970, 1973, 1979, 1984) has had a larger impact on the way that modern psychotherapy is practiced with eating-disordered patients than any other writer. Not only did she influence treatment approaches profoundly, as I shortly describe, but she also gave us a new theoretical understanding of anorexia nervosa, the prototype of all psychologically determined eating disorders. Before Bruch, anorexia nervosa was generally understood to be some form of conversion hysteria in which the refusal to eat symbolically expressed a repudiation of sexuality, especially fantasies and wishes surrounding oral impregnation (e.g., Lorand, 1943/1964; Masserman, 1941/1964; Moulton, 1942/1964; Thoma, 1967; Waller, Kaufman, & Deutsch, 1940/1964). In contrast to this drive–defense model entailing refuted oedipal wishes, Bruch emphasized preoedipal development, observing that anorexic patients display major deficits in the sense of self-identity and autonomy. In her view, anorexic symptomatology represents a defensive reparative maneuver against the underlying sense of powerlessness and ineffectiveness associated with major deficits in the personality development of the individual. She further traced these deficits to the failure of the mother to respond appropriately (in a reasonable and consistent fashion) and affirmingly to child-initiated behaviors, which results in gross deficiencies in the individual's sense of initiative and active self-experience (Bruch, 1973). In other words, while earlier writers emphasized triangular, oedipal conflicts between drive and defense at the core of anorexia nervosa, Bruch focused upon psychological deficits in ego- and self-development based on early distortions in the dyadic, mother–child relationship, in which the mother is experienced as controlling and intrusive by the young child.

With respect to psychotherapy, Bruch (1973) eschewed interpretation in favor of what she called a "fact finding, noninterpretive approach" (p. 336). She coined the phase "constructive use of ignorance" to describe her therapeutic approach to anorexic patients (1970, p. 56); by this Bruch meant that the therapist should listen closely to discern the patient's story, should treat the patient as a true collaborator, and should not act in such a way as to mislead the patient into thinking that he or she has a secret store of knowledge that is being purposely withheld. Bruch (1970, 1973, 1978) advised the strict avoidance of theory-based interpretation of unconscious wishes in the drive–defense configuration. Rather, she counseled a "naive" stance, which emphasizes listening to the patient and helping him or her (most often her) define her internal experiences as they unfold in treatment. The goal, of course, is to help the anorexic recognize what she really thinks and feels, an opportunity that she has lacked in earlier development. In short, Bruch recommended what I would consider a "clarifying" approach to the anorexic, in which primary emphasis is placed on assisting the patient to articulate what she experiences at a preconscious level. In contrast, she shunned an interpretive approach in which the primary aim is to uncover mental contents residing at an unconscious level. She felt that interpretation is often experienced by the anorexic as a recapitulation of early trauma in which she was told what she thought and felt by a superior other. She believed that interpretive interventions only confirm the anorexic patient's sense of inadequacy, and interfere with the development of trust in her own self-awareness and self-expression (Bruch, 1970, 1973).

BEYOND BRUCH: INTERPRETATION, TRANSFERENCE, RESISTANCE

My thesis is that while Bruch's noninterpretive, clarifying approach did undoubtedly represent a major step forward in the treatment of anorexic patients, her excessively narrow prescriptions regarding technique have unfortunately caused contemporary therapists to greatly underemphasize the importance of interpretive work, especially interpretation of transference and resistance phenomena, in the psychotherapy of anorexics and bulimics. Her writings represented an important advance because they served as a necessary correction to the excessive preoccupation with instinctive aims that characterized psychoanalysis in its formative years. She was patently correct in asserting that early and direct interpretation of unconscious wishes (e.g., the wish to be impregnated by the father) is experienced by the patient as an intrusive assault that damages the working alliance and the spontaneously developing positive transference. On the other hand, I think that the very cogency and brilliance of her arguments have unfortunately engendered a damaging overcorrection in which the "baby" of empathic, tactful, well-timed interpretation of transference and resistance has been thrown out with the "bath water" of unempathic, tactless, and ill-timed interpretation of id-driven wishes. My views about the importance of interpretative work in psychotherapy, especially the interpretation of transference, have been greatly influenced by the writings of Merton Gill (1979, 1982, 1985).

In essence, Bruch recommended clarification *instead* of interpretation. I believe that she would have been correct if she had stressed clarification *before* interpretation. Basically, what Bruch did was to abandon the "topographical" approach in which the therapist begins at the surface and moves slowly to the depths (Fenichel, 1941). In this method, the conscious and preconscious are addressed before the unconscious, resistance before content, and ego before id. Instead, Bruch recommended that interpretations be discarded wholesale while confrontation and clarification be preserved. Boris (1984) contends that Bruch did not really object to interpretive work per se, but rather objected to *poor* interpretive work. However, my reading of Bruch does not support his assessment.

In describing her treatment approach, Bruch declared that "interpretations are strictly avoided" (1970, p. 51). However, a close examination of her work reveals that this was not in fact so. Her last major report on psychotherapy (1979) contained several interpretations of content and defense in the case material, though they are not identified as such. At a critical juncture in her work with Annette, an adolescent anorexic, she made the following interpretation:

> "Yesterday you said not once but twice that one cannot squash a sister, indicating a double blind dilemma. When you experienced her rejection you must have felt extremely angry at her; but you lived also with the rule that one must love a sister. Therefore you were unable to protest or make your own demands." (1979, p. 31)

This was clearly an interpretation of content, or, more precisely, an interpretation of intrapsychic conflict between an angry wish and an equally powerful moral injunction to "love thy sister," leading finally to a state of paralysis. Later in the therapy Bruch offered an interpretation of defense, telling Annette that her self-punishing attitude was related to her angry feelings at her sister (1979, p. 32).

In *Eating Disorders* (1973) Bruch made an indisputable interpretation of transference, though a displaced, not a direct one. She pointed out to Felice, an anorexic in treatment with another therapist but being interviewed by Bruch in consultation, "that an increase of symptoms during the past few months could be understood as a vengeful message to her therapist that he, too, had failed her" (p. 354).

Along with explicitly discarding interpretation, I believe that Bruch also mistakenly underemphasized the roles of resistance and transference in treatment. There is little mention of resistance in her work, and, to my knowledge, no explicit reference to transference phenomena. For example, she wrote, "Much of what is termed 'resistance' may be the result of discrepancies in meaning and verbal usage, even though it may sound like ordinary words being exchanged. This makes a demand on the therapist that his communication be simple and unambiguous, free of professional jargon" (1973, pp. 337–338). In other words, she suggested that resistance may be largely artifactual, arising from a discrepancy between what the therapist says and the patient hears. The antidote to this is "simple and unambiguous" speech on the part of the therapist. Although it is undoubtedly true that poor technique greatly heightens resistance, it is equally true that resistance is inherent in any therapy. After all, resistance is only the part of the patient that resists change—that opposes the work of therapy and, in doing so, defends the status quo. Although Bruch was a psychoanalyst and a psychodynamic therapist, she appeared not to accept a precept absolutely crucial to her school: namely, that there are forces *for* and *against* change residing within the patient, and that these forces are in constant conflict throughout much of therapy.

Actually, I do not believe that Bruch's view of resistance phenomena was simple. Although she explicitly minimized it, several passages in her work implicitly suggest that she thought it important. As was apparently true of her outlook on interpretation, she appeared to be of two minds about resistance. For instance, Bruch asserted, "Patients will cling to their distorted concepts and let go of them only slowly and reluctantly" (1979, p. 27); and "patients will adhere to their distorted concepts, the false reality with which they have lived, since it represents their only way of having experiences . . ." (1978, p. 136). Bruch also noted that "They [patients] also deny that there has been anything troublesome in their relationship to their parents. Everything is perfect . . ." (1984, p. 15).

Furthermore, she (1978) warned therapists of the danger of "pseudo-agreement" on the part of anorexics. That is, the patient will seem to accept interpretation, and even elaborate upon it, but in actuality it means nothing to her on an affective level; in other words, it is just a "phony intellectualization" (p. 13). Although she did not use the term "resistance" to describe these striking clinical observations, they certainly sound like clear-cut manifestations of resistance.

I have much the same criticism of Bruch's neglect of another important technical consideration, transference. In her writings, she did not pay heed to it. Bruch apparently felt that if the therapist employs the proper stance vis-à-vis the patient—a nonintrusive, noninterpretative, fact-finding approach—a milieu is created in which the anorexic patient flourishes and the curative process unfolds *sui generis*, without transference issues' being an important concern. To put it slightly differently, my reading of Bruch leads me to conclude that she believed that if the therapist helps the patient accurately clarify what she really thinks and feels, the stalled process of separation–individuation will be reinitiated, and sufficient growth will occur within the patient to allow her to abandon her symptomatology. This viewpoint runs strikingly counter to the contemporary belief that psychotherapy is always, to one degree or another, an emotional struggle between the patient and the therapist (Blos, 1984), in which transference wishes, attitudes, and enactments play a pivotal role. My experience is that transference phenomena are ubiquitous in treatment, no matter how empathic the approach. This is compatible with the outlook of a number of recent observers (Boris, 1984; Fischer, 1989; Rizzuto, 1988) who have noted that resistance to involvement in the transference is one of the principal problems in treating anorexics. That is, anorexic patients tend to remain aloof from the therapist and not to invest themselves in treatment for long periods of time.

Later in this chapter, I describe the 2-year psychodynamic psychotherapy of a bulimarexic college student (which is still in process) that highlights such interpretive interventions. My approach has not been singularly or relentlessly interpretive. Other forms of intervention, such as clarification, confrontation, and education, have all had consistently large roles to play. Above all, throughout the therapy I have striven to create a "holding environment" (Winnicott, 1965) in which this late adolescent coed could feel secure and free to share all parts of herself, including those that she experienced as ridiculous, self-destructive, perverse, deeply embarrassing, and the like (Sandler & Sandler, 1983).

Besides the interpretation of resistance and transference, I also want to emphasize another theme: the multilayering of psychopathology, in which issues related to both preoedipal and oedipal development (i.e., deficit and conflict) are intricately interwoven. While I agree with Bruch

(1973) and Johnson and Connors (1987), among others, that failures in the phase of separation–individuation (roughly 12–36 months of age) are pre-eminent in the genesis of both anorexia nervosa and bulimia nervosa, this does not mean that conflictually based oedipal material is nonexistent or unimportant. The fact that the patient has deficits in the ego system and self-system due to failures in the preoedipal period does not indicate that the patient is preconflictual (Panel, 1988) or that oedipal themes are superfluous.[1] Of course, the opposite is equally true: The fact that an individual is torn about instinctive wishes and urges does not lead to the automatic conclusion that the person is deficit-free in the realms of ego and self. Human psychology is simply too rich and too complex to be encompassed by unidimensional statements.

JESSICA: THE CASE OF THE CONTRADICTORY STUDENT

Jessica, a 19-year-old undergraduate, consulted me shortly after the beginning of the academic year because of a 20-pound weight loss in the preceding 2 months. The consultation was really at the behest of her parents, who were alarmed about the velocity of her weight loss, and were well aware of the context in which it occurred—a 5-year history of regular bingeing and self-induced vomiting.

In the space available, I present some of the main themes of this complicated case. At this writing, the psychotherapy has extended over 2 years, and the patient has been seen *en face* on a twice-weekly basis. As will be obvious, the treatment is not yet completed, but there are encouraging signs that Jessica is making progress. I especially want to highlight the often baffling intermixture of preoedipal and oedipal themes in the psychology of this late adolescent; the playing out of these themes in the context of resistance and transference; and the value of attempting to reduce these themes by interpretation at critical junctures. Not that I was always successful in the last-mentioned endeavor! As Loewald (1960) and Fischer (1989) have noted, transference enactments of developmental deficits and lags are often not easily interpretable. At such times, the task of the therapist is predominantly to avoid fulfilling a distorted counter-transference role in response to the patient's transference enactment. For instance, by responding neutrally and empathically to a patient's provocations, one hopes to act as a "health-promoting" new object, fostering the resumption of ego development.

A few words are in order about my own brand of psychodynamic psychotherapy with this patient population. Like Bruch, I primarily seek to help the eating-disordered individual clarify her own unique inner thoughts, feelings, and attitudes. Befitting the youth of the population I see, my style is rather active. I place special emphasis on understanding and explaining, in collaboration with the patient, the salient aspects of her intrapsychic and interpersonal worlds as they emerge in the "here and now" of the treatment encounter. For example, in relationship to transference, I emphasize (as does Gill, 1979, 1982, 1985) the relatively early interpretation of transference as it develops in the immediate "here and now" of therapy, while minimizing the "there and then" aspect of transference phenomena, which links current treatment experience with archaic childhood figures ("reliving of the past in the present"). I typically choose the former, more contemporaneous route because it is more immediate and real—and thus more meaningful—to the patient. I would not object if someone described me as an interpersonalist with a strong commitment to psychodynamics.

Early Treatment; Background Information

In retrospect, I considered the first 4 months of Jessica's treatment to represent an initial "symptomatic phase," in the sense that concerns about her restrictive dieting, weight loss, and precarious health status overshadowed all others. At a surface level, Jessica was initially delighted by the materialization of her anorexia nervosa. She remarked, "I have been dieting my entire life; this is the first time I have been successful!" As Boris (1984) has so aptly stated, for the anorexic patient the anorexia is the solution, not the problem! My problem was to successfully redefine anorexia as a problem for her; in the beginning it seemed to be more my problem than hers.

Although she came to therapy regularly during the first 6 weeks, her resistance to treatment was obvious, as she quickly lost 13 pounds. This ballistic rate of weight loss culminated in a brief hospitalization at my insistence, during which Jessica managed to gain enough weight to restore her health. Future hospitalizations proved not to be required, as she has managed to maintain a medically stable but below-average body weight throughout psychotherapy. During this early phase, Jessica showed intense resistance to involvement in treatment and equally intense commitment to anorexia nervosa.

My reaction was to internally debate how intrusive I should be about her weight and eating habits before finally deciding upon the course just outlined. I would practice a sort of "benign neglect" for the time being if she managed to avoid health complications. To be "too forward" in this domain, I believe, would have been experienced as intrusive by Jessica; on the other hand, being "too permissive" might have been experienced as an abandonment by me to her own self-destructive tendencies. Largely, I attempted to act as an ancillary ego for Jessica during this difficult period.

To briefly review her symptomatic history, Jessica began bingeing and purging at age 15 following a cross-country move. As is true of the great majority of bulimic patients, she had made multiple unsuccessful attempts at dieting. Jessica was an attractive, tall young woman with a graceful, athletic physique. For years she had longed to look like a fashion magazine model, but had never been able to sufficiently reduce her caloric consumption to approach this ideal until shortly before she entered therapy. It appeared that her success in dieting was triggered by her return to school and what she experienced as a momentous decision, the choice of a major. I speculated to myself at the time that this must indeed be a difficult decision if an individual has little confidence in her capacity to choose wisely on the one hand, and on the other must be perfect in whatever she does. Her anorexic stance was founded on the following logic: "If I am unable to feel in control of my life, I will compensate by exerting total control over my diet in pursuit of perfect thinness!"

The Unfolding of Resistance and Transference

At the start of each session, Jessica always chose the chair most physically distant from me. Her eyes were constantly averted, as if eye-to-eye contact was excruciatingly painful. As the therapy unfolded, it became clear that her eye aversion had multiple meanings. Initially, it appeared to be simply an identification with other family members, particularly her father, who habitually avoided or minimized eye contact. Further inquiry revealed that it was reflective of her profound sense of shame: Jessica experienced herself as so wanting in so many domains that she literally preferred not to be seen. At a deeper level, reconstruction suggested that the eye aversion was an attempt to avoid a traumatic recapitulation of her early relationship with her mother. This was disclosed in the context of the transference relationship, when she told me that to make eye contact was to become imprisoned by me. By this she meant that she would be compelled to "cue off" me; to read my facial expressions for signs of, say, approval or disapproval; to assess my body postures to see whether I was interested or uninterested—in short, to compulsively *react* to me. By avoiding eye contact, Jessica believed that at least she had the hope of being free, of being herself, of *acting* instead of *reacting* for the first time in her life. This transference attitude was eventually linked to early failures in the process of separation–individuation from her mother through the mode of repeated interpretation and working through. From transference material we were able to reconstruct together her earliest perceptions of her hyperemotional mother as an intrusive, dominating, and needy caretaker. In order to insure the survival of the relationship, she had to march to her mother's beat. Too much independence ran the risk of maternal withdrawal and abandonment (Masterson, 1977).

Silence was the major manifestation of resistance in the first part of psychotherapy. Jessica had great difficulty with the idea and practice of free association. In a flash of insight she stated, "I am used to saying what I *should* say, but I have no idea of what I *want* to say." Nonetheless, silence pervaded many of the early sessions. Beneath her silence raged an internal struggle between holding back and keeping secret versus letting go and sharing, reminiscent of a toddler struggling fiercely with anal issues. To Jessica's categorical way of thinking, to share just a little was equivalent to "total vulnerability," and the terrifying self-perception that she was becoming a "giant liquefying Jell-O," without boundaries or definition. In contrast, keeping secret and silent meant security, but at the exorbitant cost of utter emotional isolation.

With further work it also became evident that her silence had enormous transference implications. We were able to clarify that Jessica feared that if she shared deeper parts of herself, I would be silently contemptuous and disapproving. This was linked to present and past perceptions of her aloof, methodical father. What really galled Jessica was her belief that the contempt was silent and secretive—poisonous, as it were. She said it would be so much better if the contempt was in the open; then she could at least deal with it. Her father and I were both too much gentlemen, too "professional" to openly express our arrogant deprecation of her, but she knew what we really felt. I responded to this accusation on two levels. First, I admitted that I did not know the reality of her father's feelings toward her, so her judgment of him might well be accurate as far as I knew. Second, I made a defense interpretation: Perhaps because it was too painful an awareness, she was attributing to me her own destructive tendency to be excessively self-critical.

This interactional set heralded the development of a full-blown, very complex negative father transference, which I believe had both oedipal and preoedipal components. Her silences now had a new meaning: They were a way of controlling her "blind rage" at me for failing to respond to her in a warm, human, truly caring way. In reality, her father's personality and profession played a large part in sowing the seeds of this transference reaction. He was a research scientist at a major university, and when I interviewed him I found him to be much as Jessica described— hyperrational, methodical, and emotionally unexpressive—though I did not feel that he was without care or concern for his daughter. To Jessica, however, he was a compulsive scientist both in his laboratory and at home. It was as if he could never let go and be a real father. When problems arose at home, he responded like the scientist he was: He calmly gathered data, he generated hypotheses that he shared with his wife and children, he suggested new methods of approach, and so on. However, this only infuriated Jessica because there was no fire; he seemed to give nothing of his personal self to her or the rest of the family.

Jessica interpreted my therapeutic stance of an interested, sympathetic observer to indicate that I was a hardheaded scientist—"You don't really care, it's just a job to you." While she agreed that I might be more attuned to her inner needs than her father, the real difference was so negligible to be insignificant. The overriding facts to her mind were that we were both middle-aged males who heartlessly pursued our work. Her father had failed her, and I was in the process of failing her once again.

This negative transference reaction appeared to be determined by unresolved oedipal issues. (Shortly, I describe another segment of the transference in which preoedipal themes predominated.) I surmised that Jessica had unsuccessfully negotiated the oedipal phase primarily because her father had failed to lovingly affirm both her personhood and her femininity. He had never had a nonincestuous phase-appropriate "love affair" with his daughter, which would have drawn Jessica away from her mother's orbit and confirmed her identity as a valued, advisable young woman. Her hostile, provocative attitude that I had no personal feeling or concern for her seemed to be constructed to elicit two countertransference reactions typical of the oedipus: a provoked *enemy* retaliating in kind, or a solicitous *lover* full of good intentions. To my modest credit, I managed to avoid both reactions in favor of empathically interpreting her wish that I would be the loving father that she never had. I also made it clear that while I could not give her *now* what she had needed *then*, I could help her come to terms with her father's emotional noninvolvement. I held that if she experienced, understood, and mastered this disappointment, she would be strengthened and better prepared to move on with her life.

This transference "reliving of the past in the present" had to be worked through many times before the strength of the underlying forces was reduced. Not only was there a strong wish to receive what she never got (her father's emotional involvement), but there was an equally strong desire to punish him for his failure. The strength of her rage at times terrified Jessica: She was worried that during one of her self-described "witchy" moods something "vile and destructive" within would be released, and that I and the therapy would be immediately destroyed.

Pre-Oedipal Components of Transference

I would like to shift gears here and describe a preoedipal aspect of Jessica's transference, which was ultimately linked to her mother rather than her father. In a fascinating account, Fischer (1989) has described a "pull–push" dance in the transference–countertransference engagement with a young anorexic patient, which he related to preoedipal development. I saw much the same transactional pattern with Jessica. By "pull–push" Fischer refers to an intense, frantic, circular interaction pattern in which the patient gives conflicting signals in rapid succession. In his case the patient conveyed the following contradictory messages: "I feel helpless and alone; you must help; if you do, I will feel even more helpless and overwhelmed; you must help." This sort of erratic "to-and-fro" activity Fischer attributes to a poorly negotiated rapprochement phase of the separation–individuation process as described by Mahler, Pine, and Bergman (1975).

To briefly review, the rapprochement phase refers to a period in the second year of life (approximately 16–24 months of age) during which rapid maturational development along a number of lines results in the youngster's for the first time having a keen cognitive awareness of both her separateness from the mother and her exquisite vulnerability and smallness when alone. She is caught on the horns of a mighty dilemma: On the one hand, she wants to exercise her newfound independence in the volitional and motoric spheres, but, on the other hand, when she does so she acutely feels the loss of the mother's protective wing. The behavioral manifestation of this internal conflict is "pull–push" or "to-and-fro" activity—for instance, "darting" away from the mother at one moment in joyful self-assertion, yet in the next instant clinging, literally "shadowing" her mother in an attempt to reassure herself that she is still protected by parental omnipotence.

At about the end of the first year of treatment, there was a set of pull–push transactions that illustrated the preoedipal component of Jessica's ambivalent, often negative, paternal transference. (Or perhaps it would be more accurate to say that there was a switch from a paternal to a maternal transference.) Jessica abruptly announced that she was going to spend the next quarter in Japan studying in her recently chosen major. This announcement was sprung within a matter of weeks of her scheduled departure date. She had finalized plans to study abroad some time ago, but had purposely kept me in the dark. She very boldly said, "You can't butt into my trip to Japan if you don't know anything about it." She told me that she hated her dependency on me and her mother, that she would have to stand on her own two feet overseas, and that she wouldn't have our shoulders to "cry on." In the next few days she suffered a period of truly harrowing panic attacks that required the brief prescription of alprazolam. Her declaration of independence had caused an upsurge of unconscious abandonment anxiety, which was experienced as blinding, incapacitating panic states. Eventually we were able to clarify what she did experience internally and to link it interpretively to her enmeshed relationship with her mother. Interestingly, this theme re-emerged in the session just before she left for Japan. She wanted to know my feelings about the trip. I sensed that she wanted a "vote of confidence" in what she was doing; there was a need to utilize me as a supportive, affirming parental object. I told her that my primary job was to help her understand the psychological meanings of the trip to her, but, yes, I would have objected if I thought the trip was self-destructive or unwise. I thought she was ready to handle the 10 weeks abroad and that it seemed like a great opportunity. We would have much to talk about when she returned. She was clearly relieved by my words. She smiled and said, "I guess I'm ready to set out and conquer the world." Just in case her confidence flagged, however, she requested a small prescription of alprazolam to take with her. I think this was an instance in which medication was more valued for its properties as a transitional object than for its attributes as a potent neurochemical agent. As it turned out, she never needed the alprazolam, but its presence in her travel bag was greatly reassuring to her.

Current Status

With the continued working through of the transference as it unfolded in the "here and now" of our sessions, there has been a softening in Jessica's attitude toward both her father and me. This has taken the form of a perceivable shift from ambivalence with a withholding, hostile tone to a mildly idealizing stance. I construe this as a very good sign. Numerous authors (e.g., Adatto, 1966; Blos, 1980; Chused, 1987; Ritvo, 1971) have commented on the importance of idealization, including idealization in the transference, in late adolescent development. The idealization of adults is seen as an important step in the process of internalizing identifications and building psychological structures: The adolescent literally takes in the admired qualities of a special adult and makes them "her own." In fact, this is believed to be so crucial in adolescence that Chused (1987) contends that the use of the therapist as an idealized mentor is a highly salutary development, and that transference reactions interfering with this idealization should be interpreted, not the idealization itself. This was well illustrated when Jessica learned that I would be speaking on a local radio show about adolescent depression. She nervously vowed to listen, but her greatest fear was that I would make a complete fool of myself. When I managed to sound reasonably competent over the airwaves, she was greatly relieved. Maybe I did really know what I was talking about, and maybe I did really have the skills and energy to help her. She also began to experience loving feelings toward her father for the first time in memory. She began to recognize his transparent vulnerabilities, and her accompanying wish to care for and protect him.

After 2 years of treatment, her eating disorder symptomatology has decreased sharply. Within the first 6 months of treatment, in fact, her anorexia nervosa remitted and has not reappeared. Jessica remains bulimic, however, though the frequency of bingeing and purging has been reduced by roughly three-quarters since admission. The meanings, origins, and purposes of her bingeing–purging cycle need to be more fully explored. This has been an area in which she is fiercely protective about revealing herself. There is much shame and guilt surrounding the whole sequence; her associations suggest that it has been eroticized to a large degree. To her mind, it is the one wild, crazy, excessive, free part of herself, and she wonders out loud whether she will ever be able to completely give it up.[2] For now, it is her "black-hearted friend"—a behavioral sequence that is alternately calming and deliciously relieving, but that extracts a mighty price in shame, suffering, and guilt.

She has begun to date, a large step forward, but intimacy with males remains conflicted and problematic. She will soon be making applications to graduate school, and her professional prospects are excellent. We both understand that the treatment is not yet complete, though good progress has been made. Jessica, an amateur sailor, used the following metaphor to describe her perception of the treatment experience: Before treatment she had a "boat" and a "sail," but no "keel" and "rudder" to steady her in the constantly shifting winds and currents of life. Treatment has given her the missing psychological keel and rudder, and though she might not always be adroit in how she handles her craft, she nonetheless manages now to remain upright and secure in heavy waters.

CONCLUSION

In my view, Hilde Bruch remains the seminal contributor to the practice of psychotherapy with anorexic and bulimic patients. Although I disagree with her on several major points, I find much more in her work to praise and emulate. For instance, she wrote, "The therapeutic task is to help an anorexic patient in her search for autonomy and self-directed identity by evoking awareness of impulses, feelings, and needs that originate within her" (1979, p. 27). I could not agree more fully. Interspersed throughout her psychotherapy writings are a number of suggestions related to what Stone (1981) has called the "attitude and setting" of psychodynamic treatment that are extraordinarily valuable:

1. Interventions should be based on the clinical encounter, not theory.
2. The therapist should make the patient an active participant in the process, a true collaborator.

3. The therapist should display genuine warmth and honesty in his or her dealings with the patient.
4. The patient should be "educated" about the goals, purposes, and methods of psychotherapy.
5. The tone of the sessions should not be somber. There is room for lightness in a "friendly, well-meaning way" (1970, p. 142).
6. Patience is important. It requires time to repair the developmental deficits that the eating-disordered patient brings to treatment.

In fact, one could make the case that Bruch's greatest contribution has been in transforming the attitudes of therapists toward anorexic patients. By stressing such treatment principles as empathic listening, collaboration, supportive helpfulness, nonintrusive concern, and the need to confirm the inner reality of the patient, she was, in effect, creating the sort of therapeutic setting that Winnicott (1965) called a "holding environment"—a safe, secure place, free from threat, wherein habitual, maladaptive ways of coping could be held in abeyance and new methods tried out. Most therapists would agree that the creation of a "holding environment" constitutes the *sine qua non* of any successful therapy: Without it, there is simply nothing! Bruch was clearly rebelling against classical psychoanalysis as practiced in her era—the austere, remote analyst, acting as a "blank screen," making interpretive statements from "on high" about profoundly embarrassing instinctual wishes (Stone, 1984). Moreover, these interpretations in her view were predominantly founded on theory and only weakly corroborated by clinical material, if at all.

Nonetheless, I do have some significant disagreements with Bruch. Although she did greatly improve the tone of the attitude and setting of psychotherapy, she unfortunately minimized or neglected crucial technical skills and considerations, such as interpretive interventions and adequate attention to resistance and transference phenomena. To recapitulate, I believe that Bruch failed to distinguish between interpretation of id impulses and interpretation of resistance, defense, transference, and content (e.g., identifications and intrapsychic conflict). While I agree with her that interpretation of id wishes is a hazardous proposition that often has very negative ramifications for the treatment relationship, I believe that she erred by proscribing interpretation entirely. In doing so, she discarded a powerful tool for dealing with the ubiquitous treatment phenomena of resistance and transference, among others. In contrast to her, I also contend that resistance is inherent in treatment, and not largely an artifact of poor technique. I have likewise described my view that Bruch neglected the importance of transference phenomena in the treatment of eating-disordered individuals. I believe that many contemporary psychotherapies of adolescents and young adults, including eating-disordered patients, could be enriched by greater attention to resistance and transference phenomena as well as their interpretive reduction (Swift & Wonderlich, in press).

As we enter the last decade of the 20th century, the world seems to be changing in rapid and marvelous ways. Many new developments in the recent past have improved our ability to treat the heterogeneous pathologies included under the rubric of the eating disorders. I count among these pharmacotherapy, cognitive and behavioral therapies, group approaches, family therapy, and the interpersonal Sullivanian approach exemplified by the work of Hilde Bruch. My concern is that in our headlong rush toward modernity, we will give short shrift to the eternal verities of intrapsychic life (unconscious motivations, conflict, defense, etc.) and the doctor–patient relationship (resistance, transference, and countertransference) described by Freud and his disciples earlier in this century. It is our duty to meld the best of the old and the new as we lay the groundwork for clinical and research efforts in the 21st century. Do our current and future patients deserve anything less?

Acknowledgments. I wish to thank Dr. Stephen Wonderlich, University of North Dakota School of Medicine, for his comments on an earlier version of this chapter. The expert assistance of Mr. Donna Littel in manuscript preparation is also appreciated.

NOTES

1. To briefly review, preoedipal themes are generally manifested by *deficits* in such important areas of the personality as self-concepts, object constancy, signal anxiety, body image, affect modulation, and impulse control (Pine, 1988). All of these vulnerabilities can ultimately be related to the faculty structuralization of the ego system and self-system. In contrast, oedipal themes are primarily marked by *conflict* among the different agencies of the mind (e.g., the clash between supergo standards and powerful sexual and aggressive wishes). Typical clinical presentations include success anxiety, excessive guilt and inhibition, and triangular enactments—in the case of a woman, exaggerated rivalry with other females and libidinal wishes repeatedly directed toward "unavailable" or "forbidden" men. Of course, oedipal and preoedipal issues are often intermixed in clinical reality.

2. I think that there is much to be said for Wilson's (1986) suggestion that bulimics be asked to "interrupt" or suspend their habit for a discrete, mutually agreed-upon period of time, so that they can begin to experience fantasies, feelings, and conflicts habitually warded off by the frenetic activity of bingeing and self-purgation.

REFERENCES

Adatto, C. (1966). On the metamorphosis from adolescence into adulthood. *Journal of the American Psychoanalytic Association, 14*, 485–509.

Blos, P. (1980). The life cycle as indicated by the nature of the transference in the psychoanalysis of adolescents. *International Journal of Psycho-Analysis, 61*, 145–151.

Blos, P. (1984). The contribution of psychoanalysis to the psychotherapy of adolescents. In M. Sugar (Ed.), *Adolescent psychiatry* (Vol. 11, pp. 104–125). Chicago: University of Chicago Press.

Boris, H. N. (1984). On the treatment of anorexia nervosa. *International Journal of Psycho-Analysis, 65*, 435–442.

Bruch, H. (1970). Psychotherapy in primary anorexia nervosa. *Journal of Nervous and Mental Diseases, 150*, 51–66.

Bruch, H. (1973). *Eating disorders: Obesity, anorexia nervosa, and the person within*. New York: Basic Books.

Bruch, H. (1978). *The golden cage*. Cambridge, MA: Harvard University Press.

Bruch, H. (1979). Island in the river: The anorexic adolescent in treatment. In S. C. Feinstein & P. L. Giovacchini (Eds.), *Adolescent psychiatry* (Vol. 7, pp. 26–40). Chicago: University of Chicago Press.

Bruch, H. (1984). Four decades of eating disorders. In D. M. Garner & P. E. Garfinkel (Eds.), *Handbook of psychotherapy for anorexia nervosa and bulimia* (pp. 7–18). New York: Guilford Press.

Chused, J. F. (1987). Idealization of the analyst by the young adult. *Journal of the American Psychoanalytic Association, 35*(4), 839–859.

Fenichel, O. (1941). *Problems of psychoanalytic technique*. Albany, NY: Psychoanalytic Quarterly.

Fischer, N. (1989). Anorexia nervosa and unresolved rapprochement conflicts. *International Journal of Psycho-Analysis, 70*, 41–54.

Gill, M. (1979). *Psychoanalytic psychotherapy, 1954–1979*. Paper presented at the Symposium on Psychoanalysis and Psychotherapy—Similarities and Differences—A 25-Year Perspective, Atlanta, GA.

Gill, M. (1982). *Analysis of transference: Vol. 1. Theory and technique*. New York: International Universities Press.

Gill, M. (1985). The interactional aspect of transference. In E. A. Schwaber (Ed.), *The transference in psychotherapy: Clinical management* (pp. 87–102). New York: International Universities Press.

Johnson, C., & Connors, M. E. (1987). *The etiology and treatment of bulimia nervosa: A biopsychosocial perspective*. New York: Basic Books.

Loewald, H. (1960). On the therapeutic action of psychoanalysis. *International Journal of Psycho-Analysis, 41*, 16–33.

Lorand, S. (1964). Anorexia nervosa: Report of a case. In M. R. Kaufman & M. Heinman (Eds.), *Evolution of psychosomatic concepts* (pp. 298–319). New York: International Universities Press. (Original work published 1943)

Mahler, M., Pine, F., & Bergman, A. (1975). *The psycholigical birth of the human infant*. New York: Basic Books.

Masserman, J. H. (1964). Psychodynamisms in anorexia nervosa and neurotic vomiting. In M. R. Kaufman & M. Heinman (Eds.), *Evolution of psychosomatic concepts* (pp. 320–351). New York: International Universities Press. (Original work published 1941)

Masterson, J. F. (1977). Primary anorexia nervosa in the borderline adolescent. In P. Hartocollis (Ed.), *Borderline personality disorders* (pp. 475–494). New York: International Universities Press.

Moulton, R. (1964). A psychosomatic study of anorexia nervosa including the use of vaginal smear. In M. R. Kaufman & M. Heinman (Eds.), *Evolution of psychosomatic concepts* (pp. 274–297). New York: International Universities Press. (Original work published 1942)

Panel. (1988). Anorexia nervosa: Theory and therapy—a new look at an old problem. *Journal of the American Psychoanalytic Association, 36*, 153–161.

Pine, F. (1988). On the four psychologies of psychoanalysis and the nature of the therapeutic impact. In A. Rothstein (Ed.), *How does treatment help?* (pp. 145–155). Madison, CT: International Universities Press.

Ritvo, S. (1971). Late adolescence: Developmental and clinical considerations. *Psychoanalytic Study of the Child, 26*, 241–263.

Rizzuto, A.-M. (1988). Tranference, language, and affect in the treatment of bulimarexia. *International Journal of Psycho-Analysis, 69*, 369–387.

Sandler, J., & Sandler, A.-M.. (1983). The "second censorship," the "three box model" and some technical implications. *International Journal of Psycho-Analysis, 64*, 413–425.

Stone, L. (1981). Notes on the noninterpretive elements in the psychoanalytic situation and process. *Journal of the American Psychoanalytic Association, 29*, 89–118.

Stone, L. (1984). *Transference and its context: Selected papers on psychoanalysis*. New York: Jason Aronson.

Swift, W. J., & Wonderlich, S. A. (in press). Interpretation of transference in the psychotherapy of adolescents and young adults. *Journal of the American Academy of Child and Adolescent Psychiatry*.

Thoma, H. (1967). *Anorexia nervosa*. New York: International Universities Press.

Waller, J. V., Kaufman, M. R., & Deutsch, F. (1964). Anorexia nervosa: A psychosomatic entity. In M. R. Kaufman & M. Heinman (Eds.), *Evolution of psychosomatic concepts* (pp. 245–273). New York: International Universities Press. (Original work published 1940)

Wilson, C. P. (1986). The psychoanalytic psychotherapy of bulimic anorexia nervosa. In S. Feinstein, A. Esman, J. Looney, A. Schwartzberg, A. Sorosky, & M. Sugar (Eds.), *Adolescent psychiatry* (Vol. 13, pp. 274–314). Chicago: University of Chicago Press.

Winnicott, D. W. (1965). *Maturational processes and the facilitating environment*. New York: International Universities Press.

∴ *4* ∴

Reflections on Boundaries in the Psychotherapeutic Relationship

WILLIAM N. DAVIS

Center for the Study of Anorexia and Bulimia, New York

This chapter is addressed especially to those therapists in the eating disorders community whose working orientation is either psychodynamic or psychoanalytic. In saying this, I do not intend to ignore clinicians in the field who approach the treatment of anorexia or bulimia from another vantage point. I hope that my remarks will have relevance and impact in these quarters as well. However, I expect that the several therapeutic issues I am going to explore will be particularly meaningful to those who were trained to think and to act as I was. My first contact with an eating-disordered patient was in 1977, shortly after I completed my psychoanalytic studies at the William Alanson White Institute in New York City. For me, analytic training was thoroughly in keeping with, and represented a deepening of, the broad tradition of psychodynamic psychotherapy that shaped my initial experiences as a clinician. Ever so simplified into the fabric of ordinary workaday sessions, the basic rules were to inquire and interpret, keeping alert to the vicissitudes of the therapeutic relationship. Out of this amalgam, judiciously and sometimes fortuitously applied, insight and change would occur.

At this writing, 13 years later and after many thousands of sessions with anorexic and bulimic patients, I am still a psychodynamic and in some ways a psychoanalytic thinker. Yet what I actually do, and how I understand the treatment of eating disorders, have changed considerably. My original 1977 therapeutic contact was a dismal failure, in that I could not prevent a hospital admission due to the effects of malnutrition, and could not appreciably help my patient (either symptomatically or characterologically) upon her discharge. Currently, I believe I do a much better job of helping people with anorexia or bulimia, but not only because I apply the basic rules with a skill born of experience and increased understanding. What intrigues me is the possibility that my therapeutic effectiveness depends in part upon a willingness to bend and go beyond the time-honored traditions of clinical work. This brings me to the title of the chapter. My purpose is to discuss boundaries in the psychotherapeutic relationshp, especially as these apply to and affect the treatment of severe eating disorders. By "boundaries," I am referring to the explicit and implicit assumptions that guide and limit the behavior of therapists as they seek to relate to and help their patients. In the following sections, I focus first on more general aspects of the process of psychodynamic psychotherapy. Then I turn specifically to the treatment of eating disorders.

One final word of introduction. In my experience, the treatment of severe anorexia or bulimia is a long, difficult process, and frequently an intensely absorbing struggle. Where the outcome has been successful, I have felt invigorated and positively confirmed in my role as therapist. Quite obviously, it is very exciting to enable someone to feel open and to act alive once again. On the other hand, far too often I have felt the treatment bog down into impasse, or seen it fail altogether. It was at these times, when I felt frustrated and inadequate as a therapist, that I began to challenge traditional boundaries. I did so uneasily and self-consciously, unsure of what I was doing and what I would precipitate. Nevertheless, the idea was, and still is, to find something that might actually work— something that might turn my patients away from their symptomatic preoccupations and toward the therapy. Consequently, the reasoning that follows is very much post hoc. It attempts to assemble and think through a jumble of personal experiences derived from a continuing series of therapeutic struggles. I do not imagine that I am presenting a systematic answer for the psychotherapy of anorexia or bulimia. However, I do believe that the issues addressed here deserve serious consideration if the aim of treatment is to provide eating-disordered patients with genuine help instead of reliable but ineffective method.

BOUNDARIES AND PSYCHODYNAMIC PSYCHOTHERAPY

There is no question but that boundaries are essential for the practice of psychotherapy. Therapists need to know how to think and what to do when they work with patients. Indeed, all training in psychotherapeutic interaction can be said to derive from a gradual accumulation of those particular thoughts, feelings, and behaviors deemed to represent therapy from the universe of available options. As a result, the course and content of any psychotherapy will be governed by a number of explicitly defined or implicitly accepted rules and assumptions. However, all of these boundaries can be only relatively appropriate, and none of them are necessarily rational. Boundaries "work" and can be helpful not because they are right or reflect the truth, but because therapists and then patients are trained to accept a common set of beliefs and values about psychotherapy. Initially, the culture at large joins therapists and patients in a similar construction of reality, and then the psychotherapy subculture socializes both to share a similar understanding of what is and what is not psychological treatment. Where this is not the case—as, for example, when therapist and patient come from radically different cultures that promote conflicting world views—it is difficult at best to conduct psychotherapy.

Commonly held boundaries usually benefit and protect both therapists and patients, because they reduce potential anxiety and conflict over the contents and procedures that are appropriate to psychotherapy. For example, since the culture and the mental health professions regard it as pernicious for psychotherapy to include sexual intercourse, patients can reasonably assume that their psychological needs will not serve as an opportunity for physical exploitation, and therapists can reasonably assume that their interventions will not lead to an attempted seduction or a challenge to their impulse control. Similarly, therapists and patients understand that psychotherapy can create painful feelings, and both know that therapy is paid for by the session, each of which lasts for about 45 minutes. These and many, many other boundaries constitute the fabric of psychodynamic psychotherapy—guiding, restraining, and restricting therapists and patients as they pursue the contemporary vision of psychological treatment.

However, boundaries are not always helpful and beneficial; they can also be a hindrance to psychotherapy, serving inadvertently to frustrate and confuse therapists, and to forestall psychological growth in patients. The problem is that the boundaries of psychodynamic psychotherapy do not represent established fact or immutable truth. At best they are clinical hypotheses, either shared by therapist and patient, or taught by the former to the latter. Since boundaries can reflect only relative or consensual truth, they will be ameliorative only to the extent that they include or do not exclude what in any actual therapy will genuinely be curative. Furthermore, as with any institutional form, the assumptions and rules that guide the operation of psychotherapy can become ossified or reified. This raises the possibility that psychotherapy's boundaries will come primarily to serve themselves, and will be out of step with and disconnected from the experience of therapists and the needs of patients. As a result, therapists, or therapists and patients, may believe they are doing the "right thing" in the clinical work, yet nothing of real consequence seems to happen and the treatment ends in failure. I imagine this is often the case when eating-disordered patients complain that therapy taught them something about themselves, but didn't really help; or when therapists report in frustration that they knew what was going on with a patient, but offering the insights didn't seem to have any impact on the symptom.

Similarly, any particular treatment failure is often examined from the point of view of how either the therapist or the patient was inadequate to the therapeutic task. Thus, it might be concluded that the therapist was too supportive, provided untimely interpretations, or was overwhelmed by countertransferential material; or that the patient was too resistant, unmotivated, or lacking in impulse control. None of these explanations challenge the assumptions that underlie and guide the treatment process. It is as if the boundaries are reliable, sure to generate change when therapist and patient are faithful to them. Treatment failure indicts the therapist or the patient for inability to utilize the boundaries, but does not indict the boundaries themselves.

Questioning the boundaries of psychotherapy instead of the separate participants can produce new and surprising perspectives on the treatment process. For example—and this is especially relevant to the treatment of eating disorders—consider one of the assumptions inherent in almost all training in psychodynamic psychotherapy. Therapists are taught that patients will grow psychologically to the extent that they are enabled to separate and individuate. Psychological fulfillment or maturity will be reached when the therapist has helped the patient to achieve autonomous selfhood. However, some contemporary thinking about the psychology of women (Gilligan, 1982; Surrey, 1985) suggests that female development proceeds by means of establishing increasingly complex, mature attachments. In other words, it may be that men, but not women, reach psychological fulfillment via successful separations. This perspective implies that developmental theory in general, and the clinical theory of psychotherapy, may be inadequate and one-sided. In the context of psychotherapy training, it suggests that therapists are being taught to regard all patients as if they possessed a male psychology, primarily in need of attaining autonomous self-sufficiency. Put another way, contemporary training practices may be inadvertently constructing all patients to be of the male gender. Consequently, patients with eating disorders, the vast majority of whom are female, may be undergoing treatment wherein inappropriate assumptions are being made about their psychological needs. In this circumstance the implicit boundaries of the treatment, not the therapist or patient, may contribute to unhelpful and perhaps damaging therapeutic interventions.

There are other assumptions built into the history and fabric of traditional psychotherapy that deserve thoughtful examination for their relationship to the treatment of eating disorders. Perhaps the most basic one of all is the conviction that accurate and determined analysis will finally generate change. This assumption has been and continues to be bedrock for the workaday clinical world, even in spite of the contemporary emphasis given to the concept of relationship and its vicissitudes. For it seems to me that the contribution of relationship to clinical work is ultimately subsumed by analysis. That is, the component parts of a therapeutic relationship—therapist and patient—are examined in the light of psychodynamic hypotheses in order to generate an explanation of their interaction. The concepts of transference and countertransference are the *sine qua non* of such explanations. Their point is usually to uncover a proper understanding of the relationship in order to find an appropriate direction for further inquiry and interpretation.

In its quest for answers derived from analysis, the traditional methodology tends to force reductionistic solutions. Doing this dilutes the spontaneity and power of the clinical interaction. Relationships lose their relatedness and their "ongoingness" when they are analyzed from a transference–countertransference paradigm, because transference and countertransference are essentially organizing concepts. As such, they generate interpretations and explanations but simultaneously grind the relationship to a halt, separating the people involved into separate psychodynamic parts. This is strikingly apparent when one compares clinical presentations of psychotherapy, either oral or written, with more informal collegial discussions. In the former the emphasis is almost always placed on the analysis of the case, the unspoken assumption being that it is proper and correct to utilize analytic concepts when trying to describe the essence of psychotherapy. On the other hand, it seems to me that in casual discussion of treatment there is less of a need to appear analytic. Consequently, case descriptions tend to take on the character of unique art forms, where the full flavor and color of the relationship and the people involved are more apparent and more engaging.

My intention here is certainly not to call for an end to analytic thinking, or to claim that it has no place in psychotherapy. Rather, I want to suggest that our deeply embedded urge to deal with the psychotherapy relationship from a primarily analytic perspective may have inadvertent consequences for the process of treatment—consequences that may be detrimental with regard to the treatment of severe eating disorders. For it seems to me that an emphasis on analysis and analyzing predisposes the therapist (and patient) to an interest in explaining what is, rather than in creating what might be; in observing psychological experience, rather than participating in its expression; and in reacting to the psychodynamic *status quo,* rather than acting to impose or stimulate novel permutations of available psychic resources.

In general, my experience has been that these predispositions, flowing naturally from and entwined within the analytic perspective, can impede the treatment of anorexia and bulimia. They anchor therapist and patient into separate, separated roles, keeping the therapist relatively passive, and preventing the therapist from engaging in a more personal relationship. In contrast, it appears to me that many eating-disordered patients require an interpersonal "shock," or indeed multiple shocks, in order to get better. They do not need a treatment relationship grounded in reductionistic reflection, but one that creates a dramatic, captivating engagement. Something new and different must *emerge* during the sessions, so that therapist and patient are joined in a manner that *transcends* the past and forces attention to the present and future. To put it another way, a new and vibrant connection must be forged, one that enables the patient first to sense and then gradually to participate in an interaction that is actually novel to her experience. In my own work the persistent application of the analytic mode, even at its very best, has too little and too subtle an impact to accomplish this end. As I describe in more detail shortly, the typical "resistance" of the eating-disordered patient is simply too powerful for the time-honored prescription of "inquire and interpret." As a result, not only should traditional boundaries be extended, but therapists must look for ways to break them in order to enhance the treatment process. This is not to advocate "wild" analysis or psychotherapy. Obviously, therapists should be judicious and responsible when they risk overstepping typical therapeutic rules and assumptions. My concern is with the attitude and thought process of all of us who have been wedded to analytic technique. In other words, the natural tendency in difficult or ambiguous clinical situations will be to search for new and better or different forms of inquiry and interpretation. In fact, this may be particularly the case with eating-disordered patients. The weight and solidity of the analytic position make it an especially comfortable haven to retreat to when faced with patients like severe anorexics or bulimics who easily generate doubt, uncertainty, and a sense of therapeutic inadequacy. Instead of this understandable tendency, I am suggesting that therapists would do well to resist their inclination and focus upon ways to unsettle, unhinge, or disequilibrate the ordinary patterns of the psychotherapy relationship. Once again, the general point is to establish, nourish, and maintain an emergent connection that takes the therapist–patient interaction beyond the confines quietly exacted by traditional treatment asssumptions.

ANOREXIA AND BULIMIA REVIEWED

Before discussing some specifics about my own experience with over-stepping boundaries, I want to summarize my current understanding of the eating-disordered person. In particular, what is it about her psychological state that has led me to try to create a different kind of treatment experience? It is by now well established that anorexia and bulimia are multidimensional disorders, displaying across individual cases a wide variety of etiologies, precipitants, symptomatic patterns, and character structures (Garfinkel & Garner, 1982; Johnson & Connors, 1987). Nevertheless, the broad function served by eating-disordered symptoms, and their developmental course, seem to be relatively similar. Especially in severe anorexia and in cases where bulimia follows from anorexia, it has been my clinical experience that the symptoms represent an effort to maintain a psychological status quo. Directly and phenomenologically, this is expressed and experienced as a fear of fatness and a craving for thinness. Symbolically, the symptoms express and often achieve—for a multitude of idiosyncratic reasons—a dread of change and an inability to move ahead with one's life. As such, eating-disordered symptoms are by intent both self-protective and self-constructive, although by consequence they may become self-destructive.

The symptoms develop initially in response to some real or perceived fear or inadequacy that seems to be psychologically overwhelming. First, they tend to comfort and calm the vulnerable person because they enable distraction, engender denial, and produce a temporary sense of increased control, competence, and well-being. Since this process tends to be self-reinforcing, the symptoms become more and more preoccupying. Over time the symptoms and their vicissitudes can become the dominant psychological force in an eating-disordered person's life. As a result, personal and social relationships become fragmented and fraught with conflicts involving food, weight, and dieting. Furthermore, the original connection with life-related fears and feelings of inadequacy is usually lost. In other words, the symptoms become functionally auto-nomous, assuming the status or role of a deeply engrained habit rather than a defensive response to a specific developmental conflict or in-adequacy. Finally, the severe anorexic or bulimic is quite alone in-terpersonally, separated from her previous relationships and attachments. At the same time she is obsessed by the wax and wane of her symptoms, increasingly involved in, responsible for, and responsive to their intricate, idiosyncratic patterning. Where malnutrition is present, the psychobiology of starvation adds to the compulsive, ritualistic, narrow-minded nature of her thoughts, feelings, and behavior. Often it is not too much of an exaggeration to say that the eating-disordered person comes to define herself and to be defined by her relationship to her symptoms. In this sense, Sours's (1980) title for his work on anorexia—*Starving to Death in a Sea of Objects*—is apt but incomplete. Although fundamentally alone vis-à-vis people, the severe anorexic or bulimic is actually intensely, obsessively involved in a relationship with her own unique perspective on food, weight, and dieting. Thus, she "talks" to her symptoms and they "talk" to her (the internal voices of the eating-disordered person). Her moods and behavior are dramatically affected by her understanding of the state of her symptoms (joy, peace, or sudden conviviality if she ate, exercised, or vomited "properly"; despair, dread, and irritable withdrawl if she made a "mistake" or had a lapse of control). My point is to suggest that eating-disordered people develop an extraordinarily complex *intrapersonal* relationship with their symptoms that resembles, both in process and content, the concept of object relationship. In short, within the psychological experience of a severe anorexic or bulimic, her primary object relationship is with her own symptoms. Typically, where an eating disorder is deeply entrenched, this relationship is characterized by an almost sadomasochistic quality. An anorexic or bulimic may feel anguished, enraged, or abused by her symptoms, yet may live in abject fear of "crossing" them or "disappointing" them. And even in spite of their tyranny, being connected to them or acting in harmony with them brings a sense of familiarity, safety, and relative calm.

It is this kind of psychological circumstance that faces the therapist as he or she prepares to treat an eating-disordered patient. Whether voluntary or not, whether complaining of distress or not, the patient is not an ordinary one. The traditional notion of resistance pales in comparison to the actual situation. For successful treatment means much more than uncovering the source of hidden conflict, and more even than accepting the need to gain weight or to stop purging. It is tantamount to losing the only "real" relationship in the patient's life. As such, it represents a kind of self-destruction or self-abandonement.

The ordinary boundaries of psychodynamic psychotherapy do not offer the therapist very effective weaponry in this kind of clinical war. When the rules encourage role separation, passive reflection, and timely interpretation, the stage is set inadvertently for a whole host of outflanking, manipulative maneuvers. Although terribly threatened, and particularly so at first, the patient can rather easily settle into compliant noncompliance, outright deception, and overt hostility. Whatever small skirmishes may be lost, the outcome is rarely in question, and thus the anorexic or bulimic retains her treasured, feared, hated relationship with her symptoms. As I have mentioned, what seems required here is a different kind of approach, one that recognizes the unique form and strength of the patient's resistance. In turn, this means a willingness to try to create something new with the patient, which is to say a new, emergent relationship in the here-and-now treatment experience. What is needed is not just to observe, explain, and organize what is or has been, but to risk intruding and attaching in a way that will generate a powerful captivating impact. Simply put, I think this necessitates breaking traditional therapeutic boundaries. Perhaps it follows that for an anorexic or bulimic to step over the rules and assumptions that have come to rule her life, so must the therapist attempt to overcome the constraints that have governed his or her professional behavior.

Now, how have I actually broken boundaries in my work with anorexic and bulimic patients? I am going to discuss three aspects of the treatment process in this regard. They include the initial engagement, the management of the treatment, and most particularly the expression of personal and caring feelings. Although I focus on these three areas, and offer some rationale for their selection, I want to emphasize one major point. The overall purpose of my remarks is not necessarily to produce justification for some new treatment techniques. Rather, it is to address the general, analytically bounded attitude that accompanies most of us into our sessions. I want to suggest that this attitude with all of its ramifications may hinder our therapeutic efforts as we struggle to help eating-disordered patients. Thus, the three aspects of treatment are intended more to be representative examples of a different therapeutic perspective than a carefully delineated and articulated exposition of what will work better with anorexia and bulimia. Similarly, I am by no means suggesting that all of treatment could or should proceed along the lines that I describe here. Again, I am interested in conveying the importance of a certain therapeutic outlook that can, I believe, enhance the thinking of any therapist when dealing with severe anorexics or bulimics. In point of fact, traditional psychodynamic analysis and analytic behavior are undoubtably appropriate for all of these patients some of the time, and perhaps even for some of them all the time. Certainly this has seemed to be the case in my own work. Yet, as I have alluded to above in more abstract form, there have been and continue to be moments when I feel uncomfortably encased in the analytic mode, overseeing a treatment that feels wrong, unconnected, and heading nowhere. It is especially in relation to these moments that I want to offer the possibility of consciously resisting what can so easily be taken for granted, and risking another way to be therapeutic.

THE INITIAL ENGAGEMENT

The initial session or sessions with an eating-disordered patient frequently constitute a critical phase of the treatment. At this time, during first impressions, it is extremely important for the therapist to demonstrate an ability and a willingness to really engage the patient. Ideally, this lays a groundwork for the future treatment relationship, causing the patient to register (even if briefly) that something new and different can happen in her life. Where there is little significant impact during the beginning sessions, the therapy will all too often trail off into early impasse, or plod along in protracted, superficial compliance. The anorexic or bulimic who does not have her attention and interest drawn to the therapist is not going to feel much of a strain on her relationship with her symptoms. She may experience contempt, relief, and even desperation as the treatment proceeds, but her symptoms and her deep connection with them are likely to remain powerfully entrenched. Thus, the task of the initial engagement is, however temporarily, to unsettle the anorectic's or bulimic's resistance—to create, as it were, a window of opportunity, so that the therapist can establish a genuine relational presence and so that the patient can feel some hope.

I focus shortly on the patient's hidden, often subjugated and frightened interest in recovery. For the moment, however, my point is that I have been most successful in generating initial impact by going beyond traditional boundaries. Unfortunately, I do not know how to describe this process in any systematic manner; instead, perhaps, I have come upon a few general principles. Once again, I am referring to a certain attitude or perspective more than anything else—one that emphasizes innovation and newness rather than continued dependence on the traditional tried and true. In a sense I believe I am talking about a type of art form, and one that actually may be practiced routinely by many good therapists as they begin to treat almost any kind of patient. However, in spite of its ambiguous and complicated implications for both supervision and training, I would like to legitimate the form rather than relegate it to private reverie or informal collegial discussion. As suggested above, published material, relying as it so often does on analytically derived exposition, may reinforce an escape into traditional assumptions in the face of difficult clinical situations such as those presented by severely symptomatic anorexics and bulimics.

Regarding general principles, it has been my impression that the therapist can best unsettle the resistance of eating-disordered patients by adopting an active, rather personal, quite expert, and fully responsible stance during the initial sessions. The idea is quite simply to attract the patient's attention in a way that will cause her to feel interested in the therapist and the treatment. In other words, the therapist should not gather information by means of traditional inquiry, but instead should give the patient information about himself or herself, his or her work, and possible goals for the treatment. Instead of cautious reflection and rel-

atively passive neutrality, the therapist should look for and create opportunities to be intriguing, knowledgeable, dynamic, and distinctive. The
patient should not be pursued for data, or invited to offer explanations
about herself. Pursuing is often unattractive and boring; furthermore, it
invites a power struggle, since it implies that the patient is needed to do
the therapist's work. On the contrary, the therapist should create a tempo
that suggests confident, comfortable expertise. This may be done by
talking to the patient about her symptoms and about how the therapist
imagines they have affected her life, explaining to her how eating disorders usually develop, and indicating that she does not have to be this way
forever. When the therapist senses a reaction, a shift, or a nuance of
feeling, he or she should try not to ask the patient about it, but should
instead offer his or her own thoughts. The therapist may invite a relationship, perhaps focus on its importance, but assure the patient that he or
she will be responsible for its success or failure, as well as for the
treatment as a whole. As seems appropriate, the therapist may engage in
some self-revelation—perhaps some talk about his or her life or experience with others who have been eating-disordered. Work, as it were,
should proceed on impulse and intuition rather than as a result of carefully reasoned analysis.

Throughout, the overriding objective is not a specific content, type
of therapeutic alliance, or method of producing insight. The objective is
for the therapist to demonstrate willingness and ability to offer a new
relationship for the patient—one that piques her interest and forces her
attention, thereby distracting her to some extent from a single-minded
obsession with her symptoms.

MANAGING THE TREATMENT

Traditionally, the idea of "managing" psychotherapy is a rather alien
thought. True, it is by no means uncommon to devise and then try to
follow a treatment plan, but "manage"? The word itself is rarely a part of a
therapist's lexicon. Frequently, psychodynamic psychotherapists are uneasy with, even loath to see themselves in, the role of manager. It
conjures up images of control and manipulation, of passing judgment and
making explicit consequential decisions.

Management, in the sense of taking overt action to guide and enhance a patient's well-being, is usually left to the patient. In keeping with
traditional boundaries, it is her job to exercise and make use of the fruits
of the treatment. Indeed, it should be her job since, ultimately, autonomous fulfillment is the unspoken goal of the whole endeavor. When
patients are unable to do the work they are assumed to be responsible for,
further analysis is usually the prescription, as, for example, is subsumed

under the concept of "working through." Notice, however, that this line of thought does not call the boundaries into question, but instead focuses upon the not yet sufficiently analyzed aspects of the patient, or perhaps of the therapist. Management is also eschewed for its short-circuiting quality. To much active intervention may alter and interfere with an appropriate unfolding of the transferential relationship, which in turn may do damage to the therapy process and jeopardize the ultimate success of the treatment. Again, by implication, the boundaries are inviolate, and therapy is only hindered by undue management. Sometimes, perhaps even frequently, it may also be that management issues are anxiety-provoking for therapists. The type of character structure that merges well with the quiet and privacy of the consulting room does not necessarily at the same time comfortably embrace a treatment style that includes active, public interventions. In this case, analytically oriented therapists actually may be protecting themselves rather than helping their anorexic or bulimic patients when they choose to avoid managing the treatment.

More specifically, by "management," I am not referring to making isolated decisions about how often to see a patient or whether to schedule a family session, and not even to explicitly suggesting how to construct a meal plan or what to do during a holiday meal with the family. At the risk of belaboring my point, I am referring to a certain attitude or perspective that the therapist can adopt vis-à-vis the patient and the treatment. This attitude is certainly inclusive of and just as certainly not limited to the decisions and suggestions mentioned above. It is that the therapist can convey a willingness to be in the center of events, both internal and external, that swirl around the patient's life. Furthermore, the therapist can accept primary responsibility for overseeing and directing these events in a way that he or she hopes will be in the best interests of the patient. In short, the perspective implies that the therapist assumes and provides leadership for the treatment, and in that capacity manages its many complicated vicissitudes.

If all this sounds as if I am advocating an attitude that, in combination with related behavior, will promote the actual and realistic power of the therapist, that is indeed the case. At the same time, I am not lobbying for therapists to become dictatorial, harsh figures in their patients' lives. Almost always this would be counterproductive, stimulating endless struggles for control. Instead, the image I have in mind is that of a kindly, benevolent, yet firm and steadfast parent or counselor; one who knows that he or she is more powerful, more skilled, and wiser than any child/patient; one who is willing to take the necessary action to demonstrate that this is so; and one who is prepared to assume responsibility for such actions.

This image is quite obviously far removed from that of the traditional psychodynamic psychotherapist—at least from the stereotypic picture of this person. Again, I imagine there is more artistry implied by my comments about management than there is opportunity for systematic, trainable technique. Yet the concept of managing the treatment seems worthy of attempting to legitimate. Certainly, it is worth exploring as an alternative to the relatively passive, reactive, and neutral stance that we grow accustomed to relying upon in our everyday clinical activity. In my own work, truly managing the treatment has been difficult. Really guiding a patient's parents or nutritionist, actually attempting to direct her inpatient experience, firmly encouraging a topic for a particular session— all these management behaviors, and many other similar ones, have caused me considerable discomfort from time to time. I continue engaging in such behaviors, and indeed look for ways to further establish my managerial skills and capacity, because in fact my patients often make progress when I lead the treatment.

My own assumptions about the nature of eating disorders suggests a rationale and an explanation, albeit post hoc and therefore self-justifying. Because severe anorexics and bulimics are beset by, yet entrapped within an essentially sadomasochistic relationship with, their symptoms, they are profoundly alone and excruciatingly self-reliant in an interpersonal sense. Living only with their symptoms, and turning only to them for guidance and support, they are often quite literally tyrannized by their former protectors, compelled into agonizing accountability for their every move. This is a dreadful, painstakingly burdensome, and stagnant existence. Understandably depressing, it can also be very frightening. To be "normal" again often seems so far away, like a distant surreal dream. Secret thoughts about getting better, feeling better, and being happy are constantly intruded upon by the harsh reality of their lives. Ironically, the anorexic or bulimic who originally turned toward dieting and weight regulation to avoid the threat of an uncertain future finds herself, in relation to her symptoms, saddled indefinitely with crushing, relentless responsibilities and a chronic sense of deep inadequacy.

In this context, the therapist who manages the treatment offers the eating-disordered person a relationship that is tempting and over time difficult to resist. In fact, it provides a facsimile of what she sought out originally when she developed a relationship with her symptoms—that is, a distracting, compelling safe haven where she is absolved of responsibility, freed of challenges to her adequacy, and enabled to form a protected, dependent connection. Perhaps, then, progress takes place—a loosening of the symptomatic stranglehold and a reawakening of genuine interpersonal interests—because the therapist provides a more gratifying version of what the patient needs and wants. In effect, when the treatment generates improvement, perhaps it is because the therapist creates a psychotherapy relationship that competes successfully with the patient's symptoms.

EXPRESSIONS OF CARING

The expression of personal and caring feelings is an issue that stimulates enormous ambivalence and unease among psychodynamic therapists. On the one hand, I imagine that few would object to the statement that it is important and helpful for therapists to care about their patients. Yet to express or act upon these caring feelings is frequently regarded as a serious treatment mistake. Even in the present era, where the use of one's countertransference has been accorded more and more validity, there is marked resistance to such behavior. Stunned disbelief, supportive or not so supportive calls for more supervision or analysis, outright criticism for having been too grandiose or exploitive—all of these are potential responses to a therapist who acknowledges some form of overt caring for a patient. In spite of the significance ascribed to the relational aspects of treatment, and regardless of a therapist's personal feelings, the boundaries of analytically oriented psychotherapy are quite clear on this issue. Truly successful treatment will not, indeed should not, include any explicit positive regard for patients. Only implicitly, by virtue of their ongoing, consistent presence, can therapists communicate their interest and concern, or their liking and admiration. The analytically grounded rationale is that overt caring will drastically interfere with the development of the appropriate transferential relationship. That is, it may overly gratify or overly stimulate patients, leading away from analysis and toward a relationship that seems to promise more than it can deliver, or one that may become charged with complicated sexual tensions. Furthermore, it may unneccessarily confuse or threaten patients, causing a temporary or permanent disruption in the treatment process. Finally, expressing caring feelings may unduly involve the therapist in the lives of patients, thus diminishing his or her capacity to make appropriate therapeutic judgments, or to take actions that ultimately will be in the service of successfully concluding the treatment. Typically, the force with which any or all of these relationales are applied, and hence the potential stridency of objection to caring behavior, is a function of its consistency and directness. That is, the more durable and open the caring, the more forcefully the rationale applies. Actual physical contact, as an expression of caring, is particularly objectionable and most especially so if continued over time. Indeed, it may not be to much of an exaggeration to say that physical contact treads upon a psychotherapeutic incest taboo.

No doubt the analytic point is frequently well taken. Certainly we have all heard, and sometimes read about, therapeutic horror stories in which the expression of caring has led to extremely unfortunate consequences—be they psychological, marital, financial, or legal—for either therapist or patient, or both. So caring behavior can cause serious, dangerous problems.

Again, however, I want to argue for a consideration of a different perspective. First of all, please notice that the rationales supporting the exclusion of caring behavior from psychotherapy inadvertently reinforce a reliance on the analytic mode. That is, when a treatment process is complicated or irretrievably damaged by the expression of caring behavior, it is the therapist (or occasionally the patient) who is held accountable. Rarely are the boundaries themselves called into question. The assumption is that all would have been well and the treatment would have proceeded if only the rules had been followed, rather than the possibility that the constraints fostered by the rules may have acted as a catalyst for the trouble that ensued. Thus, boundary breakdowns tend almost exclusively to generate analytic explanations that indict therapist or patient, without much consideration for the psychological impact of traditionally prescribed therapeutic limits. More important, the assumption that all will be well when the expression of caring is avoided leads all too neatly to the conviction that such behavior is never important to, or necessary for, patient recovery. Worse than this, from my point of view, is the fact that the *exclusion* of caring behavior is seldom considered when the question of what went wrong in any particular treatment is raised. That is, it could be that many psychotherapies flounder on, or end in failure, precisely because caring behavior is *not* part of the therapist's thinking or activity. From this perspective the avoidance of caring actually may contribute either to treatment impasse or to unsuccessful termination. I believe our almost instinctive, phobic-like response to caring behavior has far too often precluded a thoughtful examination of this possibility.

Ironically, caring behavior is a kind of final frontier for psychodynamically oriented therapeutic activity. Orthodox neutrality on the part of the therapist has given way gradually to an exploration of the positive and negative impact of expressing feeling. Although still subsumed within an analytic frame—that is, the concept of using one's countertransference in the session—there is increasing acceptance of the idea that therapists can enhance the treatment via interventions that reflect their own emotional response to patients. Yet we who espouse and value the psychological benefit of intimacy and authentic caring in the lives of our patients are still enormously reluctant to legitimate this particular type of behavior in our own professional lives. Even so, I suspect that explicit caring behavior finds its way into more consulting rooms than the literature and formal presentations would have us believe. Where this is the case, the potential problem may be not only the damage that caring behavior can inflict, but instead the damage inflicted by being unable to discuss comfortably and thoughtfully the therapeutic ramifications of overtly liking, touching, or hugging one's patients.

Now, with regard to the treatment of eating disorders, I have suggested that severe anorexics and bulimics need something new and different in their psychological lives in order to disengage from their symptoms. Furthermore, in the context of psychotherapy, I have argued that this "something" must emerge from within their relationship with a therapist, and that this "something" must enable therapist and patient to transcend previously established relational patterns. Finally, I have stated that in my own clinical experience the traditional analytically grounded mode of relationship frequently does not have the power to accomplish these ends. Analysis and the analytically bounded relationship offer explanation and psychological consolidation, but the instruments of the analytic mode's own strength—careful reflection, and relatively passive, reactive, and reductionistic thinking—undermine its ability to help severely eating-disordered people. Impressionistically speaking, there is not enough motion or turbulence in the treatment process to have an impact on the anorexic or bulimic. Interpersonally, the analytic mode does not encourage new forms of relatedness. Rooted in the separateness implied by transference and countertransference, its definitions tend to restrict any movement beyond these boundaries, and so it limits the potential for therapist–patient attachment.

However, it seems to me that new attachments are precisely what severe anorexics and bulimics are most in need of—attachments that offer more than is provided by the encapsulated, entrapping, and tyrannizing world of relating to symptoms. Caring behavior on the part of the therapist, expressed comfortably and openly, is an excellent counterpoint to the experience of living with the relentless rituals that surround food, weight, and dieting. Whereas managing the treatment can help to absolve the eating-disordered patient of her crushing responsibilities to her symptoms, expressions of caring can help the frightened and desperate child within her to feel hopeful, valued, and nurtured once again. The key point is to create and demonstrate a genuinely nurturant atmosphere, because over time this will be compelling. In the shadow of her symptoms, the anorexic or bulimic is often not aware of the light cast by the traditional psychotherapy relationship. It is too dim, paled by her own internal relationships. She requires a richer, deeper hue, capable of attracting her attention, and then stilling her fears when she attempts to move out of her self-induced darkness.

Perhaps I am saying only the obvious—that starving, stagnant people need to be fed in order to eliminate their symptoms and live again. I would agree, but I want to underline the fact that these people may need more real, overtly expressed, and consistently demonstrated feeding.

Saying that one likes a patient, complimenting her appearance, touching her in reassurance, hugging her in turmoil, rejoicing in her accomplishments, or sharing in her disappointments—all these behaviors, repeated and repeated, *can* enhance reattachment. I believe this because it seems to have happened both in my own practice and in that of my colleagues. Yes, there are risks—in my own work, more of the "promising what you can't finally deliver" variety—but they are not worth throwing out the proverbial baby with the bath water. A therapeutic perspective that is open to the use of caring behavior can be an invaluable treatment asset, because it can shift the therapeutic focus from more and better analysis to more rewarding, growth-enhancing relatedness.

The risks that attend the expression of caring behavior are not limited to patients. As mentioned, therapists can find themselves unduly and perhaps nontherapeutically involved in their patients' lives. However, it should be clear that what I am advocating in fact requires a therapist to risk a greater degree of involvement than would ordinarily or traditionally be the case. In a very basic sense, therapists need to permit themselves to actually feel what they feel about the eating-disordered people they are treating. In other words, with regard to caring, the therapist needs to risk really liking someone, in addition to wanting to understand her and to help her. By implication, the therapist also has to risk attachment to the patient, beyond the traditional roles prescribed for the participants in a professional psychotherapy relationship. Obviously, this is an extremely complicated endeavor. In sessions, the therapist must, in effect, be a person with personal feelings who is also a therapist, rather than a therapist who is only a person outside the office. Not only does this situation raise the danger of undue involvement; it also exposes the therapist to the stresses and strains, the emotional vulnerabilities that accompany any close or intimate relationship. But to express caring behavior in any other guise—through inherently distant calculation, for example—would seem to beg the point. If the goal is to create something vital and different, significant enough to attract the attention and attachment of a severe anorexic or bulimic, then the therapist would seem to have to risk doing just that. That is, the therapist must risk establishing, developing, and maintaining an attached, more personal relationship that differs from the organization and explanations offered by transference and countertransference, because therapist and patient derive definition and meaning from their immediate, ongoing, and conjointly created interaction. I imagine that this kind of interaction in general, and the expression of caring behavior in particular, have helped to promote therapeutic progress with many of my own patients. As time goes on, perhaps caring behavior will be accorded more thoughtful respect, making it possible for future publications to clarify and better conceptualize what here is only initially outlined.

SUMMARY

In this chapter I have attempted to raise questions about the efficacy of traditional psychotherapeutic boundaries as they affect the treatment process in general, and the treatment of severe anorexia and bulimia in particular. My major point has been that boundaries can become institutionalized, and then both ossified and reified. While this provides the workaday clinical world with a set of rules and assumptions to guide psychotherapeutic work, it is not correct to state that the truth about the method for psychodynamic treatment is known. In fact, habitual retreat to the analytic mode in publications, formal presentations, and anxiety laden clinical encounters tends to reinforce traditional boundaries while precluding other, potentially significant perspectives. With regard to eating disorders, I have described three aspects of treatment—the initial engagement, clinical management, and the expression of caring behavior—for which it seems appropriate to consider breaking traditional boundaries. My purpose here has not been to describe specific new techniques or treatment methods that should supplant the old, but to argue that a close and respectful examination of fresh perspectives is eminently worthwhile if we are to move ahead with our goal of helping severe anorexics and bulimics to recover.

Acknowledgments. I would like to acknowledge the work of Steven Levenkron and Sara Davis. Each has made a significant contribution to my thinking in this chapter.

REFERENCES

Garfinkel, P. E., & Garner, D. E. (1982). *Anorexia nervosa: A multi-dimensional perspective*. New York: Brunner/Mazel.

Gilligan, C. (1982). *In a different voice*. Cambridge, MA: Harvard University Press.

Johnson, C., & Conners, M. E. (1987). *The etiology and treatment of bulimia nervosa*. New York: Basic Books.

Sours, J. S. (1980). *Starving to death in a sea of objects*. New York: Jason Aronson.

Surrey, J. L. (1985). *Self-in-relation: A theory of women's development*. (Works in Progress No. 13). Wellesley, MA: Stone center for Developmental Services and Studies, Wellesley College.

⠈5⠈

Managing Opposing Currents: An Interpersonal Psychoanalytic Technique for the Treatment of Eating Disorders

STEVEN STERN
Northwestern University Medical School

This chapter is an extension of my previous efforts to understand the treatment of anorexic and bulimic patients in developmental terms (Stern, Whitaker, Hagemann, Anderson, & Bargman, 1981; Stern, 1986; Humphrey & Stern, 1988). Specifically, I would like to propose a set of technical principles, derived from a variety of theoretical sources, that I have found useful in therapeutic work with eating-disordered patients. These principles are not intended to define a comprehensive theory, but to delineate a conceptual approach, which may be readily integrated with other psychodynamic models of therapy.

MANAGING OPPOSING CURRENTS

The central idea that organizes this technical approach is that a key element in doing psychotherapy with anorexics and bulimics is the *management of contradictory interpersonal currents* in the patient's communications to the therapist. The concept of "opposing currents" comes most directly from the interpersonal school of psychoanalysis (Sullivan, 1957; Havens, 1976; Gustafson, 1986). Havens (1976), in his explication of

Sullivan's interviewing techniques with severely disturbed patients, noted that Sullivan placed great emphasis on separating the patient's genuine feelings and perceptions from operations that were principally for the benefit of significant others in the patient's family and broader social environment. Sullivan felt that it was impossible to gain an "accurate account" of the patient's real difficulties without clearly identifying the influence of "the other people in the room," appreciating the value of these other people to the patient, but then gradually differentiating the patient's actual experience from the impingements of the introjected others. Havens termed this back-and-forth movement between acknowledging the influence and value of "the other people" and encouraging the patient's own true feelings and perceptions "managing the opposing currents."

Sullivan's implicit theory of character pathology here has much in common with, and was probably the precursor of, such contemporary ideas as Winnicott's "false-self" organization (Bacal & Newman, 1990). It also presaged the work of family systems theorists (such as Selvini-Palazzoli) who have been interested in the opposition between individual needs and family system requirements (Gustafson, 1986). Havens (1976), and more recently Gustafson (1986), have brought Sullivan's ideas about technique into line with contemporary clinical–developmental theory, and suggested that the techniques may have more universal applicability than has been appreciated. They argue that the structure of many neurotic and characterological disorders involves contradictory motivational currents that must be identified and responded to if the patient is to become unfrozen and move forward. They provide many case examples of the application of this technique, including one bulimic woman treated by Gustafson (1986, pp. 230–235).

It has been my experience that many anorexic and bulimic patients suffer prominently from this kind of paralyisis. They are frozen developmentally, caught between opposing motivational currents. Typically, the opposition is between legitimate needs of the self (such as needs for emotional nourishment, affect containment, empathic mirroring, or support for separation–individuation) and some form of characterological self-denial, self-sacrifice, or self-distortion that has its roots in early (and often continuing) requirements imposed by the family system—especially the mother–child dyad. Thus at one level (usually unconscious) the eating-disordered patient is seeking a missed developmental experience that is necessary for the growth of the self, while at another (often more conscious) level there is an apparent disavowal or repudiation of these needs, and of the kind of object (or self-object) relationship necessary to meet them.

What I would suggest is that the success of therapy with this type of patient often hinges on the therapist's ability to track the various currents, gauge their meaning to the patient, and support each of them as they become prominent in the patient's communications to the therapist. This process, I would argue, takes precedence over interpretive work, particularly interpretation of the transference and transference resistances, at least in the early stages of treatment. Indeed, explicit reference to the transference relationship often results in increased resistance and disalliance. The reasons for this, I believe, relate to the underlying character structures of many of these patients, in which dependency needs have become dissociated due to early traumatic frustration in this area. Thus, acknowledging the importance of the therapist is too threatening to the patient's fragile self-organization. Working the opposing currents is essentially a mirroring or strengthening technique that promotes a greater sense of control and integration, and paves the way for more direct transference work at a later stage in the patient's development. These dynamics are discussed more fully later in the chapter.

OUTLINE OF THE CHAPTER

For purposes of exposition, I have organized the material in the chapter as follows: First, I give a relatively straightforward case example in which a discreet "balancing" intervention appeared to effect a significant shift in the patient's integrative capacities. With this clinical material as a reference point, I discuss the theoretical framework within which I understand the technique's efficacy. Then, to consolidate both the practical and theoretical aspects, I present a second, somewhat more complex case; the chapter then concludes with a summary of the core concepts.

CASE EXAMPLE 1

L. was a 26-year-old single woman with a 10-year history of mixed symptoms of anorexia nervosa and compulsive overeating. When she was 16 years old her weight had dropped from 135 pounds to 85, and she had had extreme weight fluctuatiions since then, ranging as high as 185 pounds when she was in college. Since graduating, she had been slowly losing weight; she had stopped binge-eating, but walked 6 miles per day, restricted her eating, and engaged in "rituals" surrounding food planning, preparation, and consumption that could only be carried out when she was alone. She reported obsessing about food-related issues for 75% of her waking hours. Her primary stated reason for seeking treatment was to gain greater control over these anorexic behaviors. One impetus for this was a new relationship with a man that was encroaching more and more on her time alone (i.e., her private food rituals). She felt that it was getting to the point where she would have to "choose between him and my eating disorder."

L. was a bright, intellectually oriented young woman who was employed in a responsible position. She had graduated from a top university and was contemplating going on to study for a master's degree in her field. Except for her boyfriend, L. was relatively socially isolated, having no close friends and only distant relations with her family.

She had grown up in a very religious Catholic family and had five siblings; she was the second of the six. Her mother while nursing L. had immediately become pregnant with her 1-year younger sister. L. described "never having completely connected" with her mother, and "always feeling that I had to do everything for myself." She felt that she had to excel to get any recognition from her parents and described both of them as "ungiving." Thus L. learned to "not need things" from her parents.

L.'s general personality style, as it emerged in the first few months of therapy, had both obsessive–compulsive and schizoidal features. She preferred to spend time by herself; yet she became tense if she had a weekend of unplanned activity, and would compulsively structure her time with lists of activities and chores. She was perfectionistic, often repeating tasks until they were executed exactly to her standards. These symptoms, however, were ego-dystonic, and were clearly identified as tendencies she deplored in herself and wanted to change.

Less ego-alien was L.'s tendency to be self-depriving. She had a conscious, long-entrenched stance of depriving herself of even minimal comforts and gratifications. Thus she would walk several miles home from work on a blustery winter day rather than take the bus, allegedly because she did not want to give in to the greater comfort of public transportation. She adhered to this philosophy in many spheres—especially her eating, where her diet was calculated to minimize pleasure in her food. She was able to associate this self-controlled, self-depriving position with her experience growing up in her family, where she had learned that "not needing" was the best way to contain her frustration, rage, and depression.

These characterological defenses were evident from the beginning in the therapeutic relationship, over which L. exercised near-militaristic control. For example, she did not set a first appointment until she established over the phone that I could see her at her preferred time, and at a particular reduced fee. Nor was frequency of sessions negotiable: She would come once a week—and I felt that finances were not the only determinant here. However, once this structure was established, she was able to engage in therapy surprisingly readily. She talked openly and freely about herself and her feelings, and seemed to form an attachment to me and develop a good working alliance within a few sessions. Although she was generally open to my comments and interpretations, she was decidedly not interested in any comments I made about our relationship or interpretations regarding her possible feelings toward me, and she became irritated with me whenever I tried to make such interventions. Her feeling was that I exaggerated the importance of our relationship and that, in any case, she was not open to exploring it. My understanding of this position was that with me, as in all of her relationships, it was necessary "not to need too much." Thus she sought to keep the therapy on as impersonal a basis as possible. In terms of the kind of analysis I am proposing, one could say that there were two opposing currents in the transference. On the one hand, there was the rigid control she exercised over the structure and the emotional distance of the relationship. But then, within these parameters, she was relatively open, connected, and spontaneous. However, these currents in the transference could not be directly commented upon without causing some disruption in the process and the alliance. I was only able to address them in the context of her outside relationships.

I would like to focus on a particular juncture in the treatment when the tension caused by L.'s opposing currents reached a crisis point. As noted earlier, an issue from the beginning was the conflict she felt between her wish to have a relationship with her boyfriend, Andrew, and the threat this posed to her private anorexic rituals. About 2 months into treatment, her complaints about this problem began to become more urgent. She found herself feeling increasingly resentful toward Andrew for not being satisfied with the time she allotted him. She saw him on weekends, which included both eating with and sleeping with him on at least one evening. She enjoyed their sexual relationship, but sharing meals was very difficult for her, since she had to forgo her rituals as well as eat more enjoyable foods in greater quantities. She considered doing this on weekends a sacrifice. When Andrew pressed her to start seeing him during the week as well, she flatly refused and became increasingly enraged at what she perceived as his increasing demands. In therapy she described the tension this conflict engendered in her. On the one hand, she liked being with Andrew and felt it was "healthier" for her to be in a relationship. On the other hand, she could not tolerate the pressure to see him more and give up her anorexic position.

L.'s resolution of this dilemma occurred as follows: She began, over several sessions, to describe a cold, indifferent feeling toward Andrew and the wish to get rid of him. She said that these feelings scared her but that they were very strong. She was feeling increasingly that she might act on them and wanted to know what I thought. I was aware of two dominant currents in this material, each having its own complex determinants. There was the current of wanting the relationship with Andrew, which I understood to be motivated primarily by a healthy developmental drive toward heterosexual intimacy and bonding. But equally strong, if not stronger, was the opposing current that strictly regulated L.'s awareness and gratification of her interpersonal needs, and preserved her private anorexic world. The latter current I assumed to be a characterological adaptation to unmanageable early deprivations, which served both security-maintaining and self-cohesive functions.

Thus, although my hope was that L. could stay open to the relationship with Andrew rather than isolate herself completely, my actual intervention was to pose both of the opposing currents back to her by empathizing with her dilemma: On the one hand, she obviously cared about Andrew and wanted to be able to have a relationship with a man. I agreed that in the long run this would be good, since it was what she wanted. But her feelings of wanting to get rid of him were quite strong, and it might be that she would have to act on these in order to preserve her private space. She seemed relieved by this intervention, and the relief seemed mainly connected with the second half of the message—namely, the "permission" to leave Andrew if that was what she needed to do.

This intervention falls in the class of what Sullivan called "double statements" and Havens termed "balancing" techniques (Havens, 1976). Explicating Sullivan, Havens wrote: " 'Double statements' are necessary to hold both interests in the mind, together with some fresh element pointing toward a future synthesis" (p. 47). In this instance I believe the "fresh element" was the implication that if L. followed the principle of acting on her own needs and feelings, however she or anyone else might judge them, she stood a better chance of ultimately reaching her goal. This injunction counteracted her characterological tendency to do exactly the opposite—namely, to distrust and disavow her needs and feelings.

In the next session L. announced that she had broken off with Andrew and felt thoroughly relieved. Indeed, she conveyed the sense that breaking up with him was an important act of self-definition and assertion about which she felt quite pleased: She had done what she needed to do for herself. My response to this development was to feel an initial twinge of concern that this was a regressive move for her, but then to feel genuinely neutral and receptive to her feelings, whatever they might be. We would see where they led.

Over the next few sessions, L. began to miss Andrew and became worried that she would break down and begin letting him back into her life. Then she came in and reported that she and Andrew were seeing each other "once every week or two" but only on a "friendship basis."

Soon thereafter she reluctantly confessed that she had started sleeping with him again but that their contact was again being rigidly confined to weekends. Finally, about 2 months after the breakup, she came in beaming, proclaiming that she was feeling totally in love with Andrew. She was seeing him much more frequently—including during the week—and was not missing her eating rituals that much. (She had not stopped these entirely, but had greatly reduced their frequency.)

In retrospect, this period in the treatment was a true turning point for L. During the subsequent year she was able to sustain her commitment to Andrew, and increasingly to relinquish her food preoccupations and rituals. There were minor reversals in both of these achievements, and there were other non-eating-related symptoms and issues that came to the fore and affected her sense of well-being. But her concern over the initial conflict between her anorexia and her wish to have a relationship was resolved to her satisfaction. No doubt in her relationship with Andrew as in her relationship with me, L. kept strict control over the emotional closeness, pleasure, and dependency that she allowed herself. But she did not identify these limitations as problems that she sought to change.

DISCUSSION

L.'s character pathology, like that of many anorexic and bulimic patients, was organized around the management of primary needs, and the tension states associated with the frustration of those needs (Humphrey & Stern, 1988). Her history suggested that early needs for emotional nurturance, holding, and caretaking (mothering) were traumatically frustrated because of the mother's limited psychological resources and preoccupation with her other children. Thus L. was forced to be largely self-sufficient in terms of providing for these basic needs. Her adaptation to this situation seemed to involve several major components. There was an identification with the need-frustrating mother, whereby L. became self-depriving as a way of feeling some degree of control over the maternal deprivation, and perhaps as a way of feeling a bond with the mother. Furthermore, by keeping her expectations low, she minimized her frustration levels and her associated tension and rage states, as well as the decompensating effects these had on her self-cohesion. Finally, she did her best to eliminate the need for other people, and sought relief from loneliness and emptiness through her private eating rituals and other obsessive–compulsive behaviors.

The impetus for treatment was that this adaptation was now impeding her developmental progress toward heterosexual bonding. Any movement toward intimacy awakened the primary needs that had been frustrated in the past (i.e., the early maternal transference) and activated states of tension and rage that in turn overwhelmed her psyche, making her feel flooded and out of control.

It seems that in entering treatment L.'s "unconscious plan" (Weiss, Sampson & the Mount Zion Psychotherapy Research Group, 1986) was to find a holding environment in which she could begin to move forward developmentally. But this holding environment needed to have certain characteristics. Most crucial, I believe, was my response as therapist to the opposition between her defensive need to control relationships with an iron hand, and her more primary needs for connectedness and emotional nurturance. Specifically, I needed to appreciate the latter while fully accepting and respecting the former. Moreover, this response needed to be demonstrated in two ways: *explicitly* with reference to the patient's relationship with her boyfriend, and *implicitly* in my management of the transference. That is, not only did I need to identify and mirror the opposing currents in the outside relationship (where the patient could acknowledge and discuss them); I also had to respond to them in the transference (where they could not be discussed) by respecting and tolerating her need to control the therapeutic relationship in certain respects. It was this combination of responses that provided the particular kind of holding environment L. needed to move forward. Thus the crucial therapeutic intervention was more a matter of *positioning* than interpretation—positioning myself evenly with respect to two powerful but contradictory motivational currents.

THEORETICAL FRAMEWORK

The theoretical framework within which I am conceptualizing both the patient's dynamics and the therapist's interventions incorporates elements from various schools and traditions within psychoanalysis. In addition to the Sullivanian interpersonal tradition already acknowledged, there are concepts from Winnicott's (1965) object relations theory, Kohut's (1971) self psychology, Weiss et al.'s (1986) "control–mastery" theory, family systems theory (e.g., Selvini-Palazzoli, Boscola, Cecchin, & Prata, 1978), and several integrative formulations (Gedo, 1979; Gustafson, 1986). The common thread that runs through these theories is an emphasis on the experiential aspects of the therapeutic process, whether these be construed as the management of conflicting currents (Havens, Gustafson), the provision of a holding environment (Winnicott), the establishment of a self-object transference (Kohut), the facilitation of the patient's unconscious plan (Weiss and Sampson), positive connotation of the patient's status-quo-maintaining operations (Selvini-Palazzoli), or direct instruction in deficient psychological skills (Gedo). Each of these models assumes that in cases where there has been significant early environmental failure, the therapist must go "beyond interpretation" (Gedo, 1979) to provide the patient with a relational experience that partially counteracts the early failure or trauma and thereby repairs the deficient self-structures and adaptive capacities.

I have argued previously that severely regressed (i.e., highly symptomatic) eating-disordered patients suffer from such early "holding environment failures" (Stern, 1986; Humphrey & Stern, 1988), and require a particular type of relational experience in order to engage meaningfully in therapy and move forward developmentally. Specifically, the therapist and/or treatment team must provide a holding environment that performs certain needed functions, such as the provision of external behavioral regulation or the mirroring of autonomous strivings, but does so in a way that is clearly differentiated from the early traumatizing responses of parental figures. Indeed, the patient can be expected to test the therapist or hospital milieu to determine (1) whether the deficient holding functions are present, and (2) whether the original traumatizing responses will be repeated (Stern, 1986). If both these tests are "passed," the patient should begin to engage in a therapeutic process.

Here I am addressing the situation of the somewhat less regressed patient whose symptoms are not so out of control that he or she requires hospitalization, and who is fully motivated for outpatient therapy. I would argue that for these patients, too, the provision of a holding environment is crucial, but that the functions being managed are at a somewhat higher developmental level. Whereas with the severely regressed, dysfunctional patient we are dealing (at least initially) with primitive self-regulatory functions, with the higher-functioning patient the central issues seem to involve more specific affect regulation difficulties and problems of dissociation and integration.[1]

The dissociative (and disregulative) processes involved are essentially similar to those described by Winnicott (1965) in his theory of the false-self organization. Prolonged frustration of primary needs calls into existence emergency strategies to manage both the frustrated needs themselves (and any associated tension states), and the external (traumatizing) interpersonal environment. The strategies are often complex, involving accommodations, identifications, trial-and-error solutions, defenses, and symptoms (compromise formations that allow partial, dissociated gratification of needs). Taken together, these strategies constitute the total characterological adaptation of the individual to an intolerable situation. As Winnicott suggested, such false-self adaptations protect the injured and vulnerable true self by working against its emergence into consciousness and its potential exposure to the old environmental dangers.

As therapists of eating-disordered patients, we are interested in the conditions necessary to facilitate the re-emergence and integration of the true self: the primary needs and developmental impulses that have been repressed, dissociated, or blunted. The general solution to this problem that has emerged across paradigms is that the therapist–patient relationship must provide the patient with a "strengthened context" (Gustafson, 1986) in which the affects associated with early injuries to the self become manageable, so that new learning (or relearning) can occur and developmental progress can resume. The method of managing or balancing opposing currents is one such strengthening technique, but one that is particularly suited to the problem of dissociated needs. In essence, this method (1) holds both of the patient's dominant motivations in mind simultaneously (the dissociated primary needs and the characterological opposition to awareness and gratification of those needs); (2) respects and empathizes with the developmental dilemma this opposition creates for the patient; (3) provides a container for both currents as they are enacted in the transference; and (4) offers the patient a "fresh element," pointing toward a possible future resolution or synthesis. It seems that the patient experiences this combination of responses from the therapist as a more complete attunement (D. N. Stern, 1985) to his or her existential position than previous caregivers have shown, and is thus emboldened to bring the hidden parts of the self into the therapeutic communication and begin the process of integration.[2]

One final comment on the utility of this method with eating-disordered patients is in order: The opposing-currents method was developed by Sullivan in his work with very disturbed patients, many of whom were paranoid in their interpersonal orientations. Sullivan felt, and Havens has convincingly reaffirmed, that with a paranoid patient it is often best to focus the patient's attention away from the therapist and the negative transference because of the potentially malignant situations that can develop. The opposing currents technique is therefore intended to be "counterprojective" (Havens, 1976); that is, it deliberately deflects attention away from the therapist to a situation "out there" that the patient and therapist may examine together—side by side, as it were.

With the exception of a few severely impaired anorexics, most eating-disordered patients are not frankly paranoid. However, many of the more disturbed anorexics and bulimics I have treated are profoundly mistrustful of other people, and are often highly resistant to entering into an avowedly dependent relationship with a therapist. Thus they tend to defend against acknowledging the importance of the therapeutic relationship or the existence of transference to the therapist, positive or negative.

Although their response to a transference interpretation may not be one of paranoid decompensation, such interventions often mobilize increased resistance and may threaten the alliance. The determinants of these resistances are complex and elusive. There are probably paranoid elements (expectations of invasion or abandonment by the therapist) as well as narcissistic elements (the need to protect fragile self-structures erected to manage early traumatic frustrations, particularly frustrations of dependency needs). Whatever the basis, these distancing and disavowal mechanisms leave the therapist little alternative but to work on transference phenomena "out there" in the patient's outside relationships. The opposing-currents method lends itself to this kind of work. It meets the patient at a distance he or she is comfortable with, stays with what is preoccupying the patient, identifies and accepts the conflicting currents in the patient's efforts to master developmental problems, and suggests a path toward possible integration.

CASE EXAMPLE 2

The second case is that of a 20-year-old bulimic woman, J., who was a junior in college when she came for consultation. She had a history of bingeing and vomiting beginning with her junior year in high school. At that time her frequency of binge–purge episodes had been five times a day, and she had been hospitalized for 1 month, apparently with some therapeutic effect: Her bulimic episodes decreased to several times per week, then fluctuated moderately over the next few years. However, during the year prior to her consultaton with me there had been an increase up to once a day, and J. now felt that she wanted to confront her problem in therapy. Moreover, she was now convinced that her eating symptoms were related to underlying emotional issues, especially as these had emerged in her relationships with her boyfriend of 3 years and with her mother. I recommended twice-a-week outpatient therapy, to which she readily agreed.

J. was from a well-to-do Protestant family that had been in the process of breaking apart for several years. Her parents had always had a conflictual marriage, and had separated in the last year. The father had moved out of state, while the mother and J.'s 16-year-old brother still lived in the family's suburban home. An 18-year-old sister had also just left home for college.

J. presented as an exceptionally pleasant, attractive, and bright young woman who was quite successful in college both academically and socially, although she was not particularly ambitious. For example, despite receiving pressure from her mother to choose a high-paying, high-status career, J. seemed quite comfortable with her current decision to go into a lower-paying social service profession. This healthy, more differentiated side of J. was evident throughout the treatment, side by side with the character problems outlined below.

J.'s relationship with her mother had been a traumatically frustrating one for as long as she could remember. The mother was described as narcissistic, superficial, controlling, critical, and at times verbally abusive. According to J., she was "consumed" with her own physical appearance and material possessions, and organized her life around her country club. Her primary concern as a parent seemed to be that her children conform to her standards of acceptability, which emphasized material, social, and physical appearances. Thus she focused on J.'s wardrobe, what sorority she pledged, and the social status of her friends, and would be openly critical if she disapproved. She had always been the dominant force in the family, intimidating everyone, including J.'s father, into compliance with her demands. The father had taken a passive and avoidant role with the mother, escaping into his work and deferring to her on all major issues, including child management. This worked to J.'s severe detriment, in that it left her undefended against the full brunt of her mother's psychopathology. J., as the most independent and defiant of the siblings, seemed to have functioned as a bad object for the mother, while her younger brother had mirrored the mother and occupied the position of good object. Thus J. had grown up feeling that very little she did or said was all right.[3]

J.'s adaptation to this family scenario had gone through several phases. There had been an acute depressive phase in early adolescence, culminating in the bulimic decompensation and hospitalization. This period had been so painful that J. did not like to think or talk about it. Later in high school she had struggled to dissociate her depression and disidentify herself with her mother, making peers and boyfriends the center of her emotional life. This was successful to a degree, but she remained highly vulnerable to her mother's demands and criticisms. Now, as a late adolescent/young adult, she had achieved age-appropriate independence in terms of her overall functioning, but remained susceptible to severe disruptions in self-esteem and narcissistic balance whenever she felt assaulted by her mother. Moreover, while J. tried to cope with this vulnerability by having as little to do with her mother as possible, in a way she kept going back for more, hoping that somehow her mother would be more accepting. What stood out in her descriptions of her visits home was J.'s near-total inability to defend or protect herself when her mother became hypercritical or verbally abusive. Not surprisingly, these contacts with her mother were associated with increases in her bulimic symptoms.

I note at this point the existence of at least two opposing currents in J.'s relationship with her mother. On the one hand, there was the "push" toward greater separation and autonomy. This probably included both a normal developmental component and a defensive component that sought to deny any identification with or dependency on the mother. On the other hand, there was the "pull" of her dissociated dependency needs that kept J. going back for more disappointment and abuse.[4]

J.'s relationship with Ted, her boyfriend, in many ways paralleled that with her mother. Ted was a depressed, narcissistically vulnerable, but controlling young man who sought J.'s unconditional loyalty and love, but was himself frightened by the prospect of sustained intimacy and commitment. Thus he had regulated their intimacy level by precipitating "breakups" when the two were closer, then seeking reconciliation when he sensed J. pulling away. Often the breakups had an abusive quality, with Ted harshly accusing J. of disloyalty, selfishness, or insensitivity. J. would feel crushed by these rejections, and would resolve to cut herself off from Ted, and try to date others. But, as with her mother, she could not seem to resist going back for more if he reinitiated contact. At the time J. began treatment, she and Ted had officially broken up but were still seeing each other frequently. J.'s stated goal was to finally separate herself from Ted emotionally so that she could seriously pursue a relationship with someone who could give her more commitment.

What I would like to focus on here is the therapeutic stance I took with J. in response to her struggle with this relationship, since that is what occupied most of our time in therapy. In contrast to the first example, where a discrete intervention was associated with a dramatic shift in behavior, in this case I felt it was the stance I maintained over many months of work that made a difference.

During the early months of treatment, I learned from trial and error that I had only a narrow band within which to work with J. Attempts to explore genetic material, such as the depressive phase in early adolescence that seemed to have prefigured the onset of her symptoms and dissociative character defenses, were met with enormous anxiety and frank resistance. Likewise, she had no interest in (and was made anxious by) looking at the vicissitudes of our relationship. It became clear that her agenda was to work on gaining mastery in her current relationships, and that my job was to help her with this process within the parameters that she allowed.

J. generally presented in sessions as either "basically doing OK," or "not doing too well." The latter state usually followed contacts with Ted (or her mother) in which she had felt abusively treated and become emotionally undone. Analysis of these depressed states revealed that she felt defeated on at least three levels: first, that she had succumbed to her wish to see Ted at all when she felt she should be dissociating herself from him; second, that she had been unable to stand up for herself during their fights; and third, that no matter how hard she tried, Ted always seemed to be unhappy with her. What actually seemed to occur in a typical fight was that J. would start out trying to defend herself rationally, but to no avail. She would then begin to doubt herself in the face of Ted's escalating accusations. Finally, in a panic, she would concede his points and promise to try to do better in the future. This masochistic submission to his controlling and rejecting position allowed her to sustain her connection with him, but at the cost of undermining her integrity and self-cohesion. Her bulimic symptoms functioned in part as a vehicle for managing the tension and affects engendered by this compromise.

The parallels between this pattern with Ted and the pattern with her mother became evident in the first few months of treatment, and J. experienced my pointing this out as a genuine revelation that gave her at least some intellectual understanding of her problem. She could see that Ted now occupied a position in her life similar to the one her mother once had (and still, to some extent, did). But her insight did not go much beyond this, and her self-destructive behavior continued unabated.

What did seem to make a difference was the way I came to respond to her two dominant opposing currents: her efforts to separate from Ted on the one hand, and her compulsion to continue seeing him and to win his acceptance and commitment on the other. Initially, there was some temptation to ally with the current that sought autonomy from a relationship that was so frustrating and seemingly self-destructive. This was the more ego-syntonic and ostensibly the "healthier" current. But it became evident that it was also the weaker one: For better or worse, Ted *was* the emotional center of her life. Once I understood this, I began gently to confront J. with it; although she put up some intellectual resistance ("Yes, but I know he'll never commit to me"), she became noticeably calmer with my insistence on Ted's importance to her. Thus our sessions took on a certain cadence. She would often begin by ashamedly confessing how she had succumbed once again to the temptation to see Ted, and how this had resulted in another disastrous fight. I would then say something like this: "I think you're being pretty hard on yourself. Clearly, Ted is still very important to you, and we need to try to understand this together. I assume that if or when you're ready to leave him, you will." With this she would experience an immediate sense of relief.

Exploration of her attachment to Ted revealed that, despite his manifestly abusive and rejecting behavior, J. in fact idealized him and felt he was the first person in her life who really knew everything about her and still accepted her. The prime example of this was that he knew about and accepted her eating disorder. Actually, in this realm he took the role of a controlling parent/therapist, insisting that she tell him all the details of her bulimia, and then constantly monitoring her eating behavior. J. found this overcontrol maddening, but it nevertheless made her feel accepted and cared about. (Ted's attitude was in sharp contrast to that of her mother, whose chief concerns seemed to be whether J. was too fat and how she looked in clothes. It also contrasted with that of her father, who was totally uninvolved.) Through this kind of analysis, we came to better understand Ted's significance to J.

I would describe this intervention as a variant of the technique of balancing opposing currents. Here, I was aware of two currents, but was openly supporting one of them for the time being: the one that was more ego-dystonic, yet seemed rooted in the stronger of her current primary need derivatives. At this point her need to be connected to an idealized self-object was taking precedence over her stated wish for autonomy (which felt at least partially defensive). My intervention, I hoped, would validate this dissociated but more compelling need, thereby making it more acceptable and accessible to further analysis.

This stance provided the framework for a working-through process by which J. was able to gain increasing mastery in her relationship with Ted (and, in parallel fashion, with her mother). Having appreciated the opposing currents of her needs for dependency on and autonomy from an accepting self-object, the "fresh element" that emerged was the idea that she could work toward achieving greater autonomy *within* a needed relationship. Rather than attempting to flee the frustrating relationships with Ted and her mother, which she was unable to do, perhaps she could sustain these connections without having to compromise herself so severely.

Although this concept was never explicitly spelled out, it became increasingly implicit in our work together. We spent many sessions microscopically examining J.'s interactions with Ted (and with her mother). At this level, too, we were dealing with opposing currents: the current of self-assertion, which sought an accepting response to her true self (her interests, values, tastes, feelings, needs, etc.); and the current of passive, masochistic accommodation, which sought to preserve the connection with the controlling and rejecting self-object at any cost. As described earlier, J. tended to enter new interactions with a meek attempt at self-assertion, only to revert quickly to accommodation when her initial gesture was repudiated. To oversimplify greatly, my interventions here fell into three broad categories: (1) balancing statements that appreciated both of the opposing currents (the wish to be accepted for herself, and the need to preserve the relationship at all costs); (2) validating statements that affirmed both the legitimacy of her needs and feelings, and her right to express them and have them responded to; and (3) reality-testing statements that challenged her idealization of the other person by interpreting his or her neurotic contribution to the interaction. An example of the latter was that I would point out how Ted's criticisms of her were controlling and distancing, and probably represented a transference reaction on his part (i.e., he was probably responding to J. as if she were his controlling, overly intrusive mother).

This combination of interventions proved to be of considerable help to J. over time. She slowly began to assert herself more forcefully and stand her ground longer. Of course, her efforts to do so met with escalated countermoves from the other person. But we learned to predict these, and I would coach her in responding to them. Fortunately, both Ted and her mother ultimately responded positively to the changes in J. Rather than rejecting her, they became less critical and more respectful, and Ted was even able to acknowledge his commitment to J. by admitting that they were actually "dating" each other exclusively.

J. terminated treatment at the point when she felt satisfied with her ability to manage both of these relationships. Over the course of our work, her bulimia had completely resolved, and she had been symptom-free for several months prior to termination. She felt that therapy had helped her both with her bulimia and her relationship problems, but she could not say exactly how, other than that I had been there to listen and help her validate her feelings about things. We never dealt directly with the core depression, which I assumed was still present but largely dissociated. There were, however, no manifest symptoms of depression at termination. Indeed, J. seemed genuinely buoyant and confident during the last several months of treatment, and appeared much less susceptible to narcissistic disruptions.

DISCUSSION

Like the character of L. in Case 1, J.'s character was organized around the management of primary needs and defenses against those needs. In this case, J.'s frustrated needs involved dependency on an idealized self-object for acceptance of her autonomous strivings and true self. This is the point of developmental fixation for many anorexics and bulimics, because of the parents' difficulty in responding affirmatively to the child's normal separation–individuation process (Bruch, 1973; Johnson & Connors, 1987; Stern et al., 1981). Here, J.'s mother, operating from a regressive narcissistic position, was unable to tolerate J.'s needs for autonomous self-definition and self-expression, and responded punitively by withdrawing love and retaliating like a competitive sibling. J.'s response to this situation had undergone a series of transformations, beginning with protest and defiance during latency, shifting to manifest depression in the period leading up to her hospitalization, then consolidating around a dissociative solution in late adolescence. All of these adaptations had contributed to her character structure at the time she sought treatment.

In entering treatment, it seems that J.'s "unconscious plan" was to confront and gain mastery of this developmental impasse by securing at least some of the experience with a self-object that she had been missing: namely, affirmation of her autonomous self. The ostensible battleground for this process was her relationship with T. (and secondarily, that with her mother), where she struggled to obtain acceptance, and to some extent succeeded.

My role as therapist in this process was somewhat elusive. Clearly, J. developed a provisional dependency on me in which she sought and benefited from my acceptance, empathic mirroring, and coaching. Yet my importance to her was largely disavowed. It seems my function was to be a kind of "self-object in the background," providing psychological fortification for her struggles "out there" in the extratherapeutic object world. Perhaps part of my function in this regard was to protect her still-fragile self from too much awareness of her needs, and hence too much vulnerability to traumatic states associated with early injuries. Acknowledging my importance to her might have threatened this narcissistic barrier, which was still necessary to her dissociative character organization.

Whatever the dynamic basis, the result was that my work with J. was rigidly confined to the analysis of the here and now, outside relationships. Within these parameters I was able to work in a variety of ways, as outlined above. It seemed to me that the cornerstone of these interventions was my response to her two dominant opposing currents: the "pull" of her underlying needs for connection and acceptance, and the "push" of her autonomous strivings, both healthy and defensive. Appreciating the dilemma posed by these two currents, and offering the "fresh element" of pursuing greater autonomy *within* needed relationships, seemed to provide J. with the "strengthened context" she needed to begin to integrate her opposing currents and move forward.

SUMMARY

In this chapter I have attempted to describe a technique for working with anorexic and bulimic patients who, for reasons pertaining to their dissociative character defenses and underlying self pathology, are unable to make use of standard insight-oriented techniques such as analysis of transference and genetic reconstruction. These patients have usually suffered severe early environmental failures in the mother–child dyad. As a result, they have evolved character structures in which frustrated primary needs have been actively dissociated, and some form of false-self adaptation has been necessary to control tension states and secure needed connections with self-objects. The technique itself derives from the interpersonal approach of Sullivan (as interpreted by Havens and Gustafson); however, as has been implied throughout this discussion, its efficacy can only be fully appreciated with reference to contemporary theories of personality and therapy such as object relations, self-psychology, and control–mastery theories. The essence of the technique is to identify the patient's dominant opposing motivational currents, to reflect these back to the patient, and to offer (either explicitly or implicitly) a "fresh element" suggesting a possible synthesis. In addition, the therapist's recognition and acceptance of the opposing currents must be embodied in his or her management of the transference, where the currents are enacted but often disavowed. In this regard, the technique gives the patient as much space from the therapist as he or she requires, and is content to stay focused on whatever problems are consciously preoccupying the patient. It is suggested that this therapeutic approach provides a holding environment that the patient experiences as safe, and as facilitative of his or her unconscious efforts to master early traumata and integrate dissociated parts of the self.

NOTES

1. Note the correspondence to Gedo and Goldberg's (1973) Phase I and II developmental deficits. Failures in Phase I result in deficits in the capacity to regulate stimuli, and call for measures of therapeutic "pacification." Failures in Phase II lead to deficits in self-cohesion or integration, and call for measures of therapeutic "unification."

2. It is useful to clarify the relationship between this technical approach and the classical concept of "analytic neutrality"—that is, the therapist's effort to remain "equidistant" from all sectors of the patient's personality (A. Freud, 1936/1946; Schafer, 1983). While the opposing-currents technique strives to be equally accepting of and empathic with the patient's various currents, there is an added element that increases its power. The concept of neutrality by itself pertains to how the therapist listens and responds to the patient's communications. It does not imply any particular form of action or intervention. The technique I am describing does entail a form of intervention: one that is similar in certain respects to the family therapy technique of "prescribing no change." The so-called "paradoxical" techniques of family therapy (e.g., Selvini-Palazzoli et al., 1978) try to identify the "good reasons" why change (or at least rapid change) may be contraindicated, and suggest that the family needs to address these factors before

change can safely be undertaken. The opposing-currents technique is not paradoxical, in that it does not prescribe "no change" with a hidden agenda of actually producing the change being discouraged. However, it shares with paradoxical techniques the assumption that there are "good reasons" for the currents that work against the patient's stated wishes to change. For example, in Case 1, despite L.'s stated wish to control her anorexic behaviors sufficiently to pursue her relationship, the primary intervention gave at least as much if not more support to her characterological resistances to this change. Similarly, in Case 2, it may be seen that while the patient overtly sought to end what appears to be a destructive relationship, the interventions validated the disavowed needs that held her in the relationship. I had no agenda either to prohibit or to paradoxically precipitate change in these cases, but rather to articulate and validate a central aspect of the patient's motivation that was being negatively connoted and repudiated by the patient.

3. Note that this splitting dynamic is characteristic of bulimic family systems (Humphrey & Stern, 1988).

4. The opposition between autonomy and dependency is of course a normal aspect of separation–individuation, whether in childhood, adolesence, or adulthood. For anorexics and bulimics, however, it becomes a paralyzing developmental impasse because of the parents' difficulty in responding to the normal vacillation between the two currents (Stern, 1986).

REFERENCES

Bacal, H. A., & Newman, K. M. (1990). *Theories of object relations: Bridges to self-psychology*. New York: Columbia University Press.

Bruch, H. (1973). *Eating disorders: Obesity, anorexia nervosa, and the person within*. New York: Basic Books.

Freud, A. (1946). *The ego and the mechanisms of defense*. New York: International University Press. (Original work published 1936)

Gedo, J. E. (1979). *Beyond interpretation*. New York: International Universities Press.

Gedo, J. E., & Goldberg, A. (1974). *Models of the mind: A psychoanalytic theory*. Chicago: University of Chicago Press.

Gustafson, J. P. (1986). *The complex secret of brief psychotherapy*. New York: Norton.

Havens, L. L. (1976). *Participant observation*. New York: Jason Aronson.

Humphrey, L. L., & Stern, S. (1988). Object relations and the family system in bulimia: A theoretical integration. *Journal of Marital and Family Therapy, 14*, 337–350.

Johnson, C., & Connors, M. E. (1987). *The etiology and treatment of bulimia nervosa: A biopsychosocial perspective*. New York: Basic Books.

Kohut, H. (1971). *The analysis of the self*. New York: International Universities Press.

Schafer, R. (1983). *The analytic attitude*. New York: Basic Books.

Selvini-Palazzoli, M., Boscola, L., Cecchin, G., & Prata, E. (1978). *Paradox and counterparadox*. New York: Jason Aronson.

Stern, D. N. (1985). *The interpersonal world of the infant: A view from psychoanalysis and developmental psychology*. New York: Basic Books.

Stern, S. (1986). The dynamics of clinical management in the treatment of anorexia nervosa and bulimia: An organizing theory. *International Journal of Eating Disorders*, 5(2), 233–254.

Stern, S., Whitaker, C. A., Hagemann, N. J., Anderson, R. B., & Bargman, G. J. (1981). Anorexia nervosa: The hospital's role in family treatment. *Family Process*, 20, 395–408.

Sullivan, H. S. (1957). *Clinical studies in psychiatry*. New York: Norton.

Weiss, J., Sampson, H., & the Mount Zion Psychotherapy Research Group. (1986). *The psychoanalytic process: Theory, clinical observation, and empirical research*. New York: Guilford Press.

Winnicott, D. W. (1965). *The maturational processes and the facilitating environment*. New York: International Universities Press.

SPECIAL SUBPOPULATIONS

∴ *6* ∴

Masochism in Subclinical Eating Disorders

HOWARD D. LERNER
University of Michigan

Within the patients in my private practice, there is an intriguing and poorly understood group of individuals who present the paradoxical picture of high academic achievement and enviable talents alongside some very primitive features in other areas of their functioning. Nearly one-fourth of my caseload, as well as my two most recent referrals, are patients with what I would term "subclinical eating disorder" as a presenting problem. These patients, mostly undergraduate and graduate students, present disturbances in eating, self-regulation, and control as one set of symptoms among many. While none of these patients, which include six women and two men, meet rigorous diagnostic criteria for either anorexia nervosa or bulimia nervosa, they do suffer from episodes of bingeing, occasional vomiting, a history since puberty of fluctuations in weight, excessive exercising, perfectionistic strivings, and a reliance on the body as a vehicle for expressing affect and exerting control over the environment (including other people). The basic clinical feature that these patients share is a marked unevenness in psychological functioning—that is, a certain discontinuity in maturational levels of functioning.

It was not immediately apparent to me that these patients presenting the symptomatic picture described had anything in common. And yet I could not work with these individuals in intensive psychoanalytic psychotherapy (three to four times per week) without feeling that something profoundly similar was occurring in the transference and countertransference. In the course of my work with them, I could see that the similarity derived from their having a common, specific traumatic disturbance in an essential aspect of their relationship with their mothers; that is, the needs of the mother were the dominant focus of each relationship, with very little significance placed on the feelings, needs, and competencies of the child. In what follows, I offer an early developmental formulation of this aspect of these patients. A clinical description of these individuals is presented, including the observation that the patients have in common a "false self," or ego style characterized by hypersensitivity, vigilance, passivity, and compliance; a masochistic orientation linked to the disturbed mother–child relationship and a core unconscious fantasy played out in the transference; and a vexing resistance involving a specific ego defect—a delusion of omnipotence (Novick & Novick, 1988). Aspects of the mother–child relationship; the role of magical, omnipotent thinking as a resistance; and the core unconscious masochistic fantasy are explored by means of historical data, memories, and (most importantly) transference–countertransference manifestations. The nature of this early maternal relationship is discussed, drawing heavily on the works of Jack and Kerry Novick on the "essence of masochism" (1987) and the "delusion of omnipotence" (1988). Finally, an overview of treatment issues is presented.

CLINICAL ASPECTS OF PATIENTS WITH SUBCLINICAL EATING DISORDERS

Striking in each of these patients is a passive attitude toward the environment—either an unspoken willingness to be influenced, or an inability to prevent being influenced. The patients present a constant and unremitting state of hypervigilance, heightened sensitivity, and excessive vulnerability. Their vigilance and sensitivity are used as a radar screen, insistently scanning the immediate outer environment in search of potential dangers, especially threats to their fragile self-esteem.

Accompanying the vigilance and sensitivity is a marked tendency toward compliance and accommodation in interpersonal relationships. Like chameleons, they quickly and accurately attune to the expectations of others and mold themselves, their behavior, and their feelings accordingly. This sensitivity and accommodation, however, are defensive and in the service of warding off potential dangers to their self-esteem. In this regard, they differ from the "as-if" character (Deutsch, 1942), whose compliance and imitative behavior is more related to a search for an identity—an identity that will do justice to the person's inflated sense of self. Because such accommodation in these patients is without emotional investment, other people are left with a sense that something crucially important but ineffable is missing. Reciprocally, the patients, painfully and helplessly aware of this compliance, are left feeling nongenuine, unreal, and powerless.

Intimately related to the compliance is a presentation of fragility. The fragility is disarming in that one quickly senses that the wrong word, the forgotten act, the slightest hint of disapproval will strain an already tenuous relationship to a point beyond repair. Underlying this profound vulnerability to external influences and perception of the outside world as cold, hostile, empty, and ungiving is a core defect in the cohesion, continuity, strength, and harmony of the self.

Developmentally, the chronic frustration of legitimate childhood needs to be noticed, responded to, and understood by the mother—to have an effect, to be mirrored empathically—interfered with the formation of essential psychological structures, especially those bearing on their capacity to derive gratification from their own dazzling skills and abilities. On the one hand, these were intelligent and verbally advanced children who had a rather "special" and important position in relation to their mothers. And yet, underlying this, their part of the relationship was characterized by joyless compliance and pseudoindependence. For these patients academic success and athletic talent often served as organizing features, but ones that gave little sense of gratification. Paradoxically, it was often the experience of success in these areas that precipitated panic, and consequently the outbreak of subclinical symptoms that led them to seek treatment. One can say that as individuals they are not failures in life but are failures in living. Their interpersonal relationships reflect a stream of disappointing "crushes," massive inhibitions, or painful loves that could be neither consummated nor relinquished.

Initially, each patient's nuclear self appears to lack reliable firmness, and there is a self-perception of being fragmented, unreal, and out of control. In this regard, these patients present what Winnicott (1960/1965) has conceptualized as a "false self" and what Krohn (1978) terms, "ego passivity"—that is, an attempt to disown, both internally and interpersonally, responsibility in the broadest sense for thoughts, acts, and impulses. In this connection, these patients have an uncanny ability to empathize with drive derivatives from others. These patients' hypersensitivity, vigilance, and peculiar empathy for drive derivatives in others can be strikingly disarming, as in the following example.

Recently, my office building "went condo" and it became necessary for me to purchase my unit. As I was briskly walking down the street to the bank for the closing, I became aware of feeling surprisingly good, quite confident, and particularly "grownup." I was aware of standing up straight and swinging my briefcase as if I had places to go, things to do, and people to meet. Thoughts came to my mind of how 2 years ago I had nervously and clumsily negotiated a mortgage for a home I bought. I recalled how anxious I felt, how insecure I was in terms of dealing with bankers, and how at times I felt like a little boy in an adult world. As I was walking along, I was very aware of how much had changed for me in the past few years and how I actually felt very good and quite self-assured about this closing. I felt proud of how I negotiated the loan with the banker. I could experience the purchase as an investment as opposed to a loss. I savored the moment, thinking that it was one of those times that I would remember in terms of feeling mature, masculine, and satisfied.

A few days later, I met with Miss A., a 26-year-old patient who was initially referred to me 2 years previously for depression, fluctuations in her weight with episodic bingeing, and an inability to experience sexual intercourse or pleasure in dating despite being stunningly attractive. Within the throes of becoming disillusioned with me, and holding an image of me as a frustrating, uncaring parent, Miss A. observed the following: that recently, as she was driving through town, she saw me walking down the street and she observed how masculine I looked and how confident I appeared—walking in such a brisk manner, and looking so well dressed, as if I had places to go, things to do, and people to meet. She stated that I was, in her eyes, the ideal man, successful, attractive; that I know who I am; and (in a depressed tone) that any woman would be attracted to me. She then visibly saddened and became complaining, saying that she didn't like that because it made her feel that she wasn't "special" to me, that she was just another patient. Miss A. could not tolerate feeling nonspecial in a relationship, and as such she could think of no reason to stay in treatment. When she felt special she felt "high," and when she felt "just like another patient" she experienced profound feelings of hopelessness, helplessness, and despair. Miss A., like other patients in this group, had an uncanny knack for accurately seizing the smallest cue that she was being attended to, as well as changes and fluctuations in my own moods and feeling states.

Treatment with these patients often begins under a cloak of great vigilance, with a readines to be distrustful. They are, as it were, there, but with one foot out the door. Swiftly, all aspects of the therapist, including attire, tone of voice, or shifting of body, come under careful scrutiny. If the therapist recalls an incident or memory mentioned sessions before, or responds in a particularly empathic manner, then the patient feels "together" and whole and considers the therapist as an ally. However, if the therapist cancels a session or responds with the slightest trace of irritation in his or her voice, then the patient reacts with hurt and pain and regards the therapist as hostile, distant, and uncaring. My own counterreaction with these patients has been one of being viewed under a microscope. Not only is my every movement closely monitored (often incredibly accurately), but my comments are carefully scrutinized, reconnoitered, and regarded as evidence to weigh before allowing the relationship to continue and possibly deepen. This stance evokes a marked countervigilance and hypercaution on my part. Realizing that interpretations will be met with an overreaction and taken as a personal attack, I have found myself at times less spontaneous, less relaxed, and more careful with my interventions.

Another important aspect of the clinical presentation of these patients, which I describe in greater detail later, is intense masochism. These patients are accustomed to putting their worst foot forward, and initially I tended to regard them as being more disturbed than they really were. For example, Mr. B., on his phone contact, sounded like a panicky and desperate individual. When I asked him if he felt that it was an emergency, he said yes, and I quickly arranged my schedule to see him. Mr. B. initially appeared in my office as a "nervous wreck." Through pressured speech, stuttering and stammering, he was able to tell me that he was preoccupied with his girlfriend at another university, with whom he had been unable to have intercourse because of premature ejaculation; that he was in danger of flunking out of graduate school, where he was pursuing an advanced degree in literature; and that over the past 2 years he had compiled more than five incompletes. He exercised compulsively, played basketball at breakneck speeds, jogged 5 miles a day, and would frequently binge on junk food. His speech, anxiety level, disheveled appearance, and barely coherent thought process made me worry that he was in the midst of a psychotic episode.

My worst fears were intensified when Mr. B. began to tell me about his childhood and adolescence. Between the ages of 12 and 17 he played an imaginary hockey game with a marble and pencil, in which he kept elaborate statistics and simultaneously did a play-by-play broadcast. Furthermore, he used to (and still did at this time) spend hours shooting baskets, keeping statistics involving himself against NBA superstars. My own counterreaction involved high levels of anxiety and intrusive thoughts about the need for medication and possible hospitalization of this patient.

Following this initial presentation, Mr. B. gradually let me know that he had graduated from Harvard, was cocaptain of the track team, and could speak six languages. What perhaps was most telling, and yet something that was only on the periphery of my awareness from the first session, was the impression that this patient bore a remarkable and uncanny resemblance to the tennis star John McEnroe. It was only later that many of those features that we commonly associate with John McEnroe became manifest in his treatment.

DEVELOPMENTAL CONSIDERATIONS

After long, arduous, and often confusing and painstaking clinical work with these patients, I gradually came to realize that their case histories, traumas that led to treatment, and major transference–countertransference enactments involved the playing out of what Novick and Novick (1987, 1988) refer to as "the essence of masochism"—that is, an underlying structure in which masochistic impulses are organized as conscious and unconscious fantasies that are fixed, resist modification by experience or treatment, serve multiple ego functions, and take the form (although not necessarily the content), of a beating fantasy.

> In the fantasies the subject is an innocent victim, who achieves through suffering reunion with the object, defense against aggressive destruction and loss of the object, avoidance of narcissistic pain, and instinctual gratification by fantasy participation in the oedipal situation. (Novick & Novick, 1987, p. 382)

The complex structure of the underlying beating fantasy has drive determinants from all levels of development. That is, it is composed of both preoedipal and oedipal determinants.

Novick and Novick (1988) define masochism as the active pursuit of psychic or physical pain—suffering or humiliation in the service of the adaptation, defense, and instinctual gratification at all levels of development. Masochism is a clinical concept whose observational and experiential grounding can be found in transference–countertransference reactions in the treatment situation. The patient's quest for pain and humiliation weaves its way into the transference, often in subtle reactions to interpretations. My own counterreaction has at times provided the first clue to the existence of an underlying masochistic fantasy in my patients. I have often felt the impulse to be sarcastic, impatient, or either inappropriately joking or heavy-handed, in response to these patients' subtle and often not-so-subtle provocations, frequently around treatment frame issues such as separations or threats to leave treatment.

For instance, after repeatedly experiencing Miss C. taking trips or in one way or another missing sessions either directly before or immediately after I did, I realized that this meek, willowy, and exquisitely fragile young honor student was inviting me to engage in a sadomasochistic struggle around who was in charge, who was on top, and who was going to win. Only much later did we realize that she wanted me to force her to come to sessions as a way to feel wanted and cared about.

The unfolding of masochism and its multiple functions must be dealt with within the transference context. Intimately linked to the transference of patients with subclinical eating disorders and to the underlying masochistic fantasy structure is the nature of the resistance that one encounters in doing clinical work with this population. Based on extensive clinical studies of masochistic patients and consistent with my own clinical findings, there is "a thread linking knots of fixation points at oral, anal, and phallic–oedipal phases . . . a *delusion of omnipotence* which infuses the patient's past and current functioning" (Novick & Novick, 1988, p. 5). This nonpsychotic delusion can include the wish to be both sexes; a profound sense of personal responsibility for death, divorce, and marital conflict; a wish for sexual parity with the oedipal patient; and magical beliefs about success, causality, and the dangerous meanings of sexuality and anger.

As a child Mr. B. (the John McEnroe look alike described above) imagined himself as a fleet halfback who couldn't be tackled. He could defy gravity. Although he had mastered six languages, he had become depressed when at a party someone said, "Learning Chinese is like learning five languages." Mr. B. decided to learn Chinese rather than complete his coursework. Class discussions to him became fights to the death. He had to be perfect, the best, number one. As a child his mother called him "Apollo." His incompletes were in part due to his need to turn in "perfect papers," but he never had enough time.

Through a developmental formulation and clinical data, I have investigated the relationship of the delusion of omnipotence to subclinical eating disorders. I contend that omnipotence of thought and action constitutes a major resistance that is extremely vexing in our clinical work with these patients; it is often responsible for treatment impasse, and it leads well-intentioned therapists to make heroic efforts toward working with these patients, which all too often fall short and end up in negative therapeutic reactions. Beginning with Freud and Ferenczi, and through the work of Klein and later Kohut and Mahler, there has been a consensus view that the child comes to acknowledge the reality of the external world through the repeated experience of phase-appropriate, nontraumatic disappointments, frustrations, and delays. Thus, the child gradually and reluctantly gives up a magical omnipotent system and accepts reality.

Following the Novicks (1987, 1988), I have found that all my patients with subclinical eating disorders have a pervasive delusion of omnipotence that takes the form of an ego defect significantly interfering with reality testing. These patients enter treatment with intense aggressive and libidinal impulses that have clashed with fragile defenses and a deficient superego; this clash produces the delusion that only they are powerful enough to inhibit their own omnipotent impulses, and then only by resorting to masochistic means such as deadening their feelings, starving themselves, recklessly bingeing, provoking attack or repeatedly putting themselves in dangerous situations, or even attempting to kill themselves. In the following paragraphs I would like to present a developmental formulation of the identification of these patients with very disturbed mothers and then, drawing on the research findings and formulations of Novick and Novick (1987, 1988), to sketch the developmental course of omnipotence in these patients. I illustrate these formulations with clinical material.

In attempting to trace the developmental pathway and origin of the "false self," Winnicott (1971) offers the following evocative image: ". . . the mother gazes at the baby in her arms and the baby gazes at her mother's face and finds itself therein." It is out of this symbiotic orbit, this very earliest holding environment, that a vital, alive feeling of self emerges in tandem with the mother's mirroring, approving response. It is this earliest object relationship in natural contact with his or her own primal feelings that give the infant sense of strength and provides the nidus around which a sense of self develops. This is the child's normal phase of omnipotence. From this state an omnipotent core emerges as an intrinsic component of the earliest self-concept. Through the normal course of development, this primary omnipotence is assigned to the parents. As the child develops a greater capacity for coping, and with it a greater awareness and appreciation of his or her own abilities, the need for such an omnipotent extension declines; that is, the need for all-giving and all-knowing parents gradually evaporates. However, when this process is interfered with, a way of regaining the original omnipotent self is attempted to avoid the shattering experience of helplessness and diffuse rage.

In all of my cases, the natural, narcissistic need for empathic mirroring by a caring agent has gone seriously awry and can not be integrated into the developing personality. In essence, these patients have suffered severe deprivation in the areas of narcissism and object relations, and this has had a considerable impact on the structuralization of their personalities. They have not had reliable, "good enough" mothers at their disposal during the symbiotic phase, nor "usable objects" (Winnicott, 1971) who could survive their own destructive impulses. Clinically, these patients cannot accept the reality that this loss occurred in the past and that no effort whatsoever can change that fact. The mothers of my patients have all declared their sensitivity to their children's needs, yet they are experienced as nonresponsive, distracted, or aloof. A confusion ensues. Does one believe what one is told, what is perceived, or what one wishes to perceive? The reality testing of emotional resonance breaks down.

When mothering is not "good enough," what the infant sees in the mother's eye is a reflection of the mother's internal state rather than a reflection of his or her self. Several factors can interfere with the establishment of the infant–mother preprogrammed empathic relationship: Physical illness, depression, anxiety, psychosis, or intrafamilial conflict can all disrupt the pleasurable interaction between mother and infant. There is a marked and significant disturbance in the pleasure economy from birth (Novick & Novick, 1987). In these cases, an external perception takes the place of a growing awareness of the self in relationship to the mother, and as a result the development of an internal sense of a competent, effective self is seriously impeded. Failures in mirroring, experienced as an "impingement" (Winnicott, 1971)—a dreaded sense of premature separation from the mother, accompanied by feeling intensely helpless and dangerously exposed and unprotected—seriously disrupts the continuity and harmony of the self in relationship to the mother and promotes the development of premature defenses, which crystallize in a "false self" within the context of a passive ego. The "false self" can be seen as a stable and complex compromise formation, including a defensive constellation that is characterized by compliance with the expectations of others, and coexisting with an ego defect involving the delusion of omnipotence. That is, the experience of maternal impingement is assimilated into and expressed through an exquisitely egocentric cognitive structure described by Piaget (1954) as concrete, solipsistic, and subjective. These patients exhibit a pervasive passivity of the ego; they are highly receptive and compliant, and are more than ready to assimilate any stimuli from the external world, including subtle shifts in their mothers' moods. These patients are, however, quite active in the pursuit of pain and failure, in part to maintain this assimilative relationship with an intrusive, impinging object.

The specific qualities of these disruptions in holding and empathic mirroring communicate the unique psychological makeup, present state, and active conflicts of the mother and are globally "taken in" by the infant as a self-protective response to premature separateness. They are internalized as the basic mark of the self—a "false self"—and are used as a model and foundation for the later development of object relations and other internal psychological structures. I have often heard my patients say, "I just don't know any other way," after once again experiencing frustration, undermining themselves, or provoking crises.

As Ogden (1978) notes, a particular form of identification results from maternal impingement, in which the patient attempts to create the illusion that his or her own spontaneous gestures ("true self") are characterized specifically by those qualities of the mother's pathology communicated through the impingement.

It was only through reconstructing repeated, painful, frustrating, provocative patient–therapist interactions in which I was pushed into a position of feeling hopeless, incompetent, and ineffective that I could come to understand that this was an indication of a history and relationship pattern relevant to this particular form of identification. Under the cumulative impact of empathic failures, my patients, beginning in infancy, turned away from their natural, preprogrammed capacities to

interact efficaciously with the real world. As Novick and Novick (1988)
state, they

> . . . instead began to use the experience of helpless rage and pain
> magically to predict and control their chaotic experiences. The failure of
> reality-oriented competence to affect empathic attunement forced the
> child into an imaginary world where safety, attachment and omnipotent
> control were magically associated with pain. (pp. 9–10)

These patients egocentrically struggle to maintain the illusion that
they, through their own sense of power, magic, and control, have created
the discordant moods and conflicting feelings that they are perceiving,
even though the states are originating outside of them. As one patient
said, "World hunger—my fault." As infants, my patients were made to
feel omnipotently responsible for their mothers' pain, rage, helplessness,
and incompetence. Disruptions in normal omnipotence secondary to
maternal impingement coalesced with cognitive egocentricity, so that the
intensity of painful feelings generated in each mother–child dyad represented a constant affirmation of omnipotence. Since there was an absence
of self–other differentiation, the mother was felt to own the infant's mind
and body, and therefore attacks on the self became a powerful weapon for
attacking the mother (Novick & Novick, 1987). The ongoing frustration of
the infant's age-appropriate need for competent interactions created a
feeling of intense helpless rage in the infant, which was defended against
by fantasies of omnipotent control and destructiveness. Some of the
patients in my eating disorder sample deny their hostile feelings toward
their mothers and regard any sign of hostility between themselves and
their mothers as the struggle to maintain an idealized view of the mothers
as loving and perfect. A patient's repeated failure to elicit an empathic
response and an unwillingness to sacrifice the "special" position of importance assigned by the mother leads to a split. The affective perception
is disavowed, and an illusory idealization of the relationship with the
mother results. The patient rejects the possibility of an empathic relationship, but to avoid entirely losing the relationship converts it into one that
is wished and longed for. The mother's failings and shortcomings are
invariably attributed to the patient's own aggression. Masochism, in this
context, can be seen as an attempt to protect the self against destructive
impulses from each level of development directed against the mother by
turning aggression against the body.

The persistence of the child's involvement with pain and omnipotent
thinking is a central thread going through the fabric of development,
undergoing various transformations. Entry into the phallic–oedipal phase
brings with is the sexualization of masochism. In normal development,
oedipal disappointments are cushioned by a solid base of self-esteem and

competent interactions with "good enough" parents. Aggressive infantile sexual theories of parental intercourse and the narcissistic knocks of oedipal exclusion are all modified by loving respect and empathic sexual information. Patients in my sample of subclinical eating disorders experienced the oedipal phase masochistically; that is, they were tied exclusively with their mothers and experienced the recognition of real physical differences between children and adults as yet another failure of their own, leaving them in states of helplessness and rage. Experiences such as overstimulation, inappropriate physical contact, and parental neglect were all transformed into fantasies of triumph, oedipal victory, and affirmation of the children's omnipotent power to coerce the parents into gratifying all needs. This is a common fantasy when divorce is part of the case history.

I have found traumas during this phase to be particularly salient in patients who exhibit binge-eating during the night. There seems to be more to this behavior than flirtation with the primal scene. For example, Mrs. D., an attractive yet highly anxious and vulnerable graduate student, was referred to treatment because of binge-eating during the night, fluctuations in her weight, and difficulty coming to terms with the divorce of her parents when she was 15. The father was a high-powered, quite narcissistic lawyer, while the mother, after the divorce, was in and out of hospitals in which she was treated for drug addiction. The patient, an only child, remembered lifelong difficulties sleeping and being alone. Her earliest memory was waking up at night and beckoning her parents, who would attempt to put her to sleep by first throwing exciting parties for her, replete with all kinds of food. She recalled that the intensity of her excitement at these parties often provoked her mother to drink as a way of calming herself so that she could put her daughter to sleep. The parents experienced intense fighting, and during long periods of arguing and hostility the father would leave the parental bedroom and move into Mrs. D.'s room. His packed suitcase next to the door was a constant reminder to Mrs. D. and her mother that he could leave at any moment.

Miss E., a 21-year-old student, was also referred to treatment because of binge-eating in the middle of the night and painful obsessing over losing her boyfriend, a star hockey player. The daughter of a physician father and business executive mother who subsequently divorced, Miss E. recalled always having difficulty sleeping and being alone. She recalled often sleeping with the *aupair;* she once woke up in the middle of the night and, terrified at finding herself alone, searched the house to find the *aupair* in the parents' bedroom having intercourse with her boyfriend.

The normal pleasures in latency associated with achievement did not take place in the patients of my sample. In fact, achievements in reality were a source of little pleasure for them. Rather, fantasies of omnipotent control and triumph, often occasioned by the experience of pain, characterized this period. In contrast to a system of competence based on work and achievement, which is experienced by most children, my patients established a magical omnipotent system in which any achievement, skill, or positive accomplishment was interpreted as due to their own omnipotence rather than to work (Novick & Novick, 1988). Success and achievement came to be associated with destructiveness and hostile triumph over others, and often led to provoking punishment and inhibition.

Ms. F., an overweight, 45-year-old widow, had lost her mother in childbirth at age 4. After being shuffled between different homes, sexually molested, and separated from her younger brother, she was shipped to a convent boarding school where she achieved impressive academic success. Years later, on the verge of being offered a prestigious college scholarship, she boasted to friends about her sexual exploits the previous summer with an older military officer. Word quickly spread to the nuns, and Ms. F. was promptly expelled. Several years later she was deemed the "star" of her graduate program and was academically courted by senior faculty. Panicked while taking her qualifying exam, she purposely and unnecessarily answered a question outside of her area of expertise, failed the exam, and with a sense of relief dropped out of the program.

An insistent dynamic in treatment was Ms. F.'s compulsion to make herself a victim whenever she got close to feelings of activity and responsibility. Whenever she recognized herself as an active, powerful person who made things happen in reality, she needed to destroy and spoil her chances because of enormous guilt over her own omnipotently destructive wishes. This was a vehicle for making me, in the transference, responsible for her hardships; a way of gaining control; and a quest for safety in a stoic rage, where she lived life vicariously through fantasies of my blissful life with my wife and daughter while resentfully nursing her rage alone, drinking, and binge-eating. Reality achievements threatened the magical system, and there was a need for misery and helplessness to feel magical. Pain and magic were mutually dependent upon each other.

All of my patients experienced difficulty during adolescence. The greatest threat to the fantasies of omnipotence was the experience of pleasure, especially pleasure derived from adult activities such as sexuality. As Novick and Novick (1988) would put it, the omnipotent system left no place for pleasure in reality, in that pleasure left them feeling ordinary and not special. All patients in my sample had a disturbed late adolescence, based on a failure to take ownership of their own bodies and minds and to integrate adult sexuality into their self-image (Laufer & Laufer, 1984).

A common fantasy and distortion of memory exhibited by many of my patients is that things were not that bad in their childhood. For instance, Miss G., a 22-year-old student, maintained two contradictory images of her childhood. One image, the Hollywood version, was of a happy little girl frolicking in a funhouse with her boyfriends and playing exciting games with her two older brothers and younger sister. The other image was of a lonely and confused little girl cuddled up in her bed alone, frightened of the yelling and screaming that she heard going on between her father and brothers. She was always the "good girl" in her family; she experienced a sense of specialness and power by being the only child who did not cause trouble for her parents.

Although she was stunningly attractive, sexually precocious, and multitalented, and although boys were always interested in her, Miss G.'s sexual activity, which during early adolescence was blatant and exhibitionistic, was later expressed secretly and then only when she was on drugs; still later it evolved into highly infantile and idealized crushes on inappropriate objects such as her minister. She was referred to treatment because of binge-eating, sexual inhibition with fears of being gay, a tremendous fear of and aversion to having sexual intercourse, an inability to find herself and select a career, and painful feelings of exclusion when hearing that her girlfriends were having sex. Miss G. had enormous talent as a student and athlete. She was captain of her high school swim team and was on the track team, but she derived little pleasure from her accomplishments. In fact, she managed to alienate many of her teachers and dropped out of swimming and track.

These patients need the experience of misery and helplessness to feel magical; that is, they use their masochism as a way of controlling their own omnipotent power. These patients fear success and reality, because success carries with it the meaning of annihilation and destruction of objects that are loved. The patients attribute omnipotent power to their own feelings, fantasies, and accomplishments. Inhibition and spoiling successful experiences and accomplishments become major vehicles for maintaining infantile relationships, protecting themselves against aggressive destruction and the loss of others, avoiding narcissistic pain, and gratifying instincts by fantasy participation in oedipal victories and triumphs.

Miss H., as part of a sudden act of defiance around the issue of growing up and becoming independent, decided to return home and take her Graduate Record Examinations. This sudden departure was part of a pattern of confused, impulsive, and poorly thought-out darting away from treatment, as well as a rapprochement with her seriously disturbed mother. Within our relationship, the sudden departure had a "Screw you! What are you going to do about it?" quality. Several weeks later she got the results; while anxiously telling me that her spectacular scores could get her into most graduate programs, she began to hyperventilate. She was using her body as a means of communicating feeling out of control around the separation and her success and of regaining control. She felt I did not believe her scores, and after an influential professor encouraged her to apply to his program, she proceeded to alienate him and dawdle in completing her coursework. Analysis of this revealed her intense fears of growing up; a view of commitment as a demand to limit herself; the need to stay a little girl and remain in treatment with me; and a fear that if she grew up I, like her father, would be uncomfortable with her. Her fantasies equated growing up with ruining my marriage and destroying my wife.

TREATMENT IMPLICATIONS

In patients with subclinical eating disorders, derivatives from all levels of development help form the delusion of omnipotence that is a major component of the underlying masochistic beating fantasy and that becomes manifest in treatment as a major source of resistance. I have found that working with the delusion of omnipotence as a resistance and an ego defect in reality testing as a major focus has helped me organize interventions that are mutative. During the early phases of treatment, resistance revolves around the need to control all impulses for fear that they will lead to the destruction of both objects and the self. One way of accomplishing this is by assuming an infantile position in relationship to the therapist. Many patients will project their omnipotence onto the therapist as a means of insisting that the parent/therapist take responsibility for managing issues of weight and eating behavior. This is often a preview of a deeper, more instinctualized wish for the therapist to take control of their lives in a definite and forceful way, frequently communicated by using their bodies to "pump" the therapist for information, suggestions, and ideas. Often parental collusion keeps a patient in this position. A subtle sign of this frequently involves arrangements for the fee, in which the patient will insist that the bill be sent directly to the parents. Removing the issue of money and the business aspect of treatment from the patient–therapist relationship infantilizes the patient; distorts the reality that the therapist is paid for professional as opposed to personal services; and contributes to the delusion of omnipotence, which interferes with the therapeutic task of assisting the patient in growing up.

Following the early phase of treatment, resistance focuses on the danger of pleasure and the threats that pleasure and reality pose to the omnipotent system. Here fear of success, intense guilt, and a desperate clinging to pain are prevalent. As Novick and Novick (1988) state, "pain is the affect which triggers the defense of omnipotence, pain is the magical means by which all wishes are gratified and pain justifies the omnipotent hostility and revenge contained in the masochistic fantasy" (p. 23).

With the dawning recognition and expression of libidinal and aggressive impulses comes the fear of not being able to stop. Spoiling becomes a powerful defense to convert pleasure to pain. One patient remarked, "Before the session I had such a delicious sandwich." Moments later she complained of a stomachache. She experienced a "delicious" session of hard work and insight in the same manner. What is ultimately therapeutic is pitting the omnipotent system against the reality principle. In this regard, I have found through clinical experience that many interventions based on the so-called "holding environment"—such as offering extra sessions, sending postcards during vacation, or actually calling the patient—are not only unhelpful but actually harmful. These well-intentioned provisions support the omnipotent system of infantile relationships, limitless supplies, magical control, and treatment based on personal care rather than professional competence. These interventions make a patient feel out of control. These patients require firm and empathic controls, with unwavering attention to the transference and resistance. As treatment deepens, according to Novick and Novick (1988), working with the delusions of omnipotence as a resistance reveals and brings into focus the fixed masochistic beating fantasy, which can then be analyzed in terms of an attempt to (1) maintain a preoedipal tie to the mother, (2) protect the object against destructive impulses, and (3) participate in a sadomasochistic relationship.

Working with the preoedipal object tie is quite difficult, because it involves examining the patients' pathology, especially their hostile opposition to growing up. Dealing with the preoedipal tie between mother and patient is crucial for subsequent change in a patient's underlying masochistic pathology and eating disorder to take place.

In his classic paper 'A Child Is Being Beaten,' (1919/1955), Freud outlined three stages of the beating fantasy that occurs transiently during normal development and that becomes fixed in patients with masochistic pathology (Novick & Novick, 1987). In the first phase (sadism) of the beating fantasy, a disliked sibling is beaten by the father. This is thought to gratify the child's jealousy and is driven by libidinal and narcissistic interests. The fantasy during the second phase is of the child himself or herself being beaten by the father. This is a direct expression of guilt that transforms the sadism to masochism. The fantasy is not only a punishment for forbidden impulses, but also a regressive substitute for it. This is where masochism and the beating fantasy become libidinized. Clinically, this can often be uncovered through analyzing masturbation fantasies. The third phase represents a turn toward sadism in terms of an over-sensitivity and antagonism toward father figures. In the case examples that follow, I illustrate how this fantasy structure is woven into the treatment process.

Miss C. had often lamented that her family motto was "food = love and love = food." After once again planning a trip in response to my previously announced plans to be away, she reluctantly offered the fantasy that I harbored hate for her because I disliked discussing her vacation plans. This was within the context of feeling miserable during the weekend, feeling excluded from her roommate's relationship with another woman, and feeling unappreciated at work. She did not know why this was coming up now or what it was about. When I said "I think I do," Miss C. said, "You can tell me why I hate you." I said, "Because you want me to stop you from going away." She enthusiastically said, "I should change the family motto—"force + food = love." Her associations led to how she was in a sense "force-fed" by her mother, and how she had a dream the preceding night that she planned her trip and I was glad to see her go.

After the interpretation of Ms. F.'s beating fantasy—her wish that I would force her to grow up, to lose weight, to have sex—she reported during a Friday session that she was feeling more sexual, in part because her housemate had given her a porno novel about older women and younger men, and in part because she was feeling more genuinely as opposed to mockingly attracted to me. Referring to me as the "captain of the football team," she said she was worried that if she had me she would want the whole team. Later she modified this to mean that if she had a little of me she would want all of me; it would never be enough, and this was depressing to her. She then reported a fantasy of her car crashing and me being an adulterer.

On the following Monday she reported that she drank heavily over the weekend, cooked compulsively, and binged. She recalled two dreams. In the first dream she was living in a house connected to another house by a giant moving van with detachable parts. As she went through her house, she observed scary cats with sharp teeth wrapped in bright colors. In the second dream she was driving her car; her foot got stuck on the accelerator and the brakes failed. She ended up at the footall stadium where there were 50 or 60 working-class men dressed in janitor suits. Her associations were to "raging hormones," wanting to spend more and more time in therapy with me, and the thought that love is the first step toward separation, the beginning of the end. She felt she needed inspiration to diet and lose weight—"The only inspiration I know is frustration." For this patient, the meaning of sexuality was intimately related to the death of her mother and later her husband. The fear was that once she let go she would not be able to stop. Food for Ms. F. represented instinctual gratification, protection from destructive impulses and their imagined consequences, and self-punishment, as it effectively removed her from dating.

Within the context of once again debating whether or not to stay in treatment, because she no longer felt "special" to me or felt that she had any impact on me, Miss A. lamented sadly that she felt "just like another patient." She offered several fantasies about returning to the idealized version of her childhood or a job in San Francisco where she could advance. Suddenly she felt I was not listening to her and angrily said, "I want to get up and leave right now," and I responded, "And have me come after you and force you to stay." Miss A. then said, "At least I would know you care." This interpretation opened the way for a consideration of sexual identity issues, specifically her bisexual conflict.

The next session Miss A. mentioned jogging and seeing guys playing basketball with one girl who "played like a girl," quite feminine; Miss A. said that she herself could take a jumpshot just like a guy. It was very upsetting, and as she recalled what a good athlete she was, she wondered whether there was something that she just couldn't give up in becoming feminine. Perhaps this was penis envy, but she didn't want a penis. She felt feminine sometimes—an inner wholeness, strength, calmness—but somehow could not let go of the activity, the movements like Magic Johnson, the fancy plays and slam dunks that she always liked. It was the active aggression and moving forward that she loved. It was not being able to let go of this, she felt, that prevented her from being feminine. She supposed that it also involved a commitment. There were memories of her younger brother, of how her parents would have stopped having children with her had she been a boy, and of how she identified with the boys by being aloof (unlike her hysterical sister). She had typically "male fantasies" of wanting to be admired, being like Martina Navratilova, and winning swim meets.

I wondered what was incompatible about this and about being a woman. Much of her discourse involved the differences between being a girl and being a woman: According to her, being a girl emphasized the externals of being looked at and popular, while being a woman was an inner feeling of wholeness. She felt she could not integrate the two and give up the active, aggressive aspects of being masculine. She wanted it all and could not bear letting go. She would be so vulnerable, it just wouldn't be *she*; she wouldn't know herself. She did not have an identity and felt she took refuge in being gay. She realized that women compete for men, and she dismissed this. She wondered whether there was a connection between being unable to commit to being a woman and other things. She feared that if she got more in touch with her feelings, she would be pushing buttons for nuclear war and having sex with everyone in my building.

CONCLUSION

The focus of this chapter has been on a group of patients with subclinical eating disorders who demonstrate a particular clinical presentation, style, form of maternal identification, resistance in treatment, and underlyng fantasy structure. They have identified with particular aspects of their mother's pathology; this model of identification is reflected in their "false-self" presentation, in their object relations, and in many aspects of their psychological structures. Each patient's early history was dominated by a view of a mother deeply involved in her own conflicts in which she was unable to protect the infant. This was experienced during the stage of normal omnipotence as an "impingement," a premature separation in which the mother's conflicted self was globally "taken in" by the growing child as a core sense of self. This disruption of normative omnipotence, in which vitally intimate aspects of the mother–infant relationship were embellished with pain, set the stage for the development and transformation of masochistic impulses. A common feature of this developmental course is the miscarriage of omnipotence, in which a system of magical thinking and power interferes with the normative evolution of the reality principle. All events and happenings are experienced magically as caused by the self; limits and commitments, as well as separations implying loss, are intolerable; the experience of growing up, in which pleasure is achieved in reality through work and mature relationships, becomes impossible. Development becomes uneven. Disturbances in eating, such as fluctuations in weight, bingeing, and excessive exercising, become futile attempts to achieve omnipotent perfection, reunion with the mother, protection against aggressive destruction and object loss, and instinctual gratification.

Acknowledgment. I am indebted to the supervisory help and theoretical formulations of Dr. Jack Novick.

REFERENCES

Deutsch, H. (1942). Some forms of emotional disturbance and their relationship to schizophrenia. *Psychoanalytic Quarterly, 11,* 301–321.

Freud, S. (1955). 'A child is being beaten': A contribution to the study of the origin of sexual perversions. In J. Strachey (Ed. and Trans.), *The standard edition of the complete psychological works of Sigmund Freud* (Vol. 17, pp. 175–204). London: Hogarth Press. (Original work published 1919)

Krohn, S. (1978). *Hysteria: The elusive neurosis.* New York: International Universities Press.

Laufer, M., & Laufer, M. (1984). *Adolescence and development breakdown*. New Haven, CT: Yale University Press.

Novick, J., & Novick, K. (1988, December). *Some comments on masochism and the delusion of omnipotence from a developmental perspective*. Paper presented at a Panel at the meeting of the American Psychoanalytic Association.

Novick, K., & Novick, J. (1987). The essence of masochism. *Psychoanalytic Study of the Child, 42,* 353–384.

Ogden, T. (1978). A developmental view of identification resulting from maternal impingement. *International Journal of Psychoanalytic Psychotherapy, 7,* 486–507.

Piaget, J. (1954). *The construction of reality in the child*. New York: Basic Books.

Winnicott, D. W. (1965). Ego distortion in terms of true and false self. In D. Winnicott (Ed.), *The maturational process and the facilitating environment*. London: Hogarth Press. (Original work published 1960)

Winnicott, D. W. (1971). *Playing and reality*. New York: Basic Books.

∴ 7 ∴

The Clinical Stages of Treatment for the Eating Disorder Patient with Borderline Personality Disorder

AMY BAKER DENNIS

*Center for the Treatment of Eating Disorders and
the National Anorexic Aid Society, Columbus, Ohio
and Midwestern Educational Resource Center,
Bloomfield Hills, Michigan*

RANDY A. SANSONE

*Laureate Psychiatric Hospital and Clinic, Tulsa
and School of Medicine, University of Oklahoma*

One of the most challenging and interesting areas in the field of eating disorders is the treatment of individuals with coexisting borderline personality disorder. In this chapter, we review the previous research supporting the coexistence of these two disorders and highlight our own diagnostic and treatment approach. In the area of diagnosis, we review the available diagnostic options for borderline personality and the psychostructural theory of personality organization. We have organized our treatment approach into four basic stages: (1) establishing the therapeutic milieu; (2) stabilizing the transference; (3) resolving internal themes; and (4) preparing the termination. These clinical impressions and treatment philosophy are based on our collective clinical experience with these complex individuals. We hope that this chapter assists the eating disorder specialist in the treatment of this often neglected population.

THE COEXISTENCE OF BORDERLINE PERSONALITY DISORDER AND EATING DISORDERS

A substantial minority of patients with bulimia nervosa have coexisting borderline personality disorder. This impression is supported by our clinical experience with the treatment of eating disorders, as well as several published studies that have explored this relationship (Gwirtsman, Roy-Byrne, Yager, & Gerner, 1983; Johnson, Tobin, & Enright, 1989; Levin & Hyler, 1986; Pope, Frankenberg, Hudson, Jonas, & Yurgelun-Todd, 1987; Powers, Coovert, Brightwell, & Stevens, 1988; Sansone, Fine, Seuferer, & Bovenzi, 1989; Yates, Sieleni, Reich, & Brass, 1989). However, all of the previous studies exploring the relationship between borderline personality disorder and bulimia nervosa have had a variety of limitations. Some have utilized unstructured interviewing techniques. Some have incorporated diagnostic instruments of questionable and/or simply unknown validity, specificity, and reliability. Other potentially confounding factors include subjects from multiple referral sources, small sample sizes, study populations with broad or unclassified weight ranges, lack of control groups, or unpublished revised scoring systems.

Despite these limitations, the research data consistently suggest the presence of a subset of bulimic individuals with borderline personality disorder. The published studies to date have involved a total of 262 bulimic subjects. If the Pope et al. (1987) data are revised by using the traditional cutoff for the Diagnostic Interview for Borderline Patients (DIB), a total of 80 bulimic subjects (30.5%) have had a possible diagnosis of borderline personality. This averaged percentage (30.5%) is surprisingly consistent when compared to the range of results reported (13%–44%). This percentage potentially represents a substantial minority of individuals in the bulimic population.

The research data regarding the relationship between borderline personality disorder and anorexia nervosa are less extensive than those for bulimia nervosa. Three studies have explored this relationship (Hudson, Pope, & Jonas, 1984; Piran, Lerner, Garfinkel, Kennedy, & Brouillette, 1988; Sansone et al., 1989). Based on these studies, the reported prevalence rates for borderline personality disorder in anorexic population ranges from 0% to 57%. Again, small sample sizes, the use of different diagnostic instruments, and the lack of control groups confound these results.

We believe, however, that these data translate realistically to a clinical population and that clinicians might anticipate the coexistence of borderline personality disorder in a significant minority of their anorexic and bulimic patients.

PSYCHOSTRUCTURAL THEORY

We are proponents of the psychostructural theory of personality (Chatham, 1985; Kernberg, 1984; Stone, 1980). According to this model, the human psyche is formed with a limited number of basic underlying psychological organizations. By "psychological organization," we mean an ongoing psychological level of functioning with "enduring ways of viewing the world, modes of thought, and/or strategies of processing information" (Chatham, 1985, p. 87).

Although there is a great deal of controversy among psychostructural theorists regarding the number and type of specific organizational levels, we believe in the existence of at least four—psychotic, borderline, narcissistic, and neurotic—each with its own continuum of severity. The presentation of these basic levels of personality organization is affected by individual personality styles or temperaments (e.g., obsessive–compulsive, histrionic, dependent, passive–aggressive, antisocial, etc.), as well as by constitutional factors (genetic endowment).

The relationship of the psychostructure to the personality style/temperament might be metaphorically likened to an M&M (the popular chocolate candy): The psychostructure is represented by the soft chocolate core, and the personality style/temperament is represented by the visible, exterior hard coating. The "core" organization is negotiated through the "shell or coating" of the personality style. For example, it is not uncommon to see a borderline patient (psychostructure) with an obsessive–compulsive personality style, who also has an eating disorder.

The psychostructural perspective has several clinical advantages. First, it encourages the clinician to consistently view patients from a multilevel perspective (i.e., genetic endowment, core psychostructure, personality style/temperament, family/cultural environment). This multilevel perspective facilitates better selection and timing of therapeutic interventions, given the extent of the patient's resources and the desired outcome (i.e., it improves clinical assessment and judgment). Second, by providing an organized construct, the psychostructural approach facilitates the clinician's long-term psychotherapy work with character-disordered patients.

The concept of "psychostructure" as separate from "personality style" may provide some answers to several clinical quandaries. It may explain why borderline individuals masquerade beneath a variety of pathological personality styles. It may explain why the traditional personality disorders in the *Diagnostic and Statistical Manual of Mental Disorders* (DSM) have been so difficult to discriminate from one another. The concept may also clarify the confusing overlap of psychodynamics among personality disorders (e.g., impulsivity), as well as the evolution of antisocial and histrionic styles from the same family.

The psychostructural perspective has resulted in our scrutiny of the premorbid history of all patients. In our work with eating disorder patients, we have noticed several historical features that have led us to three general clinical findings. First, global (i.e., broad-spectrum) self-regulation problems are more reflective of character disorder than of eating disorder. For example, prior to the development of anorexia nervosa or bulimia nervosa, there are often signs of general personality dysfunction in several areas of self-regulation (e.g., long-standing affective instability, interpersonal boundary difficulties, global impulsivity). Second, eating disorder behaviors in this subset of patients function as another manifestation of their pervasive self-destructive behavior. Their premorbid histories often reveal ongoing self-destructive themes that are unrelated to body or weight conflicts. Third, enhanced socialization tends to result in more sophisticated, more elusive, and better-compensated borderline pathology. These individuals tend to come from fairly socialized, achievement-oriented environments, such that they seem to have a greater ability to negotiate their psychopathology on an interpersonal level. These impressions are in part derivatives of our psychostructural orientation.

A DIAGNOSTIC APPROACH TO BORDERLINE PERSONALITY DISORDER

At present, the revised third edition of the DSM (DSM-III-R; American Psychiatric Association, 1987) is the official diagnostic classification system for clinicians in the United States. Borderline personality disorder is listed as an Axis II diagnosis, along with 10 other personality disorders in the DSM-III-R. There are eight behaviorally descriptive criteria for borderline personality disorder. Diagnostic affirmation requires that the patient meet at least five of these criteria, which are listed below. The list is condensed from that in DSM-III-R (American Psychiatric Association, 1987, p. 347).

A pervasive pattern of instability of mood, interpersonal relationships and self-image, beginning by early adulthood.

(1) unstable and intense interpersonal relationships
(2) potentially self-damaging impulsiveness
(3) affective instability
(4) inappropriate, intense anger
(5) recurrent suicidal threats or gestures
(6) marked and persistent identity disturbances

(7) chronic feelings of emptiness or boredom
(8) fears of abandonment

Despite the availability of the DSM-III-R construct, the clinical diagnosis of borderline personality disorder remains substantially variable. In part, this is due to the continuing theoretical controversies about the borderline concept, including whether or not it is truly a personality disorder or an atypical presentation or variation of an affective disorder. In addition, many have questioned the clinical adequacy of the DSM-III-R criteria, citing the lack of attention to quasi-psychotic phenomena and the psychological defenses/psychodynamic processes, as well as the strong emphasis on affect-related criteria.

As a result of this controversy, several other diagnostic tools have been developed to help the clinician verify a diagnosis of borderline personality disorder. These include the following: the Presumptive Diagnostic Elements (Kernberg, 1967); the Structural Interview (Kernberg, 1981); the DIB (Kolb & Gunderson, 1980); the Spitzer–Endicott–Gibbon Checklist for Borderlines (Spitzer, Endicott, & Gibbon, 1979); the Borderline Syndrome Index (BSI; Conte, Plutchik, Karasu, & Jerrett, 1980); the Personality Diagnostic Questionaire—Revised (PDQ-R; Hyler & Rieder, 1987); the Borderline Personality Disorder Scale (Perry, 1982, 1983); the Millon Comprehensive Multiaxial Inventory (MCMI, subscale for borderlines; Millon, 1983); the Separation–Individuation Inventory (Christenson & Wilson, 1985); projective testing (e.g., the Rorschach; Adler, 1973; Grinker, Werble, & Drye, 1968; Gunderson & Singer, 1975; Kaplan & Sadock, 1985; Singer, 1977; Arnow & Cooper, 1984; Patrick & Wolfe, 1983); the Transitional Object scale (TOS) of the Rorschach (Cooper, Perry, Hoke, & Richman, 1985); and the Personality Disorder Examination (PDE; Loranger, Susman, Oldham, & Russakoff, 1988).

This partial list is rich in diagnostic alternatives, including projective and nonprojective psychological tests, self-report inventories, retrospective clinical checklists, and structured and semistructured interviews. Unfortunately, the validity, specificity, and reliability, as well as the diagnostic overlap of many of these instruments, are unknown.

Given the available alternatives, the approach we use to the clinical diagnosis of borderline personality disorder is based upon the criteria of Gunderson, which are incorporated into the DIB. Originally designed as a research tool, the DIB is a semistructured clinical interview with known reliability and validity (Armelius, Kullgren, & Renberg, 1985; Cornell, Silk, Ludolph, & Lohr, 1983; Gunderson, Kolb, & Austin, 1981; Kroll et al., 1981; Loranger, Oldham, Russakoff, & Susman, 1984; Soloff, 1981) that explores five areas of the patient's long-term functioning. In the clinical setting, we do not use the formal interview booklet, but rather make an in-depth inquiry into the five general areas of the DIB by assessing the acronym "PISIA."

1. *P*—Psychotic/quasi-psychotic episodes. We explore for psychotic episodes that are transient and brief in nature, including fleeting hallucinations or delusions, depersonalization, derealization, rage reactions, unusual reactions to drugs, or paranoia, in which the patient usually recognizes the loss of reality.

2. *I*—Impulsivity. These behaviors are typically long-standing, self-destructive, and/or destructive toward others and can include substance abuse, promiscuity, suicidal gestures, self-mutilation, property destruction, threats or assaults, compulsive eating or gambling, and so on.

3. *S*—Social adaptation. We explore with the patient his or her achievement record at school and at work, including extracurricular activities, in order to assess overall social presentation. These patients usually display a social adaptation that is superficially intact, yet marked by significant problems in functioning in their social environment.

4. *I*—Interpersonal relationships. We examine the quality and quantity of interpersonal relationships that the patient has experienced in the past and present. We frequently find dichotomous relatedness in interpersonal relationships. Social relationships are usually superficial and lack warmth or commitment, whereas relationships with significant others tend to be intense and marked by dependency, jealousy, manipulation, anger, masochism and/or sadism, and idealization and/or devaluation.

5. *A*—Affect. The affect of the borderline patient is often chronically dysphoric and/or labile. We look for chronic anxiety, depression, intense anger, loneliness, boredom, and emptiness.

With the assistance of PISIA, we explore for the presence of specific symptoms in each area as described in the DIB. The patient must meet criteria in each area to confirm a diagnosis of borderline personality disorder. The subsequent translation of the patient's symptoms to DSM-III-R criteria is relatively easy. This approach is diagnostically focused and specific, and relatively easy to conduct. Personality disorder assessment is often difficult, but this method enables the clinician to clearly organize and effectively summarize the clinical findings.

DEVELOPMENTAL CONSIDERATIONS

To promote a deeper understanding of the ego deficits of the eating disorder patient with borderline personality disorder, we briefly review several developmental theories. The developmental approach to understanding psychopathology emphasizes experiential rather than constitutional factors (Meissner, 1984) and focuses primarily on the ability of the parent (or primary caretaker) either to facilitate or to impede the infant's successful negotiation of specific developmental tasks.

Several developmental theories suggest that borderline patients experience an extreme disruption in their early relationships that interfere with the ability to internalize and structuralize important ego skills, such as impulse control, problem solving, object relatedness, and affective modulation. We begin by describing Margaret Mahler's model of development. We believe this is an extremely useful way of conceptualizing the evolution of borderline organization, although we also recognize that constitutional factors, illness, and situational crises can have an impact on the infant's development.

Margaret Mahler and her colleagues (Mahler with Furer, 1968; Mahler, 1971; Mahler, Pine, & Bergman, 1975) have developed the separation–individuation theory of development, based upon their observations of healthy infants. They have described and labeled the successive phases of normal development as "normal autism," "symbiosis," and "separation–individuation." This sequence of phases is a continuous process (Mahler & Kaplan, 1977). Each phase is more complex than the preceding one and prepares the infant to negotiate the succeeding one (Breger, 1974). The borderline dilemma is theorized to consolidate because of the unsuccessful negotiation of the "rapprochement" subphase (16–24 months), which is the third subphase in separation–individuation. During this subphase, the toddler becomes increasingly aware of the world beyond the mother. This growing perceptual and cognitive awareness promotes an increasing sense of vulnerability (i.e., the realization that he or she is just a small person in a very big world). The deflation of the toddler's omnipotence is marked by anxiety and ambivalence. Two behaviors are particularly indicative of this stage of development: "shadowing" (i.e., clinging to the mother and being preoccupied with her every move), and "darting away" should the mother attempt to confine or hold. Mahler suggests that this represents the toddler's simultaneous desire for reunion (symbiosis) and drive for mastery and autonomy. The lack of adequate support by the mother during rapprochement, theoretically, results in a crisis and subsequent arrest at this developmental level. Clinically, this results in the individual's vacillating from clinging dependency to omnipotent grandiosity.

Another developmental influence may be an ongoing pathological style of relatedness between mother and toddler. Masterson and Rinsley's (1975) theory of the split object relations unit suggests that borderline personality organization may be the result of the mother's libidinal unavailability for the child's separation–individuation needs. In summary, the mother relates to the toddler in a dichotomous fashion, rewarding and reinforcing dependent clinging behavior, and threatening abandonment when the toddler attempts to become autonomous and individuate. Masterson (1980) suggests that maternal unavailability can be the result of illness, physical absence, or psychopathology in the mother. Clinically, these individuals demonstrate intense fears of abandonment with separation, and gain a sense of security with clinging dependence.

A final developmental theory relevant to borderline psychopathology is Kernberg's developmental model of internalized object relations (Kernberg, 1976). This complex theory centers on the intrapsychic differentiation of self and the internal resolution of splitting. According to Kernberg, borderline organization is caused by fixation at the "differentiation of self from object representation" stage (8 to 36 months), which results in primitive internalized object relations. The inability to integrate "good" and "bad" self-object representations leaves the individual susceptible to splitting, emotional flooding, and chaotic interpersonal relationships.

These three developmental theories are major cornerstones in the current conceptualizations of the borderline dilemma from a developmental standpoint. Our clinical impression is that many borderline individuals have been victims of parental neglect of a malignant or intrusive nature (i.e., sexual, physical, and/or emotional abuse). The impact of absent psychological mentoring coupled with intrusive neglect results in a primitively organized negative self-concept, a primitive psychological structure, and the ongoing need to self-inflict the abuse received in earlier times (repetition compulsion).

TREATMENT CONSIDERATIONS

The treatment of an eating disorder patient with borderline personality disorder is complex and at times fraught with setbacks and frustration. However, we strongly believe that such patients can significantly improve in their overall level of functioning and can recover from their eating disorder, particularly when the clinician understands the unique needs of the patient and carefully plans a treatment strategy.

The fundamental goals in the treatment of these patients are (1) the reparation of distortions in interpersonal relationships, such that the patients increase their capacity to relate to others in a more realistic way; (2) the reworking of a primitive negative self-concept; and (3) the development of self-regulation. These goals are attained through the development of evocative memory, the resolution of splitting, the consolidation of object constancy, and the incorporation of personal self-regulation.

To assist the clinician in planning a strategy when treating these patients, we have oulined our treatment approach below.

ASSESSMENT

The initial assessment should be designed to identify various eating disorder subpopulations, in order to facilitate the appropriate selection of treatment approaches and strategies. We strongly believe that the presence of an Axis II personality disorder significantly alters the treatment of anorexia nervosa or bulimia nervosa. However, eating disorder patients with and without borderline personality often appear quite similar at intake in mood disturbance and behavioral symptom presentation.

Johnson et al. (1989) found that there were no differences at intake between bulimic patients with and without borderline organization in age, sex, educational level, race, marital status, severity of eating behaviors, age of onset of eating disorder, dieting behavior, current weight, or medical history. However, they did find significant differences between the borderline and nonborderline bulimic patients in several other areas. Borderline patients were significantly more emotionally distressed and susceptible to affective instability. On the Eating Disorder Inventory (Garner & Olmstead, 1984), borderline patients reported a greater drive for thinness, greater body dissatisfaction, greater sense of personal ineffectiveness and interpersonal distrust, more maturity fears, and greater difficulty in identifying inner states and feelings. Borderline patients were more likely to harm themselves, attempt suicide, and abuse alcohol or drugs. They were overall less socially adjusted and reported significantly more stressful events associated with the onset of their eating disorder. The family environments of the borderline patients were marked by significantly more conflict, enmeshment, and disengagement. Finally, borderline patients were more likely to require medication and inpatient hospitalization than the nonborderline patients.

We believe that the assessment phase of treatment should include three important components. First, the therapist should gather a detailed eating disorder history, as well as a comprehensive individual, family, work/school, and social history. Second, it is important to assess the patient's level of social adaptation, the quantity and quality of interpersonal relationships, affective stability, psychotic or quasi-psychotic experiences, and the presence and extent of self-destructive behaviors (i.e., the PISIA assessment for borderline personality disorder).

Finally, during the assessment period, each patient should receive a complete physical examination and laboratory tests to uncover potential medical complications of their eating disorders, as well as any other physiological, self-abusive, or chemical dependency problems. Because borderline individuals may be arrested at a preverbal level of development, many communicate their feelings and emotions through their bodies. It is often extremely difficult to distinguish between psychosomatic/hypochondrical complaints and organic illness. The physical examination may clarify the etiology of such complaints.

PHASE 1: ESTABLISHING THE THERAPEUTIC MILIEU

Establishing the Treatment Environment

One of the most important aspects of the initial phase of treatment is creating an appropriate, stable environment in which a reparative relationship can take place. The patient with borderline personality disorder is typically rigid and inflexible, and appears to operate best in a structured, predictable environment. The smallest changes can cause disruption in the therapeutic process. The therapist should establish appointments on a regular basis at the same hours and location each week (i.e., same office), begin and end all sessions on time, establish a routine for fee collection, and try to decrease the number of different office personnel involved with the patient. Developing a rhythm for time and space with these environmental structures can help the patient feel safe and secure.

Emphasizing the Working Relationship

The development of a working therapeutic relationship is critical in the treatment of the eating disorder patient with borderline personality disorder. Relationship building is time-consuming and often extremely difficult, due to the borderline individual's defense structure, problems with trust, and inability to effectively regulate interpersonal distance. Frequently, these patients have gone through life being misunderstood or abused by people who are supposed to care about them. There is little reason for them to trust the therapist.

Although these patients have great difficulty with interpersonal relationships, they desperately want to attach and are searching for relationships that will not disappoint them. However, one of the primary fantasies that a borderline patient brings into the therapeutic relationship is the desire for intimacy without vulnerability. Developmentally, this may represent the return to the symbiotic phase of development, where the patient was fused with the primary caretaker and had no responsibility for maintaining the relationship. However, the therapist needs to provide an environment for interpersonal growth and mature relatedness.

In doing so, therapy becomes an experimental arena where the role of the therapist includes the regulation of boundaries, the modulation of affect, and the setting of limits (i.e., a holding environment).

Within the therapeutic relationship, the therapist should expect interpersonal boundaries to be challenged repeatedly. These patients have significant difficulty determining how close or how distant to be within a relationship. This inability to regulate interpersonal distance is a primary problem that will need to be addressed if a healthy working relationship is to be established. Thus, the therapist must persistently monitor interpersonal distance and continuously realign boundaries to avoid becoming overly close and indulgent or overly distant and denying. In verbally realigning boundaries, the therapist's affect needs to be well modulated. Overly negative responses may provide a patient with further "evidence" that the outer world is hostile and malevolent, whereas overly positive responses are often anxiety-provoking, as they are perceived as inconsistent with the patient's negative self-perception.

Finally, we believe that the therapeutic relationship should be one of trust and warmth, which allows closeness without fusion, separateness without abandonment, and confrontation without retaliation.

Limiting Adjunctive Treatments

As mentioned above, the development of a therapeutic relationship with these patients is critical for the initiation of treatment. Yet borderline patients find it extremely difficult to trust treatment providers. We have found that when multiple treatment providers are involved with these patients, there is often significant splitting and an increased incidence of acting-out behavior. Therefore, during the initial stages of treatment, we focus on intense individual psychotherapy and when possible avoid referral and/or multiple therapeutic relationships, including group treatment (i.e., outpatient groups or support groups).

In some cases, however, patients will need to be involved with other treatment providers to insure physical health and/or safety. For example, we usually attempt to avoid the use of psychotropic medications with this population; however, some patients may display significant Axis I (DSM-III-R) symptoms that may be more effectively managed with a brief trial of medication. To reduce splitting when referring and to increase the likelihood of consistency and continuity of care, we recommend the following procedures for the nonphysician therapist. First, the therapist should discuss with the psychiatrist the patient's symptoms and the reasons why the therapist believes medications would be a helpful intervention. Second, if both professionals agree that medication should be considered, they should develop a plan that includes (a) a clear method of communication with the patient about the therapist's concerns; (b) an established appointment date with the psychiatrist; (c) clarification of the role of the psychiatrist with the patient (i.e., the psychiatrist will not take crisis calls, see the patient for ongoing therapy, be viewed as the primary treatment provider, etc.); (d) exploration with the patient about the meaning of and fantasies surrounding a medication trial; and (e) the sanctioning by the patient of ongoing communication between the two professionals. The first and last steps include discussing with the patient the purpose for the referral to the psychiatrist and having the patient sign a release-of-information form permitting ongoing dialogue between professionals. If the circumstances permit, the therapist may attend the medication evaluation sessions with the patient and reinforce the distinction of roles, the procedures to be followed, and the consequences of misuse or abuse of the medications. If the therapist and psychiatrist present a united front that is clear and consistent, the chances of splitting should be reduced. This by no means prevents the patient from attempting to pit one professional against the other, but it certainly can reduce the chances of acting out among professionals.

As mentioned above, we avoid group therapy with these patients during the intial stages of treatment. However, once a strong therapeutic alliance has been established and the transference is stabilized (Phase 2), some higher-functioning borderline/eating disorder patients may benefit from a combination of individual and group treatment. We caution that this decision should not be taken lightly, as group treatment can promote regression and self-destructive acting out. The group should be facilitated by a therapist who is experienced with borderline individuals and group treatment. Ideally, the group therapist should be the same clinician who is currently providing individual psychotherapy to the patient.

Integrating the Family

Family involvement in the treatment of the eating disorder patient with borderline personality disorder is often necessary. However, we approach family sessions quite differently than we would with a nonborderline patient, where family therapy is often undertaken to explore systems issues that may have helped to create and maintain the eating disorder. In family sessions with the borderline patient, we focus on education, structure, and consistency. First, we attempt to educate the family about the symptoms and dynamics of the patient's negative behaviors. This can involve information sessions with the therapist, the reading of lay articles about borderline personality, and processing family events within the context of the patient's dynamics (Dennis & Sansone, 1989). Second, we stress the importance of structure and consistency within the family setting. Clearly defined parental roles and frequent and nonjudgmental limit setting by parents can promote organization and integration, thus allowing for increased autonomy in the patient's personal life management. When developmentally appropriate, we encourage gradual emancipation from the family.

Family treatment may be complicated by the presence of borderline personality in one or both parents. In this situation, we recommend the referral of parents to another professional for either individual or marital sessions. This prevents any disruption of the therapeutic relationship between the eating disorder patient and the primary therapist. Case consultation meetings should be routinely conducted with all professionals involved with the family, in order to insure consistency and continuity of care.

Maintaining a Realistic Focus

We believe that the initial primary focus should be on the development of a therapeutic relationship, rather than on immediate symptom control. Although we begin to educate patients on the social, behavioral, psychological, and physiological complications of their eating disorder, and to monitor eating behavior and weight, we do not attempt to radically change the restricting or bulimic behavior during the first phase of treatment. To do so may mobilize a primitive oppositional stance that is derived from the patients' distorted perception of control. Our focus is primarily on helping the patients begin to explore self-regulation as opposed to the elimination of the eating disorder. Once a stable therapeutic relationship has been established, symptom management and control can be more fully addressed.

Managing Projective Identification

Projective identification is an unconscious defensive process in borderline individuals, wherein unacceptable parts of the self are psychically "tossed out" and "housed" within a willing recipient. The therapist and significant others are often targets of a borderline individual's projections, despite the fact that the recipient's feelings and personal issues are genuinely different from the content of the projection. The occurrence of resonance in the recipient, itself, appears to provide some "verification" of the "reality" of the projection to the borderline individual, who responds by unconsciously identifying with this disguised piece of self. The borderline's subsequent behavioral response is a need both to control the recipient (i.e., the "harbored self") and to repetitively elicit responses that confirm the reality of the projection. There is often a confusing feeling of "who is doing what to whom" in the session. The whole process may result in a variety of countertherapeutic responses by the therapist (e.g., yelling at the patient, setting limits out of anger, terminating the patient).

We strongly encourage therapists to carefully monitor their own emotional reactions during sessions with borderline patients, in order to avoid resonating with these projections. These responses may ultimately culminate in strong countertransference reactions and need to be identified, explored, and resolved. Supervision, either formal or informal, that focuses on education, support, and self-understanding is extremely valuable in sorting out these confusing and potentially destructive issues.

Preparing for Countertransference

Treating patients with eating disorders can present the therapist with a variety of countertransference issues, but working with a patient who also has borderline personality disorder can be most challenging for even the highly skilled clinician.

Johnson and Connors (1987) have eloquently outlined the basic countertransference issues that the therapist should be aware of when treating the eating disorder patient. These include (1) the therapist's belief in and acceptance of society's norms for weight, shape, and appearance; (2) the therapist's disgust or revulsion concerning the binge–purge cycle; (3) the therapist's envy of the patient's pursuit of thinness and/or perfection; (4) the therapist's own problems with eating or weight; (5) the therapist's lack of empathy for the pursuit of thinness; and (6) the therapist's inability to discuss issues related to sex, sexuality, or other body-related issues.

In addition, we believe that the therapist should be aware of the countertransference issues that arise when treating the borderline patient. These patients do not just tell the therapist how they feel; they make the therapist feel it! This may result in anger, defensiveness, helplessness, guilt, and even retaliation on the part of the therapist.

We have found that many of our supervisees come into supervision with preconceived notions about treating the borderline patient. Clinicians who have previously had negative experiences with borderline patients should be acutely aware of their countertransference issues if they choose to engage in treatment with this population again. Gallop, Lance, and Garfinkel (1989) have verified our clinical impressions through a study of how nurses respond to the label of "borderline personality disorder." They reported that inpatient nurses responded to borderline patients with low levels of empathy and were often belittling or contradicting. They concluded that borderline patients may enter treatment with a stigma that sets the tone for a negative therapeutic interaction.

Therapists who have personal problems with self-regulation (e.g., substance abuse, promiscuity, gambling, shoplifting/stealing, impulsive spending, chronic dysphoria, etc.) may not feel comfortable treating patients who often lack affective, behavioral, and interpersonal modulation. Such a patient's chaotic behavior may initiate significant acting-out behavior in a therapist.

Some therapists are not comfortable with the intense transference and ever-present demandingness and neediness of borderline patients with eating disorders. These patients require consistency, continuity, and patience. The crisis-to-crisis nature of treatment, together with the patients' repetitive self-destructive behavior and/or unrealistic "tests of caring," can cripple the most conscientious of therapists. We have seen colleagues respond to these pressures through disorganization, chronic fatigue, franticness, guilt, chronic eating, or increased drug and alcohol use.

Unconscious attempts to rescue a patient are a common countertransference reaction to this population. The borderline patient frequently finds himself or herself in compromising situations and relies on the therapist to resolve the dilemma. If the therapist accepts the patient's helplessness and rescues the patient from crisis, this reinforces the patient's dependency and promotes further "tests of caring."

Countertransference reactions help the therapist maintain a sense of control and protect himself or herself from the whirlwind of emotions emanating from the patient (Dennis & Sansone, 1989). These reactions are often forceful, raw, and primitive, ranging from murderously angry, panicky, manipulated, guilty, or outraged to powerless, depressingly isolated, or completely indifferent.

We suggest several basic approaches to confronting countertransference issues. First, therapists who choose to treat this population must educate themselves thoroughly on the psychology of the borderline patient. It is essential that a therapist repeatedly relabel and reframe a patient's affect and behavior within the context of the borderline process. This requires that the therapist listen for the process as opposed to the content of sessions. It also allows the therapist to achieve therapeutic distance and to avoid becoming emotionally over- or underinvolved with the patient. Second, the therapist should be aware that the patient's behavior is not a personal attack on the therapist, but rather an attempt at self-protection (Dennis & Sansone, 1989). The therapist must step back from the patient and take a global view of the problem, and must avoid personalizing the patient's affect or behavior. Third, we believe it is essential for therapists to recognize their personal time constraints and limitations when treating this population. These patients often require far more contact time and attention than do eating disorder patients in general. We recommend that therapists limit the number of borderline patients on their caseloads at any one time. Fourth, therapists should balance the patients' needs with their available resources. Professionals who work within an institutional setting may be better equipped to manage more severely disturbed patients than private practitioners, who often lack rapid access to a variety of structured settings (i.e., inpatient programs, day hospital programs, 24-hour emergency mental health services). These structural supports can reduce therapist anxiety and facilitate the successful management of suicidal or self-destructive patients. Finally, and most importantly, we recommend that any therapist who works with an eating disorder patient with borderline personality disorder should participate in ongoing, regular supervision and should actively confront countertransference reactions. This will help the therapist maintain a more positive attitude toward and a more objective perspective on the patient.

PHASE 2: STABILIZATION OF TRANSFERENCE

Therapeutic Stance

We believe that the therapist needs to be spontaneous in affect, genuine, and routinely self-clarifying with the eating disorder patient with borderline personality disorder. Therapeutic neutrality can promote fantasizing and the evolution of a predominantly negative transference with these patients. However, during periods of acute slippage/decompensation or self-destructive acting out, neutrality helps to prevent the inadvertent reinforcement of these behaviors, which can occur if the therapist overreacts or underreacts.

Promoting Reality Testing

The therapist should promote reality testing by being genuine and modeling appropriate affect. This means being "real" and spontaneous within the therapeutic relationship. Although these individuals have an impaired capacity to be empathetic, they have a tendency to resonate with the moods of others, including the therapist. The borderline patient can often sense the therapist's mood and temperament, but frequently misconstrues the source of these feelings. This misunderstanding usually centers around the belief that the therapist's moods or feelings during a session are directly related to the patient. It is essential for the therapist to clarify for the patient the present reality. For example, after a therapist has yawned, the patient may say, "I guess I am really boring you today." An appropriate response might be "No, you are not boring me, I am just very tired today," or "No, I am not quite up to speed today, but it has nothing to do with you." The therapist does not have to explain the cause, or apologize for being tired, depressed, angry, or ill. It should be remembered that the goal is to present the patient with an integrated, whole person who experiences and can effectively manage a full range of moods and emotions. Denial of affective states can be very confusing for the patient and can promote fantasizing and splitting.

The general issue of the therapist's disclosure of feelings to the borderline patient is fraught with caveats, particularly when negative feelings are involved (e.g., the therapist yawns because the patient really *is* boring). The disclosure of negative feelings should only be undertaken when the therapeutic relationship has been adequately stabilized. In addition, such disclosures should not be done during times of patient crisis. Negative disclosures need to be semantically neutral (e.g., "Things feel a little slow today" rather than "You are boring me to death"). In summary, timing, affective neutrality, and semantic neutrality are crucial elements in the disclosure of the therapist's negative feelings to the borderline patient, and we advise general caution.

Another method of promoting reality testing is discouraging fantasy. The fantasies of these patients are often primitive and frightening. For example, many borderline patients believe that their anger or rage can annihilate or in some way destroy others. Helping the patients separate feelings and thoughts from behavior can reduce this fear. Patients should be taught to intellectualize and isolate these fantasies so that they do not continuously burden them.

Finally, it is not uncommon for these patients to consciously withhold important information or to lie directly to the therapist. Kernberg (1985) suggests that patients who chronically lie demonstrate serious ego deterioration and often project their own dishonesty and corrupt moral values onto the therapist. As a result, the patient–therapist relationship is often severely distorted by the belief that the therapist is foolish, incompetent, easily manipulated, or dishonest. Habitual lying demonstrates a basic mistrust of the therapist and a sense of hopelessness about the development of a genuine human relationship.

If the therapist suspects lying, he or she should investigate and confront the patient. Kernberg (1985) suggests that the "full resolution of reality and transferential implications of the patient's lying take precedence over all other material, except life-threatening acting out" (p. 201). Lying interferes with all aspects of the therapeutic process and must be explored, confronted, and resolved in order to promote a meaningful therapeutic relationship.

Encouraging Verbalization

Eating disorder patients with borderline personality disorder often have great difficulty expressing their feelings and thoughts to the therapist. It is important to remember that these patients are often developmentally arrested at a preverbal level. The end of the phase of symbiosis is the beginning of the child's development of language. Verbalization is the single developmental event that sets the child apart from the primary caretaker as a separate person.

Unfortunately, many of these patients expect the therapist to "know" what they are thinking or feeling at any given moment. Such a patient may even maintain the fantasy that the therapist can "read my mind." As a result, therapy sessions can often take on an empty, meaningless, or chronically confused flavor, with long periods of silence. The therapist should be active and directive, and should structure each session.

The purists of the psychodynamic model suggest that the therapist should not interfere with silences during the therapy session. However, with this patient population, we believe that long silences can promote fantasizing and the myth of the "symbiotic union." The therapist should encourage the patient to verbalize and explain what he or she is thinking and feeling, instead of allowing the patient to act it out. When the patient verbalizes thoughts and feelings, it allows him or her to acknowledge separateness.

Staying in the "Here and Now"

These patients have significant daily problems and crises that need the therapist's help and guidance. After gathering a complete and detailed psychosocial history from a patient, the therapist should attempt to remain in the "here and now." This allows the therapist to understand more completely how the individual solves problems and copes with daily activities. Keeping abreast of the patient's work/school and home environment, as well as his or her interpersonal relationships, will help the therapist identify potential catastrophes and possibly avert them. As patterns emerge, historical antecedents of these behaviors can be discussed to help the patient better understand what has caused and maintained these patterns.

Educating the Patient

Our approach to the treatment of borderline patients with eating disorder includes a significant component of patient education. In addition to educating the patients about the eating disorder and recovery strategies, we also progressively educate them about borderline personality.

Initially, we discuss with the patients each of the major areas in their lives that demonstrate long-term patterns of dysfunction (i.e., interpersonal relationships, work/school history, self-destructive behaviors, affect regulation). After a therapeutic relationship has been well established, we focus on educating the patients more directly on the five core therapeutic issues (Dennis & Sansone, 1989): low self-esteem, inability to modulate affect, inability to modulate interpersonal distance, inability to modulate impulses, and the primitive defense structure (i.e., splitting, primitive idealization, omnipotence, devaluation, denial, and projective identification). At this point, we tend to avoid using the term "borderline."

After the transference has stabilized (which can take several months or even years), we have found that labeling and explaining the disorder for select patients facilitates their deeper understanding of the therapeutic process. We may provide reading material and/or educational sessions to the patients as well as to mutually agreed-upon significant others and family members. Many of these patients have gone through life feeling different, alone, or separate from the rest of the world. Their chaotic thinking and behavior has often been confusing and frightening to them. Frequently, they believe that no one understands or can help them manage or change their approach to life. Explaining to these patients that their symptoms are not unique and that they can learn to live more balanced, less chaotic lives can promote renewed involvement and participation in treatment.

Symptom Management

During Phase 2 of treatment, we focus more directly on the management of anorexic and bulimic symptomatology. Patients are instructed on proper nutrition and meal planning, the identification of behavioral antecedents associated with binge-eating and purging, alternatives to restriction or binge-eating, stress management and relaxation techniques, methods to manage leisure time, relapse prevention strategies, and so forth. The management of eating disorder symptoms has been extensively detailed elsewhere (Anderson, 1985; Fairburn, 1982, 1984; Garner & Bemis, 1982, 1984; Garner, Rockert, Olmsted, Johnson, & Coscina, 1984; Johnson & Connors, 1987; Lacey, 1983; Mitchell, 1985).

Setting Limits

From the onset of treatment, the therapist should be prepared to set firm limits repeatedly with the borderline patient. Limits should be set out of compassion and concern for the patient's welfare and safety, rather than out of therapist anger or annoyance. We believe that limits should be matter-of-fact, nonjudgmental, concrete, well defined, and repeatedly clarified and discussed with the patient (Dennis & Sansone, 1989). Limits provide the patient with structure, stability, predictability, and a sense of control.

Limit setting may be necessary in a variety of areas, including (but not limited to) the boundaries of the therapist–patient relationship, therapist availability, behavior within the therapy session, self-destructive or acting-out behavior, involvement with other health and mental health professionals, and nonpayment of fees.

Most frequently, limit setting begins with the therapist's explaining to the patient what he or she will and will not manage within the therapeutic relationship. For many borderline patients, attachment to the therapist develops very quickly. Because of their impaired object permanence and poor evocative memory skills, these patients often demonstrate a significant need for contact with the therapist. This may result in numerous nonemergency phone calls between sessions to the therapist's home or office, requests for longer or more frequent therapy sessions, and constant letter writing or gift giving. To enhance the relationship-building process and reduce separation anxiety, we may see patients at least twice per week and additionally schedule a brief (10-minute) phone call during the initial stages of treatment. However, phone calls outside the appointed times are discouraged, with the exception of a genuine emergency. The nature of an emergency phone call is defined and discussed with the patients, and a list of other people/resources that they can contact to help them deal with day-to-day stress is developed (i.e., friends, relatives, crisis centers, etc.).

Again, the therapist must operate as a "boundary regulator" within the therapeutic relationship. These patients often experience difficulty regulating interpersonal distance. It is not uncommon for a patient to inquire about the therapist's personal life, family, and activities or to invite the therapist to participate in social activities outside the office. We encourage the therapist to be genuine and spontaneous, thus reducing fantasy. However, the patient needs to recognize the boundaries and limits of a therapeutic relationship. Like underinvolvement, overinvolvement can promote negative transference and reduce the therapist's effectiveness.

The therapist may find it necessary to establish limits around behavior within the therapy session (e.g., "I will not be able to have a session with you if you arrive high or intoxicated"). Aggressive acting out or continual angry outbursts should not be tolerated within the session. Once an affective storm or outburst has subsided, the therapist should process the experience with the patient and develop a plan to manage future episodes. Kernberg (1985) suggests that firm limit setting around acting-out behaviors within the therapeutic relationship reduces transference psychosis, enables the patient to differentiate the therapist from himself or herself, and prevents the therapist from retaliating on the basis of negative countertransference reactions.

Managing Self-Destructive Behavior: A Cognitive–Behavioral Focus

Ongoing self-destructive behavior is frequently present in patients with eating disorders and borderline personality disorder. It may be manifested as self-mutilation (e.g., cutting, burning, biting, bruising oneself), drug and alcohol abuse/dependence, promiscuity, accident-proneness, excessive risk taking, suicidal gestures, and bona fide suicide attempts. The eating disorder patient with borderline personality may dynamically condense the majority of self-destructive drives into food-, body-, and weight-related issues. Therefore, at intake, the patient's repertoire of eating disorder behaviors may appear similar to that of the nonborderline patient, even though dynamically the behaviors serve very different purposes (i.e., self-destructive acting out vs. weight, shape, and appearance conflicts). However, with many of our borderline patients, we have found broad-spectrum self-destructive behavior that began prior to and extends beyond eating disorder themes (promiscuity, cutting, shoplifting, drug abuse, etc.).

Following the diagnostic confirmation of borderline personality, the therapist needs to unobtrusively explore the patient's current repertoire of self-destructive behaviors. Each behavior is then assigned a priority in a mental hierarchy, based upon its lethality. Compared to other populations of borderline patients, individuals with eating disorders tend to be better socialized and higher-functioning; therefore, their self-destructive behavior is often less graphic and acute. However, acute and dangerous behaviors can occur and need to be stabilized as soon as possible.

If the acute self-destructive behavior is occurring in the context of an Axis I disorder (e.g., suicidal ideation secondary to major depression), the Axis I disorder needs to be stabilized and resolved. If the acute self-destructive behavior is arising out of Axis II pathology, we recommend initial stabilization with behavioral and cognitive approaches.

Behavioral approaches fall into two general categories: (1) anticipatory crisis intervention plans; and (2) behavior-specific substitution interventions. Crisis intervention plans frequently take the form of a written contract between the therapist and the patient (Silver, 1985). Such contracts are varied and individualized, but often clarify the role of phone calls to the therapist; the availability of and indications for additional appointments; the use of emergency services and hospitalization; the utilization of medication; the guidelines, if any, that will prevent termination and referral to another therapist; and so on. A contract can reinforce a neutral stance and document the therapist's desire to continue working with the patient. It can also provide a safety net for the patient and offer him or her structure and predictability.

Behavior-specific substitution interventions range from "trading down" from a more lethal behavior to a lesser one, to attempts at sublimation. Indeed, some behavioral techniques in the treatment of bulimia nervosa employ both the "trading down" and sublimation concepts (e.g., contracting for increasing "free" days coupled with encouraging calling a friend during high-risk times). Although a variety of successful substitution behaviors are described for borderline patients in the literature (Ross & McKay, 1979; Feldman, 1988; Leibenluft, Gardner, & Cowdry, 1987)—for example, painful exercise (Rosen & Thomas, 1984), squeezing rubber balls (Rosen & Thomas, 1984), or drawing on paper the self-destructive desire—most are anecdotal and have not been systematically reviewed to see whether indeed they are effective. This should not discourage their use, but rather should encourage further study of therapeutically induced substitution behavior in a borderline population.

Most cognitive approaches advocated for the mangement of self-destructive behavior in borderline patients suggest that change is most effectively promoted within the context of the therapeutic relationship (Gunderson, 1984; Kernberg, 1984; Kroll, 1988; Silver, 1985). We utilize a cognitive restructuring approach developed by Gunderson (1984), which focuses on clarifying the responsibility for, the interpersonal meaning of, and the consequences of self-destructive behavior. First, during an acute crisis, we acknowledge our legitimate inability to be or feel responsible for a patient's self-destructive behavior. Next, we attempt to explore with the patient what he or she is trying to ask for or communicate through their self-destructive behavior. Third, we clarify with the patient that self-destructive behavior impedes the effectiveness of psychotherapy. Finally, it is important that the patient recognize that a therapist's response to crisis is governed by legal and ethical concerns, and that we choose to demonstrate "caring" in healthier ways than rescuing him or her from self-destructive drives.

Following the acute crisis, we (1) discuss the patient's reaction to the intervention; (2) reinforce the ongoing need for mutual understanding of the patient's self-destructive drives; and (3) clarify that the therapist's availability during crises is limited. Consistent wording is extremely important in providing an effective environmental or therapeutic cue.

Reflecting the Positive Psychological Aspects of the Patient

Extremely important aspects of stabilizing the transference are the therapist's identification, appreciation, and reflection of the positive psychological aspects of the borderline patient (e.g., sense of humor, personal resilience, perseverance). This serves a variety of therapeutic functions. It enables the therapist to focus on and maintain a healthy, balanced perspective of the patient. This balance promotes the patient's gradual integration over time via incorporation and helps the therapist cope with predictable periods of stress and devaluation. The reflection of the positive self by the therapist also promotes an unique level of "here-and-now" interpersonal reality that stabilizes the transference over time.

However, we caution the therapist that premature reflection of the positive aspects of the patient may result in the patient's questioning the credibility or perceptual abilities of the therapist (e.g., "I know I am a black sheep, and everyone has always told me that"). Positive feedback can be perceived as dishonest or superficial. We also caution about the content of the feedback. Commenting on physical aspects of the patient (e.g., attractiveness, eyes, hairstyle, clothing) rather than psychological aspects may mobilize extreme anxiety and/or erotic fantasies, thus potentially blurring a previously determined boundary and promoting a quasi-psychotic transference.

PHASE 3: RESOLVING INTERNAL THEMES

Promoting Object Constancy

Object constancy is the attainment of stable mental representations of others (McDevitt, 1975), such that the individual has the capacity for constancy in his or her relatedness with others (Burgner & Edgcumbe, 1972). It is usually significantly impaired in borderline patients. The clinical significance of this impairment is often profound. Without the development of stable representations of others, an individual has a reduced capacity to differentiate himself or herself from others (i.e., poor interpersonal boundaries). In addition, the absence of stable internal representations prohibits the individual from utilizing an internal repertoire of meaningful others for psychological soothing. The impaired ability to soothe oneself internally emerges clinically as the intolerance of stress and the continual seeking of external soothers (e.g., food, drugs, alcohol, self-damaging behaviors, relationships, etc.). Individuals with poorly developed object constancy have a chaotic, extremist style of interpersonal relatedness, which precludes relationships with healthier, better-organized individuals.

Two areas of clinical intervention in the object constancy dilemma of borderline patients are (1) the strengthening of evocative memory (i.e., the ability to evoke the image of another when absent), and (2) the resolution of splitting. We first examine evocative memory, its assessment, and an approach to treatment.

Strengthening Evocative Memory

In borderline patients, a variety of clinical indicators suggest impairments in evocative memory. One indicator is the borderlines' exquisite intolerance of the therapist's absence. This dynamic may become particularly evident between appointments, during illness and vacations, and throughout the process of termination. During these absences, borderline individuals may act out, enlist other therapists, become disorganized, and/or experience fragmentation in their recall of the therapist. Even during the routine course of treatment, borderline individuals will frequently attempt to increase their contact with the therapist through extra appointments, phone calls, prolonged sessions, and crisis behaviors.

Another indicator is borderlines' overinvestment in concrete transitional phenomena (e.g., appointment cards, educational materials provided by the therapist). These objects function as tangible reminders of the ongoing existence of the therapist, and thus as external sources of soothing. In a variation of this theme, borderline individuals may also engage in frequent gift giving, a projection of their own need for concrete reminders of others.

In our clinical experience, the identification and subsequent therapeutic strengthening of evocative memory promote a patient's stability outside of session. We have successfully utilized several approaches to achieve this: (1) a structured increase in the contact time between the patient and therapist; (2) the incorporation of concrete transitional phenomena into the treatment arena; (3) the utilization of cognitive exercises; and (4) the use of several general psychotherapy techniques and maneuvers. These approaches may be skillfully integrated into the treatment process in various combinations.

The first approach is an increase in therapist–patient contact time. To be successful, this intervention must be an offensive rather than a defensive maneuver. An offensive position facilitates an affectively neutral, calculated, structured intervention that acknowledges the therapist's awareness of the patient's needs. It allows the therapist to remain in control of the situation and to clarify the limits (e.g., duration, availability) of a given intervention. Specific interventions may include increasing the frequency of regular appointments, providing extra appointments as indicated, and scheduling telephone contacts.

A second approach is the incorporation of transitional phenomena into the treatment process. Concrete transitional phenomena function developmentally as adult "transitional objects" (Winnicott, 1965). At any time, they give the patient a sense of concrete and tangible access to the therapist—an access that is not internally available.

We suggest that effective adult transitional objects for borderline patients should be uniquely personal, yet should satisfy therapeutically legitimate purposes. In other words, they must maintain a personalized meaning between the patient and the therapist, yet should have a valid and recognizable role in the treatment process. Examples of concrete transitional phenomena include (but are not limited to) the following: appointment cards written out by the therapist, not a receptionist (i.e., personal, yet legitimate); an educational article for the patient, specific to eating disorders or a current therapeutic issue, with an attached explanatory note by the therapist. Other therapeutic vehicles that might be personalized and provided by the therapist could include pamphlets, food records, journals, or the like. These items should be personalized in some way in order for them to take on transitional properties for a patient. If the chosen vehicle is not truly therapeutically legitimate, it may promote an unstable, potentially psychotic transference.

There are several general suggestions to follow when incorporating transitional phenomena into the therapy process. Multiple phenomena should be introduced into the treatment process, as they tend to have a broader stabilizing effect. Transitional phenomena are most effectively utilized by a patient when introduced in a noncrisis situation, and may help the patient ward off an impending crisis. During acute crises, patients appear to have extreme difficulty accessing and utilizing transitional phenomena.

As the transference stabilizes, we have found that more dynamic transitional phenomena can be effectively integrated into the treatment process. However, we strongly caution the therapist on the uses of these vehicles. The integration of more dynamic transitional phenomena must be carefully timed to avoid fostering an unstable transference. Dynamic transitional phenomena can include cassette tapes of important therapy sessions, relaxation tapes narrated by the therapist, and neutral greeting cards acknowledging specific behavioral gains (e.g., a "congratulations" card acknowledging the patient's first week free of bingeing–purging). Other examples might include postcards acknowledging return dates from vacations or patient–therapist photographs taken in the treatment setting.

The third approach to the strengthening of evocative memory is the integration of specific cognitive exercises. Most of these exercises masquerade as focused tasks, but the underlying process is the stimulation of the emotional "memory plates," specifically the recall and thus internal availability of the therapist. These exercises may include having the patient (1) write a letter to the therapist; (2) keep a journal or diary in which the patient and therapist exchange dialogue; and (3) think about or verbally role-play the therapist's reactions to "outside" situations, such that the therapist functions as an "internal companion." Another cognitive technique that we occasionally use in sessions with very stable patients is visual imagery, where the goal is to strengthen the internal visual image of the therapist.

Our last approach really encompasses a potpourri of several psychotherapy techniques and maneuvers. One simple technique that may be utilized early in the treatment process is the colloquial identification of impairments in object constancy (e.g., "You seem to have trouble with absence"). At some point, the therapist can also develop a working metaphor to quickly access this dilemma in therapy (e.g., "failed memory plates"). On a cognitive level, the therapist can define and describe the process for the patient and can even use interpretation to neutralize the valence of the patient's behaviors as they relate to object constancy. Paradoxically, at times it may be necessary to place limits on the frequency or type of contact (e.g., phone calls) with the patient to further stimulate the internal processes.

As stated before, the preceding approaches to strengthening object constancy may be utilized in various combinations at various times. The therapeutic focus on object constancy parallels other therapeutic work throughout the treatment process. As expected, it tends to fragment under stress but to be ever-resilient with continued treatment. Unfortunately, there is no known method for measuring or assessing object constancy in patients, and much of the available information is from clinical rather than research sources.

Resolving Splitting

The second area of clinical intervention in the consolidation of object constancy is the resolution of splitting. "Splitting," by definition, is the active separation of thoughts and feelings into the extremes of good and bad. In healthy individuals, splitting normally persists up to approximately age 2 and resolves during the rapprochement subphase of separation–individuation. In borderline individuals, splitting is all-pervasive in their psychological processes and persists throughout life. Splitting functions dynamically in borderline individuals to eliminate ambivalence at any given moment and to allow the individuals to experience pure perceptual and feeling states. Unfortunately, it compromises an accurate perception of reality.

Two clinical indicators of the presence of splitting in patients are valent self-expression and vacillating cognitions. Valent or emotionally charged self-expression may appear in both the expressed content and the affect of the individual. Valent content sounds extremist and judgmental (e.g., "She was a very, very evil person" or "Sometimes I am a good person but sometimes I am very bad") and may be perceived as one-dimensional, dichotomous, or rigid. This content is often expressed through intense affect, which is suggestive of both poor affective regulation and an extremist or valent communication style. The overall interpersonal Gestalt may appear somewhat histrionic.

The second clinical indicator of splitting is vacillating cognitions. Borderline individuals appear intolerant or unaccepting of ambivalence and often vacillate from one cognitive extreme to the other. This vacillating or oscillating quality becomes acutely apparent in their decision-making processes (e.g., "I must go into the hospital . . . there is no way I will go into the hospital"). It also emerges in their perception and presentation of self: They appear omnipotent, narcissistic, and grandiose in their sense of entitlement at times, and describe themselves as valueless, worthless, and despicable at other times. Both valent self-expression and vacillating cognitions are ever-present in sessions with borderline individuals and suggest a poorly integrated perceptual/cognitive process (i.e., the presence of splitting).

There are several clinical approaches to splitting. From the onset of treatment, the therapist may simply colloquially identify the presence of splitting (e.g., "That sounds really extreme to me" or "That's very black and white"). The therapist can Socratically explore the impact of splitting in various situations (e.g., "If you hate him so much, how will this affect you at the prom?"). The therapist can also clarify the implied consequences of extremist thinking (e.g., "good" people vs. "bad" people and the patient's ongoing response to them), as well as the compromises inherent in reality (e.g., "Can anyone truly be all good or all bad?").

As therapy progresses, the official term "splitting" can be introduced into the treatment vernacular to facilitate the patient's semantic and emotional access to the dilemma. Occasionally, in higher-functioning patients, exaggeration and humor can be employed to demonstrate the impractical compromises of chronic splitting. This, of course, needs to be carefully executed to insure that a patient does not misinterpret or projectively distort the therapist's intent. Once the process is intellectually understood by the patient and he or she has some sense of its consequences and compromises, deeper and more abstract understanding may be achieved through interpretation.

Throughout treatment, an important role of the therapist is to model integration. This can be done by "thinking out loud" about issues in session and contemplating the variables. This enables the patient to directly observe and experience ambivalence and the subsequent integration of perceptions and cognitions.

In our work with borderline/eating disorder patients, we have found the following guidelines quite helpful. First, it is important to anticipate and "hear" splitting in the therapy session. This enables an active and continual monitoring of the process on multiple levels—cognitive, perceptual, expressive, and interpersonal. It also enables the therapist to hear and understand what is really being perceived by the patient.

Second, it is useful to plan ahead for splitting. As stated previously, this may include initially limiting all adjunctive therapies, as well as restricting the patient's contact with "recruitable" therapists. Multidisciplinary team members and consultants need to reinforce their prescribed roles and boundaries with the patient and to set limits neutrally when the patient challenges the established structure. Although this directive role may be uncomfortable for some therapists, team members and consultants in general genuinely appreciate the structure.

Third, in confronting splitting, we have found it helpful to develop consistent interventions that will be employed on a repetitive basis. Consistency may be fostered by the repetitive identification of splitting, and the use of consistent metaphors and colloquial labels. In an approach to a Socratic or interpretive intervention, even repetitiveness of phraseology can be a useful cue for the patient. The therapist's consistent response functions as a stabilizing interpersonal structure for these individuals.

Lastly, splitting is an ongoing issue that requires continual attention and energy. Realistically appreciating this fact may help to neutralize the periodic frustrations of dealing with its continual re-emergence.

Managing Self-Destructive Behaviors: A Dynamic Focus

While the therapeutic relationship and the transference stabilize, we primarily use the previously detailed behavioral and cognitive methods of managing self-destructive behaviors. However, as patients move into Phase 3 (resolving internal themes), we focus increasingly on the dynamic meaning of their self-destructive behavior. Self-destructive behavior can be utilized as a method to (1) reduce anxiety; (2) punish a perceived "bad self"; (3) prevent fragmentation or decompensation; and (4) elicit nonintimate caring responses from others (Gunderson, 1984). These behaviors may also promote and maintain a pathological personal identity, as well as provide an immediate outlet for displaced anger (Favazza, 1989). The complex intrapsychic and interpersonal meaning of these behaviors may tend to cluster in predictable patterns for a given individual. Our goal is to uncover with the patients the dynamic meaning of these behaviors and help them develop healthier coping strategies.

Promoting Self-Regulation

During Phase 2 of treatment (stabilizing the transference), the issues involving self-regulation (e.g., self-destructive behavior, drug abuse, eating disorder) are approached primarily on a behavioral and cognitive level. During Phase 3, the emphasis shifts from structuring everyday dysregulation to exploring the broader theme of globally impaired self-regulation. Utilizing the central theme of self-regulatory difficulties with the patient enables the therapist and patient to shift from "examining each battle" to "overseeing the war." Initially, the therapist can identify and label specific events as indications of "impaired self-regulation." Subsequently, the therapist can neutrally and repetitively acknowledge the mutual need to understand these regulation deficits, and can encourage the development of the patient's internal self-control. These themes can be reinforced through exploration, clarification, and interpretation.

PHASE 4: PREPARING FOR TERMINATION

To date, comparatively little has been written on the subject of therapeutic termination of the borderline patient. A variety of factors may account for this. First, the extensive length of time required for effective treatment (i.e., years) may be susceptible to interruption via premature termination by either the patient or the therapist. A premature termination may be the consequence of a failed therapeutic contract or secondary to the patient's acting out (e.g., noncompliance with appointments, utilization of therapy for crisis only, impulsive change of therapists); the expense and/or time constraints of the treatment process; the therapist's exhaustion; the geographic relocation or death of either party; or some other factor. Indeed, clinical lore suggests that the treatment of the borderline patient may be a lifelong process initially consisting of intense psychotherapy, followed by less frequent maintenance sessions. Thus, for a variety of reasons, premature terminations may be a common clinical development in borderline cases.

Our awareness of patients' ongoing posttermination life experience is limited in scope. Although long-term follow-up studies of borderline patients are available (Carpenter & Gunderson, 1977; Carpenter, Gunderson, & Strauss, 1977; Gunderson, Carpenter, & Strauss, 1975; Hoch, Cattell, Strahl, & Pennes, 1962; Werble, 1970; Masterson, 1980; McGlashan, 1986; Pope, Jonas, Hudson, Cohen, & Gunderson, 1983), the length, frequency, and type of treatment are often unclear. In addition, the available studies do not adequately assess the posttreatment psychological status of these individuals in the three areas we believe are essential in resolving the borderline syndrome: splitting, object constancy, and self-destructive behaviors. Some of the available follow-up studies (Akiskal et al., 1985; Paris, Brown, & Nowlis, 1987; Pope et al., 1983; Stone, Stone, & Hurt, 1987) discuss the incidence of suicide; however, the tracking of other forms of self-destructive behavior has not been reported. Therefore, there is little information on symptom substitution or symptom "trading down" (i.e., shifting from a more intense symptom to one of lesser degree), or on the patient's overall regulation of self-destructive drives, during the posttreatment period. An additional dilemma in this area is the lack of valid and reliable psychological measures of the extent of splitting in a given subject or the presence and maturity of object constancy. Likewise, there is no detailed inventory for measuring broad-spectrum self-destructive behaviors, particularly those ranging from graphic to elusively sophisticated. Thus, due to the lack of adequate research data, the following material is again primarily based upon our own clinical experience.

We believe that a primary issue in the termination of the borderline patient with an eating disorder is timing. We base this decision on the patient's overall progress in the following areas: (1) self-regulation, particularly in the areas of the eating disorder, self-destructive acting out, mood, and interpersonal boundaries; and (2) interpersonal relatedness, such that boundaries are more stable and a rudimentary level of object constancy has been consolidated (increased tolerance for aloneness, reduction in clinging dependency with others, enhanced capacity for internal soothing, integration of splitting, etc.).

Realistically, we do not expect absolute resolution of symptoms as a requirement of termination (e.g., complete and permanent eradication of the eating disorder). We do, however, expect that occupational and interpersonal functioning will not be disrupted if momentary slips in eating behavior do occur during periods of significant stress. Moreover, patients who have attained meaningful involvement in relationships outside the therapeutic relationship have achieved an important prognostic milestone. The development of meaningful relationships, coupled with progressive involvement with healthier individuals, strongly suggests a lasting and significant psychostructural change.

Once the decision has been made to initiate a therapeutic termination, a clear and lengthy time frame (i.e., ideally 6–12 months or more) should be established. This allows for definition and predictability in the treatment experience, and provides the patient with the necessary time to experiment with separation. This experimentation will invariably be coupled with episodes of regression and possibly symptom re-emergence. These episodic regressions appear to be typical and relatively short-lived. They do not imply treatment failure or poorly timed termination. They may be likened to the healthy toddler's periodic intense clinging and dependency during the rapprochement subphase of separation–individuation. Although the acting-out behaviors of the borderline adult may be significantly more dramatic than those of the toddler, the therapist, like the healthy mother, must maintain warmth, availability, and tolerance coupled with consistent encouragement and support toward autonomy.

When acute regressions occur, they need to be confronted in a consistent manner. As in the past, behavioral and cognitive restructuring are useful approaches. We again emphasize the importance of the therapist's affective neutrality during acute regressive episodes, to reduce the pathological drive away from separation–individuation. During the stable periods of the termination, the therapist should explore, clarify, support, and interpret when indicated. Patient themes during the termination process will center almost exclusively on the fears and anxieties surrounding personal autonomy and the loss of the therapeutic relationship. It is important to remind the patient repeatedly that what has been learned and experienced within the therapeutic relationship can be attained in his or her interpersonal relationships outside of treatment.

CONCLUSIONS

Our intention in writing this chapter has been to broaden the literature about the clinical approaches to working with this subgroup of long-term, seriously disturbed eating disorder patients who do not seem to respond to standard brief interventions. We have attempted to describe a systematic approach to this complicated treatment process. Although there is significant disagreement in the field about the prevalence of borderline personality in eating disorder patients, we strongly believe that more attention and discussion should be given to developing strategies to help this subgroup manage their eating disorders and lead more productive and balanced lives. Systematic research needs to be conducted with this subpopulation to determine the effectiveness of various treatment approaches.

We have emphasized that the treatment of the eating disorder patient with borderline personality disorder is significantly different from the treatment of the non-character-disorder patient. Behaviorally, the borderline patient may enter treatment with complaints and eating disorder symptoms identical to those of the nonborderline individual (Garner, Olmsted, Davis, Goldbloom, & Eagle, 1989; Johnson et al., 1989). Only through a skillful, retrospective clinical interview (e.g., our PISIA approach) can the therapist determine whether the patient's psychological disturbances are a result of chronic dietary chaos or more fundamental deficits in psychological organization. If the patient presents with borderline personality organization, this should significantly alter the therapist's expectations and approach to treatment. Johnson, Tobin, and Dennis (1990) found at a 1-year follow-up that bulimic patients with borderline personality continued to demonstrate clinically significant levels of disturbed eating patterns, drive for thinness, body dissatisfaction, and depression. Therapists should expect to make a long-term commitment to the treatment process, and recognize that the reparation of distortions in interpersonal relationships, the reworking of the primitive self-concept, and the development of self-regulation are the fundamental goals for treatment, as opposed to the total elimination of the eating disorder.

We hope that this chapter has helped to demystify the treatment of the borderline patient. Many practitioners in the mental health field avoid labeling their patients as "borderline" or avoid treatment of this population in general. They believe that this label carries with it the stigma of lifelong dysfunction with little hope of recovery. We strongly disagree with these assumptions. We have had the privilege of long-term work with numerous extremely dysfunctional patients. Assisting them in eliminating their self-destructive lifestyle and developing healthy interpersonal relationships has been not only stimulating and challenging, but also extremely rewarding.

We caution the reader that our approach to the treatment of the eating disorder patient with borderline personality is based on our joint clinical experience and not on systematic research. Our approach is colored by our personal perception of the borderline process, the specialized eating disorder facilities that we have administered, and the patients whom we have treated. We hope that our experience is truly reflective of the experiences of others.

REFERENCES

Adler, G. (1973). Hospital treatment of borderline patients. *American Journal of Psychiatry, 130,* 32–36.

Akiskal, H. S., Chen, S. E., Davis, G. C., Puzantian, V. R., Kashgarian, M., & Bolinger, J. M. (1985). Borderline: An adjective in search of a noun. *Journal of Clinical Psychiatry, 46,* 41–48.

American Psychiatric Association. (1987). *Diagnostic and statistical manual of mental disorders* (3rd ed., rev.). Washington, DC: Author.

Anderson, A. E. (1985). *Practical comprehensive treatment of anorexia nervosa and bulimia*. Baltimore: Johns Hopkins University Press.

Arnow, D., & Cooper, S. H. (1984). The borderline patient's regression on the Rorschach test: An object relations interpretation. *Bulletin of the Menninger Clinic, 48*, 25–36.

Armelius, B. A., Kullgren, G., & Renberg, E. (1985). Borderline diagnosis from hospital records: Reliability and validity of Gunderson's diagnostic interview for borderlines. *Journal of Nervous and Mental Disease, 173*, 32–34.

Breger, L. (1974). *From instinct to identity: The development of personality*. Englewood Cliffs, NJ: Prentice-Hall.

Burgner, M., & Edgcumbe, R. (1972). Some problems in the conceptualization of early object relations: Part II. The concept of object constancy. *Psychoanalytic Study of the Child, 27*, 315–333.

Carpenter, W. T., & Gunderson, J. G. (1977). Five year follow-up comparison of borderline schizophrenic patients. *Comprehensive Psychiatry, 18*, 567–571.

Carpenter, W. T., Gunderson, J. G., & Strauss, J. S. (1977). Considerations of the borderline syndrome: A longitudinal comparative study of borderline and schizophrenic patients. In P. Hartocollis (Ed.), *Borderline personality disorders: The concept, the syndrome, the patient* (pp. 231–253). New York: International Universities Press.

Chatham, P. M. (1985). *Treatment of the borderline personality*. New York: Jason Aronson.

Christenson, R. M., & Wilson, W. P. (1985). Assessing pathology in the separation–individuation process by an inventory: A preliminary report. *Journal of Nervous and Mental Disease, 173*, 561–565.

Conte, H. R., Plutchik, R., Karasu, T. B., & Jerrett, I. (1980). A self-report borderline scale: Discriminative validity and preliminary norms. *Journal of Nervous and Mental Disease, 168*, 428–435.

Cooper, S. H., Perry, J. C., Hoke, L., & Richman, N. (1985). Transitional relatedness and borderline personality disorder. *Psychoanalytic Psychology, 2*, 115–128.

Cornell, D. G., Silk, K. R., Ludolph, P. S., & Lohr, N. E. (1983). Test–retest reliability of the diagnostic interview for borderlines. *Archives of General Psychiatry, 40*, 1307–1310.

Dennis, A. B., & Sansone, R. A. (1989). Treating the bulimic patient with borderline personality disorder. In W. Johnson (Ed.), *Advances in eating disorders* (Vol. 2, pp. 237–265). Greenwich, CT: JAI Press.

Fairburn, C. (1982). *Binge-eating and bulimia nervosa*. London: Smith, Kline & French.

Fairburn, C. (1984). Cognitive–behavioral treatment for bulimia. In D. M. Garner & P. E. Garfinkel (Eds.), *Handbook of psychotherapy for anorexia nervosa and bulimia* (pp. 160–191). New York: Guilford Press.

Favazza, A. R. (1989). Why patients mutilate themselves. *Hospital and Community Psychiatry, 40*, 137–145.

Feldman, M. D. (1988). The challenge of self-mutilation: A review. *Comprehensive Psychiatry, 29*, 252–269.

Gallop, R., Lance, W. J., & Garfinkel, P. (1989). How nursing staff respond to the label "borderline personality disorder." *Hospital and Community Psychiatry, 40,* 815–819.

Garner, D. M., & Bemis, K. M. (1982). A cognitive–behavioral approach to anorexia nervosa. *Cognitive Therapy and Research, 6,* 123–150.

Garner, D. M., & Bemis, K. M. (1984). Cognitive therapy for anorexia nervosa. In D. M. Garner & P. E. Garfinkel (Eds.), *Handbook of psychotherapy for anorexia nervosa and bulimia nervosa* (pp. 107–146). New York: Guilford Press.

Garner, D. M., & Olmstead, M. A. (1984). *Eating Disorder Inventory.* Psychological Assessment Resources Inc.

Garner, D. M., Olmsted, M. P., Davis, R., Goldbloom, D., & Eagle, M. (1989). The association between bulimic symptoms and reported psychopathology. *International Journal of Eating Disorders, 8,* 500–515.

Garner, D. M., Rockert, W., Olmsted, M. P., Johnson, C., & Coscina, D. V. (1984). Psychoeducational principles in the treatment of bulimia and anorexia nervosa. In D. M. Garner & P. E. Garfinkel (Eds.), *Handbook of psychotherapy for anorexia nervosa and bulimia nervosa* (pp. 513–572). New York: Guilford Press.

Grinker, R. R., Werble, B., & Drye, R. C. (1968). *The borderline syndrome: A behavioral study of ego functions.* New York: Basic Books.

Gunderson, J. G. (1984). *Borderline personality disorder.* Washington, DC: American Psychiatric Press.

Gunderson, J. G., Carpenter, W. T., & Strauss, J. S. (1975). Borderline and schizophrenic patients: A comparative study. *American Journal of Psychiatry, 132,* 1257–1264.

Gunderson, J. G., Kolb, J. E., & Austin, V. (1981). The Diagnostic Interview for Borderline Patients. *American Journal of Psychiatry, 138,* 896–903.

Gunderson, J. G., & Singer, M. T. (1975). Defining borderline patients: An overview. *American Journal of Psychiatry, 132,* 1–10.

Gwirtsman, H. E., Roy-Byrne, P., Yager, J., & Gerner, R. H. (1983). Neuroendocrine abnormalities in bulimia. *American Journal of Psychiatry, 140,* 559–563.

Hoch, P. H., Cattell, J. P., Strahl, M. O., & Pennes, H. H. (1962). The course and outcome of pseudoneurotic schizophrenia. *American Journal of Psychiatry, 119,* 106–115.

Hudson, J. I., Pope, H. G., & Jonas, J. M. (1984). Psychosis in anorexia nervosa and bulimia. *British Journal of Psychiatry, 145,* 420–423.

Hyler, S. E., & Rieder, R. O. (1987). *Personality Diagnostic Questionnaire— Revised (PDQ-R).* New York: New York State Psychiatric Institute.

Johnson, C., & Connors, M. E. (1987). *The etiology and treatment of bulimia nervosa: A biopsychosocial perspective.* New York: Basic Books.

Johnson, C., Tobin, D., & Enright, A. B. (1989). Prevalence and clinical characteristics of borderline patients in an eating-disordered population. *Journal of Clinical Psychiatry, 50,* 9–15.

Johnson, C., Tobin, D., & Dennis, A. B. (1990). Difference in treatment outcome between borderline and nonborderline bulimics at one year follow-up. *International Journal of Eating Disorders, 9,* 1–11.

Kaplan, H. I., & Sadock, B. J. (1985). *Modern synopsis of psychiatry, IV.* Baltimore: Williams & Wilkins.

Kernberg, O. F. (1967). Borderline personality organization. *Journal of the American Psychoanalytic Association, 15,* 641–685.

Kernberg, O. F. (1976). *Object relations theory and clinical psychoanalysis.* New York: Jason Aronson.

Kernberg, O. F. (1981). Structural interviewing. *Psychiatric Clinics of North America, 4,* 169–195.

Kernberg, O. F. (1984). *Severe personality disorders: Psychotherapeutic strategies.* New Haven, CT: Yale University Press.

Kernberg, O. F. (1985). *Borderline conditions and pathological narcissism* (2nd ed.). Northvale, NJ: Jason Aronson.

Kolb, J. E., & Gunderson, J. G. (1980). Diagnosing borderline patients with a semistructured interview. *Archives of General Psychiatry, 37,* 37–41.

Kroll, J. (1988). *The challenge of the borderline patient: Competency in diagnosis and treatment.* New York: Norton.

Kroll, J., Pyle, R., Zander, J., Martin, K., Lari, S., & Sines, L. (1981). Borderline personality disorder: Interrater reliability of the Diagnostic Interview for Borderlines. *Schizophenia Bulletin, 7,* 269–272.

Lacey, J. H. (1983). Bulimia nervosa, binge eating and psychogenic vomiting: A controlled treatment study and long-term outcome. *British Medical Journal, 286,* 1611–1613.

Levin, A. P., & Hyler, S. E. (1986). DSM-III personality diagnosis in bulimia. *Comprehensive Psychiatry, 27,* 47–53.

Leibenluft, E., Gardner, D. L., & Cowdry, R. W. (1987). The inner experience of the borderline self-mutilator. *Journal of Personality Disorders, 1,* 317–324.

Loranger, A. W., Oldham, J. M., Russakoff, L. M., & Susman, V. (1984). Structured interviews and borderline personality disorder. *Archives of General Psychiatry, 41,* 565–568.

Loranger, A. W., Susman, V., Oldham, J., & Russakoff, L. M. (1988). *Personality Disorder Examination.* Unpublished manuscript.

Mahler, M. S. (1971). A study of the separation–individuation process and its possible application to borderline phenomena in the psychoanalytic situation. *Psychoanalytic Study of the Child, 26,* 403–424.

Mahler, M. S., with Furer, M. (1968). *On human symbiosis and the vicissitudes of individuation: Vol. 1. Infantile psychoses.* New York: International Universities Press.

Mahler, M. S., & Kaplan, L. (1977). Developmental aspects in the assessment of narcissistic and so-called borderline personalities. In P. Hartocollis (Ed.), *Borderline personality disorders: The concept, the syndrome, the patient* (pp. 71–85). New York: International Universities Press.

Mahler, M. S., Pine, F., & Bergman, A. (1975). *The psychological birth of the human infant.* New York: Basic Books.

Masterson, J. F. (1980). *From borderline adolescent to functioning adult: The test of time.* New York: Brunner/Mazel.

Masterson, J. F., & Rinsley, D. B. (1975). The borderline syndrome: The role of the mother in the genesis and psychic structure of the borderline personality. *International Journal of Psycho-Analysis, 56,* 163–177.

McDevitt, J. B. (1975). Separation–individuation and object constancy. *Journal of the American Psychoanalytic Association, 23,* 713–742.

McGlashan, T. H. (1986). The Chestnut Lodge follow-up study: III. Long-term outcome of borderline personalities. *Archives of General Psychiatry, 43,* 20–30.

Meissner, W. W. (1984). *The borderline spectrum: Differential diagnosis and developmental issues.* New York: Jason Aronson.

Millon, T. (1983). *Millon Clinical Multiaxial Inventory* (2nd ed.). Minneapolis: National Computer Systems.

Mitchell, J. E. (1985). *Anorexia nervosa and bulimia.* Minneapolis: University of Minnesota Press.

Paris, J., Brown, R., & Nowlis, D. (1987). Long-term follow-up of borderline patients in a general hospital. *Comprehensive Psychiatry, 28,* 530–535.

Patrick, J., & Wolfe, B. (1983). Rorschach presentation of borderline personality disorder: Primary process manifestations. *Journal of Clinical Psychology, 39,* 442–447.

Perry, J. C. (1982). *The Borderline Personality Disorder Scale (BPD-Scale): Semi-structured version.* Cambridge, MA: The Cambridge Hospital.

Perry, J. C. (1983). *The Borderline Personality Disorder Scale (BPD-Scale): Structured interview.* Cambridge, MA: The Cambridge Hospital.

Piran, N., Lerner, P., Garfinkel, P. E., Kennedy, S. H., & Brouillette, C. (1988). Personality disorders in anorexic patients. *International Journal of Eating Disorders, 7,* 589–599.

Pope, H. G., Frankenburg, F. R., Hudson, J. I., Jonas, J. M., & Yurgelun-Todd, D. (1987). Is bulimia associated with borderline personality disorder? A controlled study. *Journal of Clinical Psychiatry, 48,* 181–184.

Pope, H. G., Jonas, J. M., Hudson, J. I., Cohen, B. M., & Gunderson, J. G. (1983). The validity of DSM-III borderline personality disorder: A phenomenologic, family history, treatment response, and long-term follow-up study. *Archives of General Psychiatry, 40,* 23–30.

Powers, P. S., Coovert, D L., Brightwell, D. R., & Stevens, B. A. (1988). Other psychiatric disorders among bulimic patients. *Comprehensive Psychiatry, 29,* 503–508.

Rosen, L. W., & Thomas, M. A. (1984). Treatment techniques for chronic wrist cutters. *Journal of Behavior Therapy and Experimental Psychiatry, 15,* 33–36.

Ross, R. R., & McKay, H. B. (1979). *Self-mutilation.* Lexington, MA: Lexington Books.

Sansone, R. A., Fine, M. A., Seuferer, S., & Bovenzi, J. (1989). The prevalence of borderline personality symptomatology among women with eating disorders. *Journal of Clinical Psychology, 45,* 603–610.

Silver, D. (1985). Psychodynamics and psychotherapeutic management of the self-destructive character-disordered patient. *Psychiatric Clinics of North America, 8,* 357–375.

Singer, M. T. (1977). The borderline diagnosis and psychological tests: Review on research. In P. Hartocollis (Ed.), *Borderline personality disorders: The concept, the syndrome, the patient* (pp. 45–62). New York: International Universities Press.

Soloff, P. H. (1981). Concurrent validation of a diagnostic interview for borderline patients. *American Journal of Psychiatry, 138*, 691–693.

Spitzer, R. L., Endicott, J., & Gibbon, M. (1979). Crossing the border into borderline personality and borderline schizophrenia: The development of criteria. *Archives of General Psychiatry, 36*, 17–24.

Stone, M. H. (1980). *The borderline syndromes: Constitution, adaptation and personality*. New York: McGraw-Hill.

Stone, M. H., Stone, D. K., & Hurt, S. W. (1987). The natural history of borderline patients treated by intensive hospitalization. *Psychiatric Clinics of North America, 10*, 185–206.

Werble, B. (1970). Second follow-up study of borderline patients. *Archives of General Psychiatry, 23*, 3–7.

Winnicott, D. W. (1965). *The family and individual development*. London: Tavistock.

Yates, W. R., Sieleni, B., Reich, J., & Brass, C. (1989). Comorbidity of bulimia nervosa and personality disorder. *Journal of Clinical Psychiatry, 50*, 57–59.

∴ *8* ∴

Treatment of Eating-Disordered Patients with Borderline and False-Self/Narcissistic Disorders

CRAIG L. JOHNSON
Laureate Psychiatric Clinic and Hospital
and Northwestern University Medical School

After several years of being enamored with the similarities between eating-disordered patients, clinicians and researchers are beginning to return to mapping out the variety of biological and psychological adaptations that disturbed eating behavior can serve for individuals. Emphasis seems to be turning to identifying subgroups of anorexic and bulimic patients for whom more specific interventions are warranted. Of particular interest is the subgroup of patients who present with significant character pathology. These patients usually do not respond to either brief cognitive–behavioral interventions or psychopharmacological treatment. They generally require longer-term, informed psychotherapy.

The task of this chapter is to extend some of my previous work on the treatment of eating-disordered patients with borderline and narcissistic disorders (Johnson & Connors, 1987). I begin by reviewing some of the prevailing theories regarding developmental difficulties among eating-disordered patients; I then attempt to articulate some fundamental differences in cognitive styles, defenses, and experience of self and others between restrictors and bulimics. Finally, I discuss some of the transference and countertransference issues that therapists encounter in working

with restricting and bulimic patients who have borderline or false-self/
narcissistic disorders.

DEVELOPMENTAL DISTURBANCES

Several prominent theorists have attempted to determine the specific
disruption in the early holding environment that leads to subsequent
problems such as anorexia nervosa or bulimia nervosa. Bruch (1962)
suggested that the symptomatic behavior of anorexia nervosa is an adaptation to early developmental disruptions that occur in the late symbiotic or
early differentiation subphase of separation–individuation (Mahler, Pine,
& Bergman, 1975).

Bruch argued that a central issue for anorexic patients is difficulty
with "interoceptive awareness"—a term she coined to describe problems
in identifying and articulating internal states. She further elaborated how
a child can develop this type of deficiency in interaction with a particular
type of caretaker. According to Bruch, children are active participants in
their development. Their participation involves emitting a signal related
to some need state that they initially experience as diffuse and undifferentiated. The caretaker must decode the signal and organize a

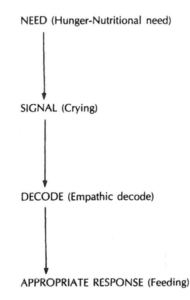

FIGURE 8.1.   Differential learning of nutritional need and feeding. From *The
Etiology and Treatment of Bulimia Nervosa* (p. 97) by C. Johnson and M. E.
Connors, 1987. New York: Basic Books. Copyright 1987 by Basic Books. Re-
printed by permission.

response. A child's increasing ability to appropriately differentiate his or her internal states is facilitated or interfered with according to the caretaker's ability to accurately decode and respond to the child's cues (see Figure 8.1).

> Appropriate responses to cues coming from the infant, in the biological field as well as the intellectual, social and emotional field, are necessary for the child to organize the significant building stones for the development of self-awareness and self-effectiveness. If confirmation and reinforcement of his own and initially rather undifferentiated needs and impulses have been absent or have been contradictory or inaccurate, then the child will grow up perplexed when trying to differentiate between disturbances in his biological field and emotional interpersonal experiences, and would be apt to misinterpret deformities in his self–body concept as externally induced. Thus he will become an individual deficient in his sense of separateness, with diffuse ego boundaries and feel helpless under the influence of external forces. (Bruch, 1973, p. 56)

Bruch further elaborated on how faulty decoding by the primary caretaker results in confusion and lack of differentiation of internal states, particularly those related to the experience of hunger (see Figure 8.2):

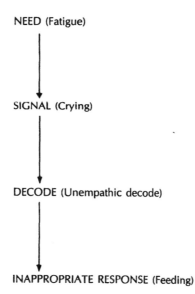

NEED (Fatigue)

SIGNAL (Crying)

DECODE (Unempathic decode)

INAPPROPRIATE RESPONSE (Feeding)

FIGURE 8.2. Interoceptive awareness difficulties: Confusion around the relationship among nutritional need, fatigue, and feeding. From *The Etiology and Treatment of Bulimia Nervosa* (p. 98) by C. Johnson and M. E. Connors, 1987, New York: Basic Books. Copyright 1987 by Basic Books. Reprinted by permission.

When a mother offers food in response to signals indicating nutritional needs, the infant will gradually develop the engram of hunger as a sensation distinct from other tensions or needs. If, on the other hand, a mother's reaction is continuously inappropriate, be it neglectful, over-solicitous, inhibiting or indiscriminately permissive, the outcome for the child will be perplexing and confusing. When he is older he will not be able to discriminate between being hungry or satiated, or between nutritional need and some other discomfort or tension. (Bruch, 1973, p. 56)

Since both restricting anorexics and bulimics appear to manifest substantial difficulty with interoceptive awareness, perhaps specific differences in the mother–child interaction predispose patients toward a restricting versus a bulimic adaptation to the interoceptive difficulties. In the following sections, I argue that both caretaker over- and underinvolvement result in unempathic decoding and may predispose children to the type of self-regulatory difficulties observed in restricting anorexics and bulimics. Furthermore, I also believe that restricting behavior is a specific adaptation to maternal overinvolvement and that bulimic behavior reflects an adaptive response to maternal underinvolvement.

It is important to note that this early attempt to differentiate restricting and bulimic individuals according to specific developmental disruptions is quite speculative. As depicted in Figure 8.3, we are talking about a normal distribution of maternal responsiveness within both groups, but with clustering along the continuum of maternal involvement. The rationale for attempting this differentiation is that if there really are differences in the nature of maternal responsiveness, then they may well suggest different treatment strategies for the two groups.

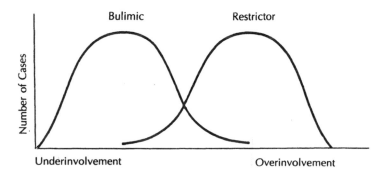

FIGURE 8.3. Disruptions in maternal preoccupation. From *The Etiology and Treatment of Bulimia Nervosa* (p. 98) by C. Johnson and M. E. Connors, 1987, New York: Basic Books. Copyright 1987 by Basic Books. Reprinted by permission.

MATERNAL OVERINVOLVEMENT AND THE
RESTRICTING STANCE

A number of investigators have observed that mothers of classic restricting anorexia nervosa patients are domineering, intrusive, overprotective, and overtly or more subtly discouraging of separation–individuation. They encourage enmeshment and often respond to the children according to their own needs rather than those of the children. This enmeshment prevents the children from acquiring a firm, independent, cohesive sense of self and leaves them dependent on the primary caretakers for self-regulation. During childhood and latency, there is minimal developmental pressure to disrupt the symbiotic attachment between mother and child. The beginning of adolescence, however, with its new demands for separation and individuation, can potentially disrupt the mother–child relationship. It is at this point that self-starvation serves a variety of adaptive functions.

Bruch originally suggested that anorexics' relentless pursuit of thinness and defiant defense of that behavior is an adaptive effort to take charge of their selves. Control of their selves is concretely represented by controlling their bodies, and the measure of control is continued weight loss. The persistent pursuit of thinness thus serves a dual function of undoing feelings of ineffectiveness by successfully achieving body control (thinness) and engaging in an oppositional behavior that, at least at a superficial level, disrupts the symbiotic relationship with the mother.

Selvini-Palazzoli (1974) suggested a slightly different adaptation in the anorexic stance. Like Bruch, Selvini-Palazzoli observed that anorexic patients experience significant self-definition and self-regulatory difficulties as a result of enmeshed symbiotic relationships with overcontrolling mothers. However, Selvini-Palazzoli argued that the changes that occur during puberty are overwhelming and engulfing to these patients (the vast majority of whom are female):

> Because of the development of breasts and other feminine curves, the body is experienced concretely as the maternal object, from which the ego wishes to separate itself at all costs. . . . The patient considers and experiences her body as one great incorporated object which overpowers her and forces a passive role upon her. (Selvini-Palazzoli, 1974, p. 90)

Selvini-Palazzoli concluded that anorexia is a form of intrapersonal paranoia that should be classified somewhere between schizophrenia and depression. The anorexic experiences food intake as an increase to a monstrous thing (the body at the expense of the central ego). The anorexic stance then becomes a desperate attempt to live, by overcoming the all-powerful, bad body that is the embodiment of the bad internal object.

Another group of observers, probably best represented by Crisp (1980) and his colleagues, have emphasized that the severe weight loss among restricting anorexic patients protects them from the psychological and biological demands that accompany puberty. The emaciation that accompanies the starvation returns an individual biologically to a pre-pubertal physical state. Endocrine changes that are directly related to weight loss, or percentage reduction of adipose tissue, eliminate second-ary sexual characteristics (breast and hip development, menstruation, etc.). This basically relieves the pressure of biological maturation and the attendant demands around sexuality and separation. Interestingly, the manipulation of body weight essentially allows the patient to control the timing and pace of puberty. Psychologically, the severe emaciation mini-mizes separation demands. Also, paradoxically, the debilitating side effects and fragility associated with severe emaciation insure further enmeshment and symbiotic attachment to the primary caretaker. It is important to note that the adaptive function of the weight loss is to protect the ego-impaired patient from developmental demands for which she is unprepared. The anorexic behavior appears to allow the patient to make a self-assertive statement while simultaneously insuring that separation expectations will be minimized.

The common denominator among these different theories is that the restricting anorexic child reaches puberty with developmental vul-nerabilities in regard to self-awareness, self-definition, and self-regulation. Furthermore, the vulnerabilities are precipitated by some degree of maternal overinvolvement. The self-starvation is a desperate attempt to assert some autonomy, defend the fragile self against further maternal intrusiveness, and protect the fragile ego from the psy-chobiological demands of adulthood. I would also like to suggest that the predominant defensive style of restrictors is paranoid in nature. They attempt to establish and maintain boundaries by utilizing rigid, over-determined, avoidant defenses. They establish a sharp inner–outer, self–other border and then utilize the paranoid defenses to protect the bound-ary from intrusive invasion. As the next section indicates, this behavior contrasts with that of bulimics, who appear to rely more upon hysterical defenses in an effort to compensate for self-regulatory deficits arising from an experience of underinvolvement with their primary caretakers.

MATERNAL UNDERINVOLVEMENT AND THE BULIMIC STANCE

In contrast to mothers of restricting anorexics, mothers of bulimic patients have been described as passive, rejecting, and disengaged. It is important to emphasize that they usually are not blatantly neglectful caretakers; on the contrary they appear superficially to attend adequately to their children's primary needs. The underinvolvement or disengagement appears to be more subtly manifested as a type of emotional unavailability. The quality of the caretaking could be characterized as form without substance. Although the primary needs are attended to, there is no warmth in the holding experience or mutually enjoyable mirroring (e.g., gleam in the eye) that facilitates the capacity for self-soothing. These mothers generally have intrapsychic deficits themselves that result in affect regulation problems. The children's infantile needs appear to overwhelm the caretakers or to provoke rageful resentment.

A primary caretaker's emotional unavailability sends a child into the differentiation phase with a very tenuous bond to her. The child's experience is one of an insecure base from which to launch individuation. Under these circumstances the child may become tentative and even clingy. The clinginess, particularly through the rapprochement phase, further taxes the mother's limited resources and may provoke increased rejection of the child's needs to be soothed and comforted. When this happens, there are a number of substitutes that the child may use. There is a strong likelihood that since soothing is unavailable from the mother, the child will begin to seek self-regulatory tools outside the mother–child unit. Since food has such powerful symbolic associations, it is likely to be adopted by the child as a self-regulatory tool. The function that the food serves can be conceptualized as being similar to that of a transitional object. In essence, it becomes something the child invests with the ability to comfort her and, more important, that she has control over.

In summary, both maternal over- and underinvolvement can result in impairment in a child's ability to self-regulate (obtain object constancy, a cohesive self, and positive self-regard). For the restrictor, self-starvation may be an adaptive effort to defend against self-regulatory deficits resulting from maternal overinvolvement. In contrast, the bulimic's chaotic eating behavior may reflect a desperate attempt to compensate for an "empty experience" resulting from maternal underinvolvement. In a sense, the fundamental difference between the restricting and bulimic mode can be thought of as the bulimic's search for something to take in, compared to the restricting anorexic's attempt to keep something out.

Since most bulimic patients regard themselves as failed restrictors, what prevents them from relying on the restricting defense? Self-starvation is a highly depriving behavior that is motivated by intense commitment or fear. Ascetics and zealots experience a spiritual purity or fanatical commitment in response to self-starvation. The deprivation enhances their sense of strength. For classic restricting anorexics, the self-starvation (control of body) may serve to defend them against the

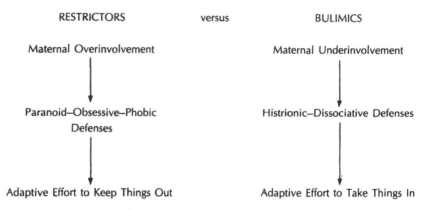

FIGURE 8.4.   Adaptive context for restricting and bulimic behavior.

threat of maternal intrusiveness. The sense of protection allows them to feel strong and safe.

Among the bulimics, however, I have found that deprivation associated with self-starvation is unbearable over time because it exacerbates the fundamental deficit in the holding environment, which is emptiness resulting from parental detachment. Consequently, in the absence of being able to sustain more paranoid/avoidant defenses, the bulimic is pushed toward a defensive adaptation that involves efforts to take in things to compensate for feelings of emptiness or dysphoria. This pursuit of emotional supplies is often frantic, diffuse, and chaotic, reflecting perhaps a more primitive hysterical defensive style (see Figure 8.4).

In the following sections, I attempt to differentiate between eating-disordered patients who present with borderline characteristics and those who present with false-self/narcissistic disorders. I also attempt to identify how restrictors and bulimics differ within these two character-disordered groups (see Table 8.1).

EATING-DISORDERED PATIENTS WITH BORDERLINE PERSONALITY DISORDER

Current research indicates that approximately 25%–35% of eating-disordered patients will also carry an Axis II diagnosis of borderline personality disorder. The percentage of patients presenting with this type and degree of character pathology is, of course, highly affected by the nature of the treatment center. Large teaching hospitals that tend to treat

TABLE 8.1. Variations in Character Pathology for Anorexic and Bulimic Patients

	Borderline	False-self/narcissistic
Restrictor (Overinvolvement)	Malevolent intrusiveness (intentional)	Nonmalevolent intrusiveness (unintentional)
	Attachment—hostile, controlling enmeshment	Attachment—controlling but less hostile and punitive enmeshment
	Separation—retaliation by other, injury to self	Separation—depletion of both self and other, injury to other
	Self—repeatedly overwhelmed in danger	Self—extension of other, without identity, ineffective, reactive
	Other—punitive, controlling, harsh, critical	Other—fragile
	Defenses—paranoid defenses used to establish and protect boundaries, splitting	Defenses—less paranoid, more obsessive, phobic
Bulimic (Underinvolvement)	Malevolent neglect (intentional)	Nonmalevolent neglect (unintentional)
	Attachment—hostile disengagement resulting in clingy dependence	Attachment—less hostile disengagement; wish for intimacy versus fear of disappointment, discovery, rejection; injury to other
	Separation—abandonment, emptiness, fragmentation	Separation—protective of self and other, pseudoautonomy, distant closeness
	Self—worthless, unlovable	Self—fraud, inadequate, destructively needy
	Other—withholding, punitive	Other—incapable of adequate holding
	Defenses—hysterical impulsive used in effort to introject, projective identification	Defenses—schizoid defenses, avoidance, denial, isolation of affect, intellectualization, suppression

Note: From *The Etiology and Treatment of Bulimia Nervosa* (p. 105) by C. Johnson and M. E. Connors, 1987, New York: Basic Books. Copyright 1987 by Basic Books. Reprinted by permission.

more tertiary cases will have a higher percentage than settings such as university counseling centers. Our preliminary research has indicated that the clinical characteristics, treatment, and course of illness with this subgroup of patients are quite different from those of patients who present with little character pathology (Johnson, Tobin, & Enright, 1989).

Clinically, these patients have significant ego impairments that result in pervasive self-regulatory difficulties. They are quite vulnerable to temporary episodes of depersonalization (breakdown of self–other or inner–outer boundaries). Phenomenologically, the patients experience this as a fragmentation of self or depersonalization. A range of impulsive behaviors (binge-eating, self-mutilation, substance abuse, promiscuity, etc.) are often used in an effort either to disrupt, to distract, or to avoid these regressions. The patients also experience intense affective instability marked by rapid fluctuation of moods, ranging from intense rage to profound feelings of emptiness, boredom, and anaclitic-like depression (Blatt, 1974). Interpersonal relationships are quite chaotic and shift from idealization to devaluation. Their experience of self and others is often laced with a sense of aggression or malevolence that results in sadistic and masochistic interactions with others.

Interestingly, our research shows that this group cannot be distinguished from nonborderline patients with eating disorders on the basis of their symptomatic eating behavior alone. In a recent survey, we found that there were no differences between borderline and nonborderline eating-disordered patients in the frequency of binge-eating or vomiting, or in the onset and duration of eating symptoms (Johnson et al., 1989). Similarly, there were no differences in current weight or weight history, in the number of dieting attempts, or in the age at which dieting was initiated. The only difference between the two groups was in laxative abuse, perhaps the most physically abusive method of purging. It is my opinion that this method of purging is preferred by the borderline patients because the function is more in the service of self-integration or self-punishment than simple weight regulation (Johnson & Connors, 1987).

Despite the homogeneity of eating symptoms, we found marked differences between the borderline and nonborderline groups on a wide array of other clinical indices. The borderline group reported significantly greater emotional distress, particularly in areas of depression, anxiety, hostility, and somatization. The borderline group also showed a general pattern of impulsive and self-destructive behaviors. Moreover, the borderlines reported a much more chaotic and unsatisfying pattern of relationships, less overall satisfaction with social and sexual relationships, and greater interpersonal conflict, particularly with women. Finally, the borderline group showed the type of conflictual and emotionally impoverished milieu characteristic of borderline families.

Preliminary research has also indicated that treatment outcome results are quite different for patients who present with significant borderline features (Johnson, Tobin, & Enright, 1989). At a 1-year follow-up, 62% of a borderline subgroup of patients were bingeing and purging twice a week or more (i.e., they continued to meet *Diagnostic and Statistical Manual of Mental Disorders,* third edition, revised [DSM-III-R] criteria), while only 21% of the nonborderline group retained this level of symptomatic behavior. Even more noteworthy, 43% of the borderline group were unchanged or worse at this follow-up, compared to 10% of the nonborderlines.

I feel confident that borderline features will continue to emerge as a powerful predictor of poor outcome among eating-disordered patients. Although this is unquestionably a difficult group to treat, they are treatable, and I have found that with long-term, informed psychotherapy the subgroup does get better. The treatment demands are simply different from those of eating-disordered patients who do not have concurrent borderline features.

In the following paragraphs I begin to contrast some of the dynamics, transference themes, and countertransference vulnerabilities between restricting and bulimic borderline patients. Once again, the similarity between the two groups is that each has experienced a level of malevolent intent from the primary caretaker. Among the borderline restrictors it is malevolent intrusiveness, and among the borderline bulimics it is malevolent withholding. The primary defensive mode among the borderline restrictors is more paranoid/obsessive, and among the borderline bulimics the defensive style is more histrionic/dissociative.

Restricting Borderline Patients

The key feature among restricting borderline patients is that they experience parental overinvolvement as malevolently intrusive. The caretakers have attempted intentionally to enmesh the children in a hostile dependent relationship. These patients perceive that their efforts to separate or differentiate will result in active punishment or retaliation. Attachment for these patients means enmeshment in a controlling, hostile, intrusive relationship. The experience of the self is one of repeatedly being overwhelmed by another who does not have the child's best interest at heart. These patients desperately erect paranoid defenses in an effort to protect the fragile self from being overwhelmed. It is within this group that I have found many patients who have been sexually or physically abused.

Body image distortion among these patients is a central feature to their psychological adaptation. Research has consistently demonstrated that patients who persisted in their body image distortion had the poorest outcome (Garfinkel & Garner, 1982). It has been our clinical experience that those patients who are most treatment-resistant (who have the poorest outcomes) fall into the category of restrictors with borderline personality.

I have found the specific adaptive function of the body image distortion within this subgroup to be as follows. Essentially, in an effort to protect the fragile self from intrusiveness that is experienced as malevolent, the restricting borderline patient has created a paranoid system in which fat becomes the symbolic focus of the paranoid defense. Although these patients are not grossly psychotic, in moments of perceived threat their thinking, particularly regarding their bodies, can become somewhat delusional.

These patients do not have a schizophrenic psychological system. Rather, they are more similar to paranoid-state patients, who develop elaborate defenses to protect themselves from a perceived threat. The defense of the self against the threat then provides a mechanism for structuring one's life. But the paranoid structure can be maintained only as long as the central belief or distortion is preserved. The patient must cling to the one central distorted belief, because if that belief is not true, then all subsequent behavior does not make sense. The delusional belief regarding the perceived threat and the psychological organization erected against the threat are circumscribed, however, and often do not result in complete psychological debilitation.

The restricting borderline patient initially attempts to establish a sense of self by taking charge of her body (body equals self). Fat becomes a concrete symbol of a feared feeling of hostile invasion and control. Fat then becomes a paranoid object that has many distortions associated with it, including an attribution of volition (fat has a mind of its own, goes where it is unwanted, will take over, etc.). The patient can then mobilize defenses against this threat and achieve a sense of control and safety, which is highly reinforcing.

The distorted body image allows the patient to develop an autonomous, self-derived belief system that is organized around a central perceived threat (fat). The defense of the self against the perceived threat (fat) gives the patient a sense of purpose (goal). The fear associated with the perceived threat (fat) provides motivation for the individual to avoid the threat. Thinness (avoidance of fat) then results in a profound sense of control. If she acknowledges her thinness (no fat), however, then purpose and motivation are lost. She would also experience cognitive dissonance if she did not cling to the body distortion. Rationally, emaciated individuals do not intentionally starve themselves unless they are crazy (out of control). Consequently, they must change the perception/belief about their degree of fatness in order to avoid the dissonance and preserve the psychological system. The tenacity of a patient's protection of the distorted body image is an indication of the degree of intrapsychic brittleness or fragility. It is crucial for therapist to understand that, for these patients, the disturbed belief about their bodies is a necessary distortion that allows a psychological organization to exist; it gives the patients autonomy, control, and a sense of purpose and motivation.

Transference and Countertransference Themes

Treatment of restricting borderline patients is difficult and usually requires years of patient, persistent, consistent, and caring involvement. The predominant transference themes usually revolve around issues of control (see Table 8.2). These patients usually are attentive to any indication that the therapist is trying to assert his or her will upon them. They are highly distrustful and quick to assume that the therapist is intentionally attempting to enmesh them in a hostile dependent relationship where they will ultimately be punished for autonomous behavior. The therapist's task is to create a therapeutic holding environment where patients learn that they can engage in an interdependent relationship without the aggressive/punitive control issues they are familiar with. It is important for the therapist to keep in mind, however, that the patients have experienced a level of malevolence in previous attachments that has resulted in a profound withdrawal into the anorexic stance. For these patients, the regression is more than just a fear of the psychosexual demands of adolescence: There is a deep-seated belief that the vulnerability that accompanies attachment will result in sadistic exploitation. The greater the patients' experience of malevolent intent from early significant others, the greater the resistance to relinquishing the unrelated world that is inherent in the anorexic stance. Once again, the experience of the patients is that others have aggressively and intentionally attempted to enmesh them for sadistic purposes.

The predominant countertransference vulnerability with this subgroup is being provoked into sadistic intrusiveness. Unfortunately, avoiding this can be a complicated task. Since the adaptations these patients have made (pursuit of thinness) can place them at serious medical risk because of their low weight, limit setting is often unavoidable, as is the power struggle that accompanies it. I have been struck by how often well-trained staff can be provoked into administrating whatever intrusive intervention may be warranted (nasal gastric tubes, etc.) in a more sadistic manner than is necessary. The vulnerability for this type of

TABLE 8.2. Borderline Restrictor (Malevolent Overinvolvement): Transference and
Countertransference Themes

Transference themes
  Hostile control
  Sadistic aggression
  Intent to injure

Countertransference vulnerabilities
  Feeling controlled, manipulated
  Frustration, helplessness
  Provoked intrusiveness
  Managing intention of intervention

countertransference reaction is especially high for anorexic patients who are being treated on general pediatric units. Nursing staff can become enraged when confronted with anorexic patients who appear to be intentionally trying to destroy themselves, while on the same ward there are children with leukemia, for example, who are prepared to endure extremely painful interventions in an effort to recover. The staff members generally experience the anorexic patients as manipulative and as intentionally attempting to thwart their well-intentioned interventions. Ultimately, the staff usually becomes enraged and engages in a power struggle around refeeding. This is a struggle that staff members will win at one level and miserably lose at another. They can overpower the patients and force weight gain, but these patients feel misunderstood and feel they have revealed the staff 's true sadistic/intrusive intentions, which is a replication of their primary experience of caretakers. It also reaffirms their belief that the world of others is malevolent and that they must survive by complying until they are discharged, at which time they promptly return to their anorexic stance. I have also seen well-intentioned treatment facilities attempt to avoid this trap by erring in the direction of not aggressively pursuing weight restoration. This is also a mistake, because the patients can become extremely comfortable with the adaptation they achieve with the low-weight anorexic stance.

Successful intervention with this subgroup requires maintaining the delicate balance between unambivalently intervening to restore weight and health, while simultaneously monitoring the patients' vulnerability to experiencing the interventions as intentionally malevolent. There is no question that the treatment team's actions are intrusive; what one can question with the patients, however, is whether they feel that the actions are intentionally designed to injure or thwart them. As I am writing this, I am aware that I am attempting to capture a very elusive detail; to a degree, what I am suggesting smacks of parents' intrusively setting limits on their children and then righteously feeling that it is for the children's own good. It is true that parents sometimes do know what is better for their children, and there are times when caretakers need to err in the direction of assuming a high level of control. I have come to believe, however, that the ingredient that makes or breaks this type of intervention is the extent to which the action is genuinely in the service of the patients' needs as opposed to the therapist's or treatment team's needs. If the benign/benevolent intention of the interventions are consistently monitored and communicated to the patients, then gradually this subgroup will relinquish their paranoid/schizoid adaptation and risk relatedness. It is important to note, however, that talking about the intention of the intervention may not be particularly effective in the short run. What the patients usually respond to is the "sense" of intention that is present in the spirit of the treatment team.

Outcome

Prognosis with this subgroup is guarded. Typically, they will restore their weight to slightly below menstrual threshold or just short of 100 pounds. Socially, they often return to school or work but remain interpersonally isolated.

A Variation among Borderline Restrictors: A Defense against Psychosis

I would also like to comment on a slightly different variation of borderline restrictors. There is also clearly a subgroup of patients who are attempting to ward off intrusive thoughts and feelings through paranoid mechanisms that have not been prompted by malevolent intrusion from others. Instead, it appears that they have experienced, usually near the onset of puberty, an accute psychotic episode. It appears to be less a function of the nature of the holding environment and more of a biogenetic event. The net result, however, is that the patients are overwhelmed by some affective–cognitive experience that they will do anything to avoid re-experiencing. The hypomanic and extremely focused behaviors in their exercise abuse and self-starvation are in the service of distraction and rigidly protecting against any unstructured time or space where the disorganized thoughts and feeling might reappear.

    Interestingly, these patients appear to be defending more against biologically mediated events than against extremely pathological object relations. The transference themes are often difficult to identify, because the patients are continually preoccupied by their internal state. The resistance to attachment is different than among patients who have had bad experiences with significant others. This group is more concerned about psychologically decompensating if they do anything to disrupt their precarious defenses. The defenses, resistances to treatment, and course of illness are very similar to those of the previous subgroup of patients. The central difference is the absence of sadomasochistic elements in the object-relational world. There is not the same level of hostile distrust that has to be worked through. The focus of the work with these patients is for the therapist to gradually create a sense of confidence that he or she can help the patients manage the powerful internal states that once over-whelmed them. I have found that gradually introducing medications to help titrate the depression, anxiety, pressured thoughts, and so on is a helpful adjunctive intervention. Usually, however, these patients will not agree to take medications until a credible treatment relationship has been established. Without the support of a therapeutic relationship, they can-not tolerate even the slightest shift in internal feelings created by the medication. Without reassurance, they experience the shift in the base-line experience as a harbinger that they are about to be out of control and overwhelmed by their feelings once again.

If, over time, the therapist can demonstrate to the patients that he or she can be helpful in managing these feelings, then gradually the patients usually relax their rigid defenses. There is usually, however, a critical weight level (around menstrual threshold) that creates a showdown. Essentially, there comes a point where the patients have to feel safe enough to breach this weight barrier and take the risk that they will not be overwhelmed as in the past. The pace and timing of this event are highly variable and usually need to be mostly controlled by the patients. The therapist needs to maintain the attitude of moderate upward pressure on weight toward this critical threshold, while simultaneously being respectful of the patients' need to control the pace of exposure and their fear of falling apart.

Interestingly, with this subgroup of patients there can come a point where they are fundamentally ready to confront the weight barrier, but need the therapist to take charge of the feeding. Fundamentally, they need to delegate control. This often represents a new dimension of trust and attachment in the therapeutic relationship. These patients often do not even want the responsibility of chewing food to cross the weight barrier. Although I usually disagree with the use of liquid supplements for weight restoration, this is an instance where I support their temporary use.

Bulimic Borderline Patients

In contrast to the restricting borderlines, the key feature for bulimic borderline patients is parental underinvolvement that is experienced as malevolent neglect. Most often the primary caretakers, for a variety of intrapsychic reasons, have had difficulty being emotionally available for their children. For some, the children's neediness or dependency overwhelms their own poor ego resources and threatens boundary disintegrations. Or the attention given the infants provokes regressive longing and resentment over injuries they themselves have sustained developmentally. Whatever vulnerability an infant triggers, the result is that the caretaker emotionally disengages from the child. This leaves the child without external help to regulate her internal states. Particularly for borderline patients, this disengagement or withholding has an aggressive or intentional quality that contributes to the patients' more sadomasochistic tendencies.

These patients often internalize the emotional unavailability of the caretaker as evidence that they are unlovable, worthless, and deserving of punishment. They will then mutilate themselves in an effort to punish themselves, with the body once again becoming a concrete representation of self. Interpersonally, they are repeatedly involved in sadomasochistic relationships. Attachments are marked by clingy neediness that alternates with rageful, paranoid withdrawal. Separation is terrifying because it results in profound emptiness, feelings of abandonment, and ego fragmentation. Self-mutilation often appears not only as an effort to punish the unlovable self, but as an effort to avoid depersonalization.

Bulimic borderline patients often attempt to utilize a restricting paranoid defense. The experience of deprivation inherent in starvation is unbearable, however, because it exacerbates the prevailing feelings of emptiness. Self-starvation may also be an effort at self-punishment or an effort to starve out the bad self. Ultimately, though, the bulimic borderline patients are unable to sustain the paranoid stance and must rely on frantic efforts to take in things from the outside (introject) to relieve the chaos and dysphoria.

Transference and Countertransference Themes

In contrast to the controlled, obsessive-like treatment demands of restricting patients, work with bulimic borderlines is much more active and stormy. The patients' use of primitive defenses such as splitting and projective identification often makes the course of treatment chaotic.

There are several aspects of treatment with this subpopulation that warrant comment (see Table 8.3). First, I feel that the primary form of treatment should be the management of the borderline dynamics, rather than focusing more specifically on the eating-related symptoms. This is a subgroup of patients who are usually polysymptomatic and will engage in symptom substitution if their relational needs are not managed thoughtfully. This is not to say that borderline bulimics should be denied the range of symptom management strategies that have been useful for eating-disordered patients in general, including cognitive–behavioral, psychoeducational, and response prevention techniques. However, my experience has been that these techniques are helpful only after a significant therapeutic relationship has evolved. The type of healing therapeutic relationship that is necessary with these patients takes years, perhaps decades, rather than months to develop. Consequently, the therapist needs to be careful with both his or her and the patients' ambitiousness regarding symptom remission in order to protect against the harsh, critical, often masochistic fallout that can occur from the patients' feelings of failure.

The pathway to developing a healing therapeutic relationship with borderline bulimics is simultaneously simple and quite complicated. The primary task, from my perspective, is to demonstrate to the patients over the course of time that the therapist is committed, consistent, durable, and reliable. Since I feel that the primary self-regulatory difficulty among the subgroup stems from neglect, the therapist needs to err in the direction of being actively involved in the management of the patients' lives. The objective in this strategy is quite simply to attempt to restore some faith in the ability of human relatedness to soothe and contain dysphoric affects. The ultimate goal is for the patients to be able to make use of human contact rather than substances to manage their feeling states. Unfortunately, the malevolent aspects of their early relationships

---

TABLE 8.3. Borderline Bulimic (Malevolent Underinvolvement): Transference and Countertransference Themes

Transference themes
   Durability—surviving neediness
   Reliability— containing, soothing dysphoric affect

Countertransference vulnerabilities
   Managing projective indentification
   Pacing treatment
   Managing guilt over unavailability
   Managing intent to abandon

with significant others create resistance and repetitions that often make achieving the simple task complicated.

Achieving some level of attachment is a prerequisite for any effective treatment relationship. Accomplishing attachment is, however, usually not the most demanding part of treatment with these patients. Managing the attachment over time and nudging the patients toward some modicum of separation are far more complicated. Once these patients find an adequate holding environment, they can become quite demanding about getting their needs met. Their neediness, coupled with their propensity to use projective identification, puts unique demands on the therapist.

Recently, much has been written about projective identification (Tansey & Burke, 1985). Essentially, "projective identification" is an interactional process whereby an individual unconsciously communicates his or her experiential state by provoking thoughts and feelings in others that resemble his or her own. For example, a patient who is feeling enraged may behave in a way that provokes similar rageful feelings in the therapist. Interestingly, it can be argued that through this projective defense, borderlines attempt to create an emphathic connection with others. The task for the therapist who is confronted with this defensive style is to receive the projection and avoid being provoked into enacting it. This is achieved by effectively decoding or metabolizing the projection and then attempting to achieve the empathic connection by interpreting the internal state. Managing this defensive style over the course of time is no small chore. These patients' experiences of extremely powerful feelings such as rage, emptiness, and annihilation anxiety often produce internal stress that they need to escape as quickly as possible. This leads to impulsivity, which can be infectious to the therapist and other patients who may have contact in outpatient groups or inpatient milieus.

One transference test or repetition that has to be survived by the therapist is as follows. Since the patients have experienced a sense of masochism in their caretakers' underinvolvement, the tendency is to want to create a hostile/dependent or a more frankly sadomasochistic relationship with a therapist. The unconscious goals of the patients is to provoke the therapist into withholding or ultimately abandoning the patients. Since these patients are adept at projective identification, they will often progressively exhaust an individual therapist and provoke him or her into enacting a hostile abandonment. I have found that there are several safeguards to help protect against this repetition. These include the following:

1. The therapist should be experienced in working with borderline patients or be highly supervised in the treatment of this subgroup.

2. I feel that it is very difficult to manage these patients in a small outpatient practice setting. I have found that having the patients involved in a range of interventions (group therapy, family treatment, nursing, medical management, etc.) is quite useful. This team usually allows the therapist to take breaks when necessary without feeling that a patient is going to fall apart if he or she is not immediately available. Larger hospital settings are usually best equipped to facilitate a broader institutional transference, which is a useful adjunct to the individual transference.

3. Since the therapist needs to make a long-term commitment to a very difficult treatment, he or she should not attempt to treat more than two or three of these patients at any one time.

4. I have two pet phrases I use in training our residents to work with these patients. First, when in doubt about how to respond to a demand from a patient, "Err in the direction of being human." Second, "Don't initiate anything with the patient that you are not prepared to continue for the rest of your life." The first phrase represents my sentiment that therapists have to relate to these patients in a forthright and compassionate manner. The second phrase reflects my hard-won wisdom that both a patient and a therapist need to have limits. The limits, however, will unfortunately be experienced as withholding. Therapists will undoubtedly feel guilty about being unavailable. Under the pressure of guilt and frustration, a therapist may be quite vulnerable to impulsively offering an intervention that may help in the short run. Unfortunately, it is often an intervention that he or she is not prepared to sustain over a long period of time. As the therapist gets overextended, the tendency is to abandon the case because there is no other way out. Consequently, the second phrase is an effort to remind therapists to be thoughtful in the face of demands or wishes about what they are initiating with these patients. It is undoutedly easier not to offer something to a patient than to take it back once it is apparent that it cannot be sustained.

Outcome

Although long-term outcome data are not available for these patients, my colleagues and I have the clinical impression that improvement does occur, but very slowly. Chaos remains a part of their lives. With time and a consistent treatment relationship, however, they develop better psychological tools to manage their chaos. Many of these patients continue the binge–purge behavior, but the degree to which it interferes with their lives markedly decreases, and other self-destructive behaviors such as substance abuse and self-mutilation disappear. Although they are able to work and engage in interpersonal relationships, both aspects of their lives are episodically in turmoil.

EATING-DISORDERED PATIENTS WITH FALSE-SELF/NARCISSISTIC DISORDER

Heinz Kohut (1971) and D. W. Winnicott (1965) both described a group of patients who initially present for treatment with neurotic-like life adjustment problems. As treatment progresses, however, it becomes clear that these patients have significant developmental deficits that result in self-regulatory difficulties. Winnicott coined the term "false-self organization" to describe a particular adaptation these patients make to disruptions in the early mother–child relationship. According to Winnicott, a "true self," or the normal development of a sense of self independent of another, occurs as a result of emphathic encouragement by the primary caretaker of the infant's spontaneous (self-generated) gestures. Essentially, the mother encourages, values, and responds to cues emanating from the infant. If these spontaneous gestures continue to be encouraged, they evolve into self-awareness and self-directed behavior. These individuals feel that thoughts, feelings, and action originate from within themselves and that there is a sense of connectedness to the events in their lives.

False-self organizations emerge when the primary caretaker is unresponsive to or overrides the infant's spontaneous gestures. Unempathic mothering resulting from either over- or underinvolvement disrupts the growth of the capacity for interoceptive awareness, which in turn precludes the possibility of consolidating self-regulatory skills.

The false-self adaptation occurs when an individual creates a persona in an effort to compensate for or hide the interoceptive deficits. This persona is usually reactive and accommodating. These individuals usually complain of feelings of nonexistence, fraudulence, and ineffectiveness. They often have a veneer of adequate integration and achievement, because they superficially have good social skills. Unfortunately, they discount or devalue whatever success they have experienced because they feel they are frauds. Consequently, self-esteem can never be enhanced, because any successful achievement is negated.

We believe that individuals who present with false-self/narcissistic organizations, although they can be quite disturbed, have greater ego resources than borderline patients. They do not generally experience others as having malevolent intent, as borderline patients do, and they are not as vulnerable to the more severe boundary lapses of the borderlines.

Restricting False-Self Patients

The dynamics and clinical presentation of restricting patients who present with false-self organizations closely resemble those of the classic restricting anorexics about whom Bruch (1978) and others (Selvini-Palazzoli, 1974; Sours, 1980; Swift & Stern, 1982) have written for so many years. In fact, one is struck with the similarity between Winnicott's formulations regarding "maternal impingement and subsequent false-self adaptation" and Bruch's conceptualization of how narcissistic, overcontrolling mothers lead to interoceptive awareness difficulties. According to Bruch, the pathway to anorexia nervosa begins during early childhood (the differentiation/practicing subphase), when these patients adapt to maternal intrusiveness by becoming compliant "parent pleasers." This adaptation leaves their sense of self and their capacity for self-regulation intricately tied to or dependent on their primary caretakers. Essentially, they become experts at reading cues from others about how to feel and behave. Given the dependence on external resources, they also learn to accommocate themselves freely to others, because they would be lost if the relationship were disrupted. The self-starvation, with the attendant resistance to external influence, is an attempt at assertive, independent behavior. It is an effort to establish some sense of competency, control, or identity that is independent of and often in conflict with significant others.

In contrast to borderline restrictors, the false-self restrictors do not experience the intrusiveness as intentionally malevolent or sadistic. The attachment, while controlling, is not laced with the aggression of borderline restrictors. Separation fears do not revolve around fears of retaliation or annihilation. Instead, they center more around the side effects of loss, which result in a feeling of depletion in both self and other. These patients often become very concerned about the effects their separation will have on others. They experience themselves as extensions of others without identities, and subsequently as terribly ineffective. There is a substantial discrepancy between how others see them (usually as competent) and how they see themselves. They are less paranoid than borderline restrictors and rely more on obsessive–compulsive and phobic defenses.

Treatment with this group is much less complicated than with borderline patients, primarily because they do not view the world as primarily malevolent; consequently, they are less paranoid and more engageable in treatment.

Transference and Countertransference Issues

The primary transference themes revolve around ambivalence regarding attachments and fears of depletion in both self and other should separation occur (see Table 8.4). A dynamic tension around attachment is constantly enacted with the therapist. Patients feel the need to rely on the significant other psychologically in order to regulate tensions, but when this happens they feel engulfed, without identity, and ineffective. Given this ambivalence around attachment, the therapist's task is to restrain himself or herself from intervening with the patients too quickly or too actively.

The primary theme regarding separation is that both self and other will not be able to function without the continuance of the enmeshment. In contrast to borderline restrictors, false-self restrictors do not fear rageful retaliation from the significant other for separating, but fear instead that both will experience debilitating depression. Given that these patients have generally relied heavily on others to negotiate life, they are often quite phobic about new situations.

Therapists should generally err in the direction of benign underinvolvement with these patients. The tendency to provide solutions quickly and actively when the patients are struggling with difficult decisions should be carefully avoided. Gently encouraging autonomous actions, providing neutral consultation during decision processes, and reassuring patients that their separation will not provoke disorganization in others or the therapist are important guidelines for treating these patients. Split management is also very useful with these patients to minimize the risk of intrusive overinvolvement by the therapist.

Outcome

Effective individual therapy and family treatment usually result in good outcomes with these patients. Although treatment may be relatively long, it generally does not require the very long-term commitment needed with the borderline patients. The group often fully recovers from anorexia nervosa, although throughout their lives they often remain vulnerable to relying too heavily on the thoughts and actions of others.

TABLE 8.4. False-Self/Narcissistic Restrictor (Nonmalevolent Overinvolvement): Transference and Countertransference Themes

Transference themes
  Ambivalence around attachment
  Separation anxiety

Countertransference vulnerabilities
  Overprotectiveness
  Reluctance to separate

Bulimic False-Self/Narcissistic Patients

For bulimic patients, the pathway to the false-self organization appears somewhat different, once again reflecting the nature of the deficits in the holding environment. Like their borderline counterparts, these patients have also experienced some disruption during separation–individuation that has resulted in a disengagement with their primary caretakers. Unlike the borderline bulimics, however, these patients do not experience the caretakers' unavailability as intentional or malevolent. Their ego resources are also more sophisticated, so that regressions, lability of affect, and so forth are less visibly manifested. Instead of the borderline patients' frantic defenses, these patients rely more on avoidance, denial, isolation of affect, and intellectualization. Interacting with them is similar to being with a high-level patient who has schizoid tendencies.

These patients exhibit a unique adaptation to the maternal disengagement. They respond to the unavailability of their caretakers by affecting a pseudomature adaptation. In essence, they have enough ego resources to compensate by prematurely taking responsibility for their own and often others' self-regulation. Unfortunately the caretakers, or the broader families, experience their premature adaptation as a relief, which results in the children's receiving positive reinforcement and even a sense of self-esteem for compliant, nondemanding, hyperresponsible, pseudomature behavior.

The prefix "pseudo-" is appropriate because while such a child has adequate structure to adapt superficially, she does not have adequate structure to accommodate her more infantile needs, such as being comforted and soothed when frightened, angry, anxious, or simply needy. In the absence of the caretaker's ability to respond to these dysphoric and disrupted states, the child splits them off and isolates them. Often a patient interprets these needs as troublesome, a sign of being out of control, and perhaps even destructive. Progressively, the patient feels she is two people: one whom the world sees as competent and in control of things, and another who feels desperately needy (which the patient experiences as being out of control). The discrepancy between the two states results in a self-representation of fraudulence and inadequacy. A self-defeating "Catch-22" emerges in which the patient immediately devalues any compliment or praise for successful achievement, because it indicates that the other person has been fooled or is a fool. Consequently, others who offer compliments are discredited as incompetent judges.

Attachment or the possibility of intimacy for these patients provokes a wish–fear dilemma: Their wish for someone to recognize and respond to their needs is juxtaposed against their fear of allowing someone to see their neediness. Allowing someone to see this side is frightening, because the acknowledgment of having needs might collapse the self-esteem and self-organization that has evolved as a result of the pseudomature behavior. As a result of their fear of discovery, interpersonally these patients maintain what I have called a "distant closeness." In interacting with them, one has the illusion of relating, but over time it becomes apparent that they are desperately protecting a separateness. Unlike interactions with schizoid characters, where one senses predominantly an intrapsychic vacuousness along with impoverished social skills, with these patients one senses that a range of feelings is being actively suppressed.

For these patients, food has often become their safest and most trusted ally. They will allow themselves to behave in the presence of food in a way they would not allow any person to observe or participate in. They also invest food with the ability to regulate different tension states. Some patients will actually anthropomorphize food, attributing to it such humanlike qualities as volition and the ability to relate to them. Allowing a person to help with difficult feelings would mean risking too much exposure. It also involves turning to the world of humans, who have been experienced as much less reliable then food.

Transference and Countertransference Issues

The primary transference themes with these patients revolve around issues of attachment (see Table 8.5). In contrast to the borderline bulimics, who are eager to attach but then unwittingly attempt to spoil the relationship, these patients are very cautious about involvement. Since the central developmental disruption revolves around premature separation in response to nonmalevolent caretaker underinvolvement, the therapeutic task with this subgroup is to create a holding environment that allows the patients to initially experience a regressive dependency that evolves into a mature interdependency.

Resistance from the patients to becoming involved at this level can be formidable. They appear to be continuously struggling with the wish–fear dilemma described above. The opportunity for involvement provokes a range of fears, from superego-based feelings of failure to more primitive concerns regarding being used and using others up.

At the level of more superego-based issues, I have been impressed to what extent these patients become trapped by their definition of success. This can be a very ambitious and competitive group. It appears that many within this group have taken to an extreme, or perhaps perverted, a message that has been part of the women's culture that they have grown up with over the last two decades: the message that as young women they should strive to be independent. Unfortunately, many within this subgroup have taken this to mean that they should not need anyone. Consequently, they believe reliance on others would be experienced by them and others as a sign of personal weakness and failure.

This particular definition of success/independence unfortunately

TABLE 8.5.   False-Self/Narcissistic Bulimic- Nonmalevolent Under-involvement: Transference and Countertransference Themes

---

Transference themes
  Encouraging dependency attachment: Wish–fear dilemma
    Wish—being taught and held
    Fear—discovery and overwhelming others

Countertransference vulnerabilities
    Distraction by competent performance
    Tolerating distant closeness
    Managing idealizing transference

---

reinforces the pseudomature/hypercompetent adaptation they are all too familiar with. At the family level, pseudomature behavior or becoming a lieutenant parent is either subtly or overtly applauded, because the nondemanding, help-providing behavior actually relieves the parents of responsibility and perhaps even glues the system together more fundamentally. Consequently, a patient actually accrues some feelings of self-esteem from appearing to be a competent caretaker. The cost of this adaptation, as mentioned earlier, is that the patient must split off and suppress her own needs. At a broader cultural level, this is also a young woman who appears capable, in control, and without need of others' help. So the culture admires her as well, and hence the false-self adaptation is further reinforced. The primary fear connected to these concerns is that others will discover that she is not as capable as she appears, which would result in the collapse of the self-esteem or identity that has been derived from others' admiration of her apparent self-sufficiency.

At a deeper level, part of the fear of exposure revolves around others' seeing how desperately needy these patients actually feel. At a more primitive level, it has become clear to me that this is a group who have not been adequately held as children. They have not had the opportunity to feel the full range of feelings such as uncertainty, ambivalence, fear, selfishness, sadness, and rage in a holding environment that simultaneously permits expression of these feelings and offers reassurance that the feelings are normal and manageable. In response to their disappointment, disillusionment, and sometimes cynicism about the ability of others to attend to them adequately, they have turned to nonhuman objects (food, drugs, etc.) to attempt to meet their needs. They thus express and gratify a range of longings through the ritualized eating behavior.

If the therapist is successful in getting these patients to focus more of their longings into the treatment relationship, he or she must be prepared for a voracious attachment. A principal fear these patients have is that their needs are overwhelming to others, and that if they do risk attachment they will deplete the other and eventually be disappointed once again. It becomes the task of the therapist to demonstrate to the patients over the course of time that he or she does not need protection from the intensity and range of feelings the patients experience. Furthermore, the feelings are not shameful or necessarily overwhelming events.

The wish side of the wish–fear dilemma is to be taught and held— "taught" in the sense that they wish to attach to someone who appears to know how to navigate life's challenges and who is willing to share this experience. These needs are generally met through the evolution of an idealizing transference. Once again, at a more primitive level, the longing is to be both physically and emotionally held. The wish is to be in the presence of a caretaker who is sufficiently settled within himself or herself to focus on decoding and responding to the patients' needs.

One encounters a number of countertransference vulnerabilities in working with this subgroup of patients. These patients are consummate caretakers. It must be remembered that these patients have spent their lives learning how to adapt themselves to others in order to lessen demands on significant others. Consequently, the therapist needs to be extremely attentive to communicating continuously to the patients that he or she is there to care for them as well as possible. This is not to say that the therapist should not or will not be taken care of at times by the patients. As mentioned earlier, the goal is actually mature interdependency, which implies reciprocal caretaking. Certainly, however, in the early stages of treatment the therapist needs to err in the direction of communicating to these patients, largely through a sense of confident expectation and consistent attentiveness, that he or she is there to care for the patients.

A type of caretaking can occur through the patients' being nondemanding or ostensibly compliant. The therapist has to be quite careful in responding to these patients' making gains in the therapeutic relationship. This is a particularly complicated issue, because our patients do present with specific symptoms (low weight, binge–purge behavior) for which we do have specific strategies that can help improve their symptoms. My colleagues and I have always stressed that the therapist does need to make available to the patients these structured tools. We have also always mentioned that is is imperative that the therapist be attuned to the transference implications of these structured interventions. With this subgroup of patients, the therapist needs simultaneously to respond encouragingly to the patients' doing better with their behavior, while also communicating to the patients the understanding that there is more to their struggle than simply gaining control of their symptoms. If the therapist simply focuses on the patients' competent performance with whatever task they are assigned, the patients will feel that they have fooled yet another person, and then disillusionment in the ability of others to see who they really are will increase. These patients can often take care of therapists by enhancing their egos through quick remission of symptoms. They will then quietly return to the rituals and will become more secretive and often lie about how well they are doing, because that is what they feel others want to hear.

Another transference vulnerability involves the management of the idealizing transference. If the therapist is patient enough, responsive enough, and lucky enough, the patients will develop an idealizing transference. This is a hoped-for development in the course of treatment, because this is a developmental experience that has usually been denied this patient group. It is, however, a powerful experience for both patients and therapist. The most common mistake I have seen therapists make is to interfere prematurely with the idealization. Typically, therapists become uncomfortable with the power and influence they have over the patients as the patients progressively regress into depending upon the therapists. The therapists will often start openly discouraging the patients from viewing them that way, or, more indirectly, they will emotionally withdraw out of fear of the increasing dependency longings. It is imperative for therapists to maintain the perspective that the patients desperately need to feel that someone else has the ability to be in charge, resilient, and powerful. I always reassure therapists that the other shoe will drop soon enough, since we are not omnisicient, omnipresent, or omnipotent. Our human fallibility will naturally assert itself soon enough, and the patients will acknowledge it when they are ready. In the meantime, the experience of being held by someone who is strong, capable, and responsive is quite healing for this patient group.

The other side of vulnerability is that therapists will occasionally become overstimulated with the idealization, lose perspective, and begin to believe that they are indeed omnipotent. This can result in therapists' acting out in particularly arrogant and grandioise ways. They are then surprised, often wounded, when the patients begin the process of de-idealization. This can deteriorate into the therapists' desperately attempting to restore the idealization for their own narcissistic needs, which creates very fertile ground for the patients to become caretakers once again.

Outcome

Assessing outcome with this subgroup can be quite complicated. Given their illusiveness and defensive compliance, they can easily substitute one ritualized behavior for another. I have found, however, that if the therapist remains patient and manages the idealizing transference, the wish to be taught and held eventually overtakes the fear of exposure and disappointment. The process of working through the phases of defending against attachment, developing an idealizing transference, and de-idealization usually takes several years of at least twice-a-week treatment. A lower frequency of sessions usually allows patients to effectively preserve the distant closeness that I have mentioned earlier. The less intense frequency can also allow them to create the illusion of relatedness. When the patients work through the stages of treatment, they will relinquish the bulimic symptoms. Despite the deidealization phase of treatment, the therapist needs to be prepared to gracefully and thoughtfully accept and manage how important he or she will continue to be to the patients over the course of time.

REFERENCES

Blatt, S. (1974). Levels of object representation in anaclitic and introjective depression. *Psychoanalytic Study of the Child, 29,* 40–56.

Bruch, H. (1962). Perceptual and conceptual disturbances in anorexia nervosa. *Psychosomatic Medicine, 24,* 187–194.

Bruch, H. (1973). *Eating disorders: Obesity, anorexia nervosa, and the person within.* New York: Basic Books.

Burch, H. (1978). *The golden cage: The enigma of anorexia nervosa.* Cambridge, MA: Harvard University Press.

Crisp, A. H. (1980). *Anorexia nervosa: Let me be.* London: Academic Press.

Garfinkel, P. E., & Garner, D. M. (1982). *Anorexia nervosa: A multidimensional perspective.* New York: Brunner/Mazel.

Johnson, C., & Connors, M. (1987). *The etiology and treatment of bulimia nervosa: A biopsychosocial perspective.* New York: Basic Books.

Johnson, C., Tobin, D., & Enright, A. (1989). Prevalence and clinical characteristics of borderline patients in an eating-disordered population. *Journal of Clinical Psychiatry, 50,* 9–14.

Johnson, C., Tobin, D., & Dennis, A. B. (1990). Difference in treatment outcome between borderline and nonborderline bulimics at one year follow-up. *International Journal of Eating Disorders, 9,* 1–11.

Kohut, H. (1971). *The analysis of the self.* New York: International Universities Press.

Mahler, M., Pine, F., & Bergman, A. (1975). *The psychological birth of the human infant.* New York: Basic Books.

Selvini-Palazzoli, M. (1974). *Self-starvation.* London: Chaucer.

Sours, J. A. (1980). *Starving to death in a sea of objects.* New York: Jason Aronson.

Swift, W. J., & Stern, S. (1982). The psychodynamic diversity of anorexia nervosa. *International Journal of Eating Disorders, 2,* 17–35.

Tansey, M. H., & Burke, W. F. (1985). Projective identification and the empathic process. *Contemporary Psychoanalysis, 21,* 42–69.

Winnicott, D. W. (1965). *The maturational process and the facilitating environment: Studies in the theory of emotional development.* New York: International Universities Press.

·. 9 ·.

Gender Identity Issues in Male Bulimia Nervosa

JOHN A. SCHNEIDER
Stanford University School of Medicine
and School of Medicine, University of California—San Francisco

Over the past decade, bulimia nervosa and anorexia nervosa have become established as largely gender-specific disorders. Most researchers agree that (1) eating disorder symptoms are most prevalent in women (90% to 95% of bulimia occurs in women); and (2) although the incidence of men with eating disorders is rare, a disproportionate number are homosexual. Herzog, Norman, Gordon, and Pepose (1984) found that many of their male bulimic subjects had a homosexual orientation. Yager, Kurtzman, Landsverk, and Wiesmeier (1988) found more problems with eating issues in a homosexual sample than in a heterosexual control group. Likewise, my colleagues and I (Schneider, O'Leary, & Jenkins, 1990) observed a relationship among gender, sexual object choice, and eating attitudes, finding homosexual men to have more problems with eating-related issues than heterosexual men. In other studies, up to 50% of males with eating disorders also experienced homosexual conflict (Crisp, 1967, 1970, 1983; Crisp & Toms, 1972; Dally, 1969). These findings raise the question of the relationship between eating disorders and homosexuality in males.

In this chapter I explore this apparent link from the standpoint of psychoanalytic theory, first by presenting theoretical material and examining certain aspects of early male development, and then by reviewing several cases. I attempt to show that the finding that so many men with eating disorders are homosexual relates to the psychodynamic underpinnings of the eating disorder. I will argue that these psychodynamics involve gender identity issues that are similar for both homosexual and heterosexual males with bulimia. The differences are ones of degree. I will argue further that the normal development of core gender identity[1] in boys protects against the development of eating disorders in males, leading to its lower incidence.

Many authors have concluded that something peculiar to the mother-daughter relationship contributes to the development of eating disorders in women (Sugarman & Kurash, 1982; Sperling, 1983; Ritvo, 1988). I propose that similar psychodynamics underlie bulimia in males as well, and that eating disorders for both males and females, heterosexuals and homosexuals, are symptoms related to mother–infant relationships. From a psychoanalytic perspective, bulimia nervosa, like choice of sexual object, is a manifestation of unconscious motivations, developmental issues, and object relations. To focus on a bulimic's choice of sexual object is to miss the underlying drama behind the superficial binge–purge message.

A CLINICAL THEORY OF EATING DISORDERS IN MALES

Incidence and Severity

In this chapter I focus on male bulimia nervosa rather than anorexia nervosa, although there are analogous identity problems in patients with both symptom profiles. Evidence suggests that on virtually all clinical and psychometric dimensions that have been measured, and in the organization of early psychodynamics, the different types of eating disorders are similar.[2]

The large majority of persons with eating disorders are female.[3] The question arises as to why there is a difference in incidence between men and women, and how men and women differ in their manifestations of eating disorders. At a fundamental level, there is still argument about whether male anorexia nervosa even exists as a diagnostic category. Although the first reported clinical case (Morton, 1694) was male, and the first report of treatment (Gull, 1874) referred to the disorder in males, current opinions vary.

Authors who believe the disorder occurs in males agree that it involves greater pathology than for females, is more difficult to treat (Crisp & Toms, 1972; Dally, 1969; Taipale, Larkio-Miettinen, Valanne, Moren, & Aukee, 1972), and involves psychosexual conflict (Crisp, 1967; Crisp & Toms, 1972; Deneux, Soms, Le Clech, & Messak, 1977). Sperling (1978) and Selvini (1965) believe that the complex psychopathology of the anorexia nervosa syndrome does not occur in males. In contrast, Mintz (1983) holds that the psychic conflicts for eating-disordered males and females are the same.

Eating-disordered males and females have been found to be similar on psychometric measures (Schneider & Agras, 1987). Males, however, manifest bulimia more severely, and their ego states are more fragmented (Sours, 1980). Clinical experience has been that those men who enter treatment are more disturbed and more difficult to treat than females (Gwirstman, Roy-Byrne, Lerner, & Yager, 1984; Herzog et al., 1984; Yager et al., 1988; Mitchell & Goff, 1984; Pope, Hudson, & Jonas, 1986; Russell, 1979). Eating disorders begin earlier in males than in females, in many cases before puberty (Bruch, 1971). In contrast to females, males with eating disorders were often obese and passive in childhood during the latency stage.

A possibility exists that the clinical population underrepresents the incidence and overstates the severity of male bulimia. Many male bulimics have said that they considered bulimia an adolescent girls' disorder and were embarrassed to seek help or let anyone know about their disorder until it became severe. This implies that those male bulimics with less severe dysfunction do not seek help.

Also, the predominant diagnostic criteria for male and female bulimics may differ. The usual diagnostic criteria are that the patient has difficulty controlling recurrent binge episodes; that the patient engages in purging by self-induced vomiting, use of laxatives or diuretics, strict dieting, or vigorous exercise to prevent weight gain; and that the patient evidences an overconcern with body weight and shape (American Psychiatric Association, 1987). Because cultural pressure to be thin, a factor for many eating-disordered women, may be less severe for men, clinicians, parents, and physicians may fail to identify as bulimic the many male bulimics who are overweight. In addition, bulimic men may not be readily diagnosed who, although not vomiting or restricting their food intake, exercise excessively to stay thin. It is more socially acceptable for a man to exercise to excess than for a woman; "he's just a jock." Bulimic men and women who overexercise appear to have different motivations for doing so. Men who work out excessively appear to do so in an attempt to look more masculine, in contrast to anoretic females who exercise excessively to avoid looking feminine.

These differences in diagnostic criteria may contribute to the lower incidence of identified eating disorders in males than in females. There is, however, the possibility that the lower incidence also relates to the psychodynamics underlying the disorder.

A PSYCHOANALYTIC PERSPECTIVE: UNCONSCIOUS CONFLICT IN EATING DISORDERS

What I describe in this section is how food and eating-related behaviors are used to enact unresolved conflicts from early caretaking relationships.

From a psychoanalytic perspective, symptomatic behavior is an effort to integrate the present with the unconscious past. The eating disorder symptom is an indirect response to a developmental problem, a final common pathway for psychological conflict. Hence, even though the symptomatic behavior may disappear (temporarily or permanently), the underlying problematic dynamics remain until they are addressed. The diagnosis must be made on the basis of the person's dynamics, internal object relations, and early development, all of which predate the symptom and, in some cases, remain after the symptom has ceased.

Broadly speaking, the eating disorder symptom is an expression of unconscious conflict. Within the context of treatment, it may become a desperate personal communication about the patient's fears, wishes, and fantasies presented in condensed form. It communicates what the patient has experienced but cannot express. In it is contained a fragmentary version of the patient's developmental and historical drama—a narrative in its most condensed form, containing the wish and also the fear. As in all addiction symptoms, its repetitive quality both results in and evidences a sense of hopelessness and despair.

Gender Identity Issues in Males:
A Developmental Perspective

To understand how gender identity relates to bulimic symptoms in males, it is illustrative to compare male and female gender identity development. For female bulimics, the crucial developmental issues related to the eating disorder appear to be issues of autonomy and development of an identity separate from the mother. While identifying with the mother as a female, a girl must distance herself from the mother to attain autonomy and individuality. Physical separation from the mother challenges the girl's confidence that she can survive on her own. Gender sameness helps sustain the illusion that the girl and her mother are really one, even if they are sometimes separated. Whenever boundaries between self and other are blurred in this way, individuals may rely excessively on external or transitional objects for comforting, rather than developing their own capacity for self-soothing. Because of gender sameness, this blurring is more likely in females than in males (Chodorow, 1989).

Many authors including Johnson and Connors (1987) and Sugarman, Quinlan, and Devenis (1981) suggest that the developmental issues for females with bulimia nervosa are rooted in conflicts around autonomy and separateness. Many female bulimic patients ingest food to create a sense of relatedness and then purge food to define a sense of existence in which they are separate and autonomous persons. They purge food to maintain an illusion of control over the mother—either to reject the mother as a defense against being rejected; or to express anger at the mother; or to incorporate the mother, which is then followed by feeling unworthy, and by expelling her. Disruptions in the primary feeding situation make it difficult for a girl to attain a sense of having her own clear needs and the confidence that they will be met. The primary issues in female bulimia, therefore, appear to be autonomy and authenticity. What I would like to suggest in this paper is that although this may be true for females with bulimia, this is not the case in male bulimia.

In contrast to female bulimics, male bulimics appear to have difficulty, not with autonomy, but with gender identity. I distinguish between core gender identity and gender role identity.[4] For infant boys, as for girls, the primary object of identification is the mother (Stoller, 1968). One task of a male during the preoedipal period is to transcend this primary identification with his mother and go on to a secondary identification with his father. For boys to attain a healthy sense of maleness, they must experience the normal psychological development that allows them to disidentify with the mother and counter-identify with the father (Greenson, 1968).

As a boy transfers his primary identification from mother to father, conflict results from the fact the boy has powerful loving feelings for the mother and, at the same time, desires to separate and gain autonomy from her (Mahler, Pine, & Bergmann, 1975). Closeness to the mother is valued, but excessive closeness threatens the boy's independence and gender differentiation. The father's presence during this period is important to the son's achieving a male gender identity.

We know little about the role of the father during the first 2 to 3 years of an infant's life, but we do know that a father plays an important role simply by his presence in helping the boy to move toward identification with him and disidentification with the mother. Stoller (1979) noted that the "father serves as a shield to protect the child against impulses the mother might have to prolong the mother–infant symbiosis"[5] (p. 839), and in so doing promotes gender identity.

Ogden (1989) reminds us that a boy's masculine gender identity is first introduced to him by his mother under the influence of her identification with her father, her view of her husband, and the subsequent reflection of those views on her infant son. Blos (1985) states that "gender identity formation is fostered in the boy child by his father's presence, as well as the mother's love of and affirmation of her husband's maleness. Both countervail the son's modeling of his core gender identity on the mother" (p. 16). Stoller (1975), too, believes that femininity in boys is not solely due to mother–son symbiosis; rather, "both mother and father must do their part."

Early psychoanalytic thinking gave little importance to the positive role of the father in preoedipal development, viewing the father as an intruder who disturbs the blissful dyad between mother and child. According to this early point of view (Abelin, 1971a), the father evokes fear and aggression usually associated with strangers (Diatkine, 1966; Freud, 1923/1961; Lebovici & Diatkine, 1954; Lewin, 1955; Mack-Brunswick, 1940).

More recent psychoanalytic formulations give the father a more positive and strategic role. The father has been found to be important to a variety of early ego functions, including delay of gratification (Mischel, 1958), perception (Barclay & Cusumano, 1967), and intelligence (Glazer & Moynihan, 1963). Mahler and Gosliner (1955) were first to point out that by about 18 months of age, the infant perceives the father as an important object. This concurs with findings by Piaget (1937, 1954, 1945, 1951) that in the first 18 months the child is able to form simultaneous images of itself and its objects.

Schaffer and Emerson (1964), in one of the earliest attempts to understand the father–infant relationship, found that following their first specific attachment, most infants began to select other specific objects as well. By between 7–18 months of age, nearly all the infants in their study were attached to both father and mother.

The French analysts in particular have ascribed a crucial role to the father image. Abelin (1975) introduced the term "early triangulation" to describe the infant's observation that there is a nonmother, or a different parent. This early triangulation leads to the attainment of stable mental representations comprising father, mother, and self. The father is viewed as a mediating third between mother and baby, whose role in the infant's development fosters the capacity to identify and name differences. He represents the capacity to symbolize. He presents the dialectic idea that says to the baby, "You lose something and you gain something." The father is not just spoiling the fun between mother and infant; he (or his substitute) represents the capacity to symbolize history and champions the development of knowledge as contained in symbols.

Early triangulation is a key element lacking in the early development of psychotic patients (Lang, 1958; Leclaire, 1958). Abelin (1971b) found that psychotic children were unable to comprehend or cathect the father (or "other" parent); they were also unable to form symbolic images of themselves and their objects.

This capacity for symbolization has direct relevance to eating disorders. Segal (1957) suggests that psychotic and schizoid patients in particular have not developed the capacity to communicate using symbols. These patients are unable to use symbols to overcome loss, and instead attempt to replace the original object in a concrete way. Likewise, in patients with eating disorders (although they are not necessarily psychotic or schizoid), the eating disorder symptom may stand for a dysfunctional relationship and serve as a substitute for it.

McDougall (1985) referred to a group of patients, described as neither psychotic nor neurotic, who externalize intolerable inner experiences with psychosomatic symptoms as a means of self-protection and self-survival:

> These patients attempt to make an external object behave like a symbolic one and thus repair a psychic gap. The object or situation will then be sought addictively. Basically all addictions, from alcoholism and bulimia to the taking of sleeping pills, are attempts to make an external object do duty for a missing symbolic dimension. (McDougall, 1974, p. 455)

Disturbances in the father–infant relationship may promote problems with core gender identity directly by fostering a mother–son symbiosis, or indirectly by limiting the infant's development of the capacity to symbolize. As the boy grows, the father also assumes an ever-increasing role in gender role identity, demonstrating to his son what males do that is masculine. If the infant son is overinvolved with the mother and maintains symbiosis with her, he may lack gender differentiation and never truly disidentify with the mother.

A boy may remain overinvolved with his mother because his father is absent or dead, or in some cases because his father is abusive. When the boy has an abusive father, disidentification may be short-circuited; or the boy may identify in a very pathological and terrifying way with his father's violence.

The mother is usually connected to the child in intimate, positive physical ways. An abusive father is connected to the child in intimate, negative physical ways. Violent abuse makes it difficult for the child to maintain boundaries. It results in bodily intrusion, as opposed to bodily integrity, and adds to the boy's confusion around his self-representation and gender identity.

Where abuse is an issue, the boy is in constant reaction to the environment, which he perceives to be incessantly impinging on him. Identifications are more primitive, less mature, and less differentiated, all of which make it difficult for him to feel grown up or masculine.

Development of Eating Disorders

For both males and females, the development of eating disorders is related to difficulty in the mother–infant relationship. Between 12 and 18 months of age, the emotional availability of the caregiver can foster the infant's self-awareness and affective continuity, which are then available for self-regulation (Emde, 1980). I maintain that when caregiving is not optimal, self-regulation is affected in a regressive way and becomes tied to food and the feeding connection with the mother.

If a mother is very poorly attuned[6] to the overall needs of the child, and is therefore disturbingly overstimulating and intrusive or understimulating, the child defensively shuts off critical modes of relating to the mother and concentrates his or her attention on the feeding activity. This defensive shutoff can interfere with object relations development, and the act of taking in food can become a singular and primary mode of relating. When the child would normally begin self-feeding, and learning self-soothing and self-regulation, the relationship to the mother is maintained solely by the act of being fed—a defensive concentration of the relationship in the feeding act. What the child misses in this situation is the intimate face-to-face contact in the human feeding situation and associated interactions.[7]

Stern's work with infants advances Erickson's (1959) idea that the child incorporates visually as well as orally during feeding. For Stern (1985), visual and auditory "incorporation" are equal in importance to the primary physiological need to eat as a way of taking in the world. It seems that a defensive shutoff of these activities not only may interfere with the normal mother–child relationship, but also with the child's eyes opening to look beyond the mother in the process of disidentifying with her.

According to Winnicott (1956), in normal development, the feeding situation is almost an invisible event, a naturally unobtrusive situation requiring little thought. Therefore it seems to me that when the "fit" is not right between caretaker and infant, the baby may have to bring into bold relief what ought to have been invisible, and hold on to it addictively as a concretized connection to the mother. In health development, as with synchronous mother–infant activity, the mother's need to feed and the infant's need to be fed should be inseparable.

If food becomes isolated from all other functions of object relatedness, such as the mother's holding, looking at, and touching the infant, food becomes burdened with playing an unnatural role. Typically, food becomes a symbol for the early maternal relationship. But in cases of primitive eating disorders, the eating act becomes overburdened, having to carry more than its own symbolic weight as it continues to be a concrete means of maintaining the maternal relationship through incorporation. The feeding situation becomes an attempt to make up for all the early interpersonal connections that ultimately were not there.

Food becomes overemphasized and overtaxed. The feeding takes on an endless desperation as it attempts to carry meaning that it cannot. Ultimately there is the feeling that something is missing in the feeding experience, and the situation becomes a forced effort to substitute quantity for quality. The repetitive nature of bulimia stems from this unsatisfactory eating experience because the need to be satisfied is not hunger (Ogden, 1988). As with most addictive problems, because of the ambivalent nature of early infant–parent relationships, the addiction in eating disorders is to the process of taking in and losing the food, rather than holding on to it (Krystal, 1988).

GENDER IDENTITY DIFFICULTY RELATED TO EATING DISORDERS

I have set out to explain why clinical populations of male bulimics are often homosexual. I have stated by thesis that the crucial issue is gender identity, which is related to developmental issues in infancy and to the male child's disturbed relationship with his father. I have also described how eating disorders (specifically, bulimia) may stem from developmental issues related to the infant's feeding and care by the mother. What is still to be explained is the connection between male bulimia and gender identity confusion.

Gender identity difficulty and eating disorders both represent pathological adaptations to very early development. Between 12 and 18 months of age, both male and female infants are involved in gender identity issues, and simultaneously with the processes of weaning and self-feeding. Given that functions can be disturbed most readily while in the process of development, the simultaneous development of gender identity and self-feeding creates the likelihood that disturbance in one may catalyze disturbance in the other.

From this perspective it is no surprise, and is in fact predictable, that few men with typical male gender identity become bulimic. Male infants who disidentify with the mother and identify with the father are less likely to confuse boundaries between self and mother, and are more able to develop the capacity for internal self-soothing and self-regulation. For girls, the object of identification remains the mother. Hence a disturbance in developing autonomy and authenticity does not interfere with female gender identity development.

Normally, at about 18 months—as the child develops symbolic functioning and the father becomes a representation for "thirdness"—the child moves on from the mother; both the mother and the feeding relationship, once so primary, become less prominent. If we consider hunger metaphorically as the wish to be soothed and fed, when the child is hungry the desire for mother shifts to the foreground once more, and the thinking, defining function associated with the father becomes less important. The child returns to primary-process functioning (Schafer, 1968), where the wish and the deed are one.

Correspondingly, when the infant is not possessed by the need to be fed and soothed, he or she is in a more curious state of mind—a "love affair with the world," as Greenacre (1957) has called it. He or she is discovering things like roll toys, and playing with the difference between presence and absence, between big and small, appearing and disappearing. At these times, the father becomes the content of the child's world, and the mother becomes context. In this formulation, secondary-process thinking becomes foreground and the maternal holding environment becomes an invisible background.

Of special interest to our task of linking eating disorders and gender identity problems are the findings by Neubauer (1960) and Yarrow (1964) that oral fixation is characteristic of fatherless subjects. Blos (1985) has referred to the son's "search for the loving and loved father" (p. 33); Herzog (1980) has called "father hunger" the affective state associated with this yearning in male infants; and Abelin (1977) described it as "father thirst." Blos (1985) aptly points out that both these authors use terms within the oral modality to refer to the male infant's feeling toward an absent father.

Mothers of bulimic men, for various reasons, often are overly involved with their sons and less involved with their husbands. Lichtenstein (1961) suggests that the mother's involvement with the child's gender identity is initiated through the infant feeding situation. This idea is supported by Murphy (1962) and Korner (1973), who found that mothers vary their feeding responses depending on the gender of the child. A female infant is basically similar to the mother; hence the mother identifies narcissistically with the female infant. She feels that she is the girl, and may therefore be open to feelings of sensuality during nursing and more reluctant to project her violent and hostile affects on the female child. In the case of a boy, however, the mother may be afraid to experience nursing as a highly sensual experience, and may be more likely to project her negative affect onto "that which is not female." This may contribute to boys having more severe manifestations of eating disorders and greater difficulty with gender identity.

In instances where the child also has a troubled relationship with an abusive father, the same mode of coping used earlier with the mother is applied to the father. With a physically intrusive father, the male infant may succeed in disidentifying with the mother sufficiently to develop core gender identity, but then may encounter a new problem with gender role identity. As an adaptive effort, the abused boy may prolong his clinging to the mother, or, paradoxically, may cling to the father to secure the masculinity that he has not obtained through normal means of identification.

The child's progression in the battle to move away from his mother and take in his father is stymied when there is child abuse. The reprieve from symbiosis with his mother is short-lived and followed by a battle to extrude the dangerous masculinity of his abusive father. The dilemma is how to get the father's masculinity in while getting rid of dangerous characteristics of the father. If the image of the father is frightening, attempts may be made to get rid of the fear symbolically through purging. We might posit that bulimia is an abused male's attempt to orally take in something of the father, then the subsequent need to purge it quickly because his life is in danger if he holds it in.

I suggest that in most cases of male eating disorders, there is some form of gender identity concern—sometimes more dramatic, as in cases of core gender identity problems, and sometimes less obvious, as in cases of gender role identity problems. Most bulimic men have disturbances in core gender identity and/or severe difficulty in masculine identification. We have not found bulimia in highly masculine homosexual males.

In some cases where there is a homosexual object choice, there may be an unconscious urge to "get a penis" that is felt to be missing, and therefore bulimic homosexuals may need to "fill themselves" with another's penis. Eating may be used to replace the search for the penis when a phallic sense has not been established.[8] "The unconscious fantasy of some homosexuals is that through the sexual act they will regain their alienated masculinity through symbolic introjection" (Krystal, 1988, p. 181). Many bulimic homosexuals will say, "I never come, not until I get home and masturbate by myself." Yet this is after they have spent the whole day performing fellatio on many men in succession. The sexual repetitiveness serves a desperate, narcissistic need: These men feel taken care of and defined by the sex act, which compensates for the sense of not having a valid penis. One penis is not sufficient, and thus there is the enactment of orgiastic liaisons that call for sexual acts wherein many men are used to try to fill the void left by the absent, poorly internalized father. But the sex act does not create a stable identification. Instead, it is a transitory "incorporative" episode in which something felt to be lacking internally is found in the outside world and temporarily taken in.

My argument is that the issue related to bulimia is not homosexual object choice, but rather core gender identity. Bulimic men display a range of sexual object choice, from heterosexual to homosexual, and a range of disturbances in core gender identity, from moderate to profound confusion. In some cases where core gender identity is not apparently disturbed because the father was not absent, other difficulties appear with regard to masculine identification related to abusive, frightening, or disgusting fathers.

In bulimic men, there is an effort to repair the disturbance in masculinity through incorporative and expulsive means. Bulimic men behave as though they believe that relatedness is established by eating, and separateness by purging. I argued above that such a belief results from a disturbance in the mother–child relationship at about 18 months of age. One aspect of this disturbance is the child's fear of losing his separate identity through merger with mother. Normal male gender identity, when it is reasonably secure, protects the boy against this fear. In contrast, when core gender identity is uncertain, the boy is at risk for this merger and may actively seek a concrete sense of masculinity to use as a bulwark against fears of merger and nonexistence.

CLINICAL ILLUSTRATIONS

The following cases are from my clinical practice. I have selected them to exemplify the varying levels of gender identity problems, from confusion to transsexualism, and from heterosexual object choice to homosexuality. The cases are presented in order, from the least to the most severe apparent manifestations of gender identity disturbance. In each case, I describe my patient, present some of his developmental history, and then summarize my understanding of his problems related to gender identity and bulimia.

Case 1: Mr. R.—Resignation from Life

Mr. R., age 34, was brought to the initial consultation by his mother, with whom he had been living since becoming too weak to care for himself. At the time he was 5 feet 6 inches tall, weighed 75 pounds, and was consumed by his overcoat, which appeared vastly oversized. His physical features were skeletal, just protruding bone structures, so that it was difficult for me to determine his gender or age by looking at him.

R. was suffering from general weakness affecting his mobility. At our first meeting, he let me know that the stairs to the office were too steep, and that it took too much energy for him to talk to me. He was skeptical about psychiatry, and he warned me that he would be stubborn and fearful of becoming involved with me. He was concerned because his weight had been continually dropping over the past few years. "I've pretty much wasted away, and I'm interested in what you have to offer." His condition had developed gradually over time from taking less and less food and occasional purging; the purging had recently stopped.

He was frightened of women, and his mother had been the only woman in his life. He said he had come only because his mother wanted him to be helped, but that all feelings were absent in him. All he felt was hunger and a desire for "something missing."

R. believed that he wasn't feeding himself because he was afraid of getting fat. He was also skeptical about being fed, and didn't trust anyone to feed him. He was especially concerned with the quality of the food he ate, and felt the food on which he grew up "did not keep his mind active."

R. told me that he had previously been an avid tennis player and had worked in a tennis shop for many years. His father, who died when R. was 12, had also been a weekend tennis enthusiast. Tennis had been R.'s life as well, and those were his best father–son memories.

R.'s father had been in the Navy, and hence from the time he was born, R. had moved frequently. His duties in the military had taken R.'s father away from the family for long periods of time while R. was growing up.

R. had lived with his mother until he was 20, moving out when she asked him to begin taking responsibility for some of the house-work. When he moved out, he said, there was a "dark cloud over my head."

When I asked about his father, R. immediately wanted to get out of his chair and get his mother from the waiting room to comfort him, but couldn't get up because he was too weak. I commented on his reaction, and he began to whimper and shake uncontrollably, whining that he wanted his mother.

R.'s mother came in at the end of his initial interview. She immediately began speaking of the losses of the men in *her* life: her husband, her recent boyfriend, and her father.

My understanding of R. was that he had identified with his mother's view of his dead father, giving him the appearance of a male core gender identity. However, there was an illusory quality to this identification. In a sense, R. did not see himself as a person at all. When R. was a young child, his father was absent.

R.'s mother, a very disturbed woman, confused boundaries between herself and her son, and between herself and her husband. Thus R. came to regard both his father and himself as *aspects* of his mother. With his father's death, an already shaky belief in his own existence was substantially weakened. He identified with limited aspects of his father's image, such as an interest in tennis. He reconnected with his mother, and ambivalently allowed himself to identify with her, and to be fed by her. Becoming more and more terrified as the boundaries between the two got thinner, he rejected her feeding, but was unsuccessful in taking over feeding himself. The loss of his father removed an important prop to his sense of existing as a person separate from his mother. The case thus illustrates the failure of an illusory gender identity to protect R. from the development of an extremely severe eating disorder, and points to the fact that a useful gender identity must be rooted in a sense of personal existence.

Case 2: Mr. S.—Adopting Mother's Role

Mr. S., 26 years old, came to treatment because he "felt stuck." He said, "I don't know where to turn—I'm unhappy with the environment I'm living in." He was tall and thin with a deep voice and a crew cut, looking much younger than his age.

S. had a bingeing ritual that involved eating a large breakfast and then going to several secret trails he had laid out, where he vomited and jogged. He repeated the same routine in the afternoon. He felt physically weak and drained after these episodes. Although he felt the routine was degrading, he said that he repeated it out of boredom and feelings of anger and deprivation.

S. said that he had been concerned about his body most of his life—at age 9 about having a fat stomach, by age 12 about his weight. As a child he hated school, and missed up to 14 weeks every year for various somatic complaints for which no cause was found. He looked forward to the time alone with his mother and the special meals she would make for him. (He was the youngest of several children.)

S.'s mother had a secret drinking problem that she denied, although S. felt that her personality was changed by it and that it caused problems with his father. She used heavy denial as well as alcohol to deal with her depression. His father never confronted his mother about the problem; it was S. who eventually confronted her, and he stayed out of school to try to cure her. He was desperate to stay at home, perhaps out of fear that she would die without him.

In high school he worked on bodybuilding. His first 2 years at a local college went well enough, except for his concerns about his appearance. He lost weight the summer before transferring to an out-of-state college, and felt that people were noticing his skinniness, which made him feel he was more in control than other people. While he was away at college, his eating got out of control; he went from 160 to 200 pounds in 5 weeks. He did not make a college athletic team, although he was quite skilled. He had trouble concentrating on his schoolwork, and after 9 weeks, he dropped out and returned home.

At the time of our first meeting he was also concerned about his severe difficulty in getting along with his father. He had been living with his father, cooking for him, and sporadically working odd jobs. S.'s father worked 7 days a week, 12 hours a day, at a food-related job that S. felt was menial. S. despised his father's ordinary life and "establishment" values, and said, "I never wanted to be like that and follow what the norm was." Deeply saddened by his mother's death, he was equally hopeful that he would have more time with his father. His anticipation turned to disappointment, perhaps because instead of becoming a son, he took the place of his mother in the household.

My understanding of S.'s issues is that he suffered from a severe separation anxiety that had continued throughout his life. S. identified with his mother as a means of remembering her (rather than mourning her loss), and wished to hang onto her as an undifferentiated object. His bulimia was a way of continuing his mother's alcoholism. She had also had an eating disorder when she was a child. As do many patients with separation problems, S. felt he was being left behind when all the other (and older) children left. Like some youngest children, he tried to cure his depressed mother by not separating from her.

S.'s father was a weak and psychologically absent individual who worked all the time and did not take his place to help his son "triangulate" out of his early relationship with his mother. Like his mother, who attempted to humiliate her husband for not being a "good provider," S. also had a distaste for what he perceived as his father's ineffectual masculine role, and became confused about his own gender role identity. He seemed to have assumed his mother's role in the family: staying home, cooking for his father, and being jealous of his father, just as the mother had been jealous and insisted on including herself in their father–son activities.

S.'s bulimia appeared to be his attempt to define himself as masculine in an external, physical way to counter his internal doubts and fears of merger with mother. His bingeing and vomiting were a defensive means to justify staying with the mother, a futile effort to repair his disturbance in masculinity. Exercising was a way to compensate for his passivity, and he said it made him feel "strong, masculine, and in control." His identity appeared to be in limbo: He was unable either to move away from his mother or to move toward his father and a masculine role. His life was on hold. Socially he never had boyfriends or girlfriends and was unable to enter the academic or work world, staying at home instead to keep the image of his mother alive by assuming her role.

Case 3: Mr. B.—Shutting Off Violence

Mr. B., aged 43, came to treatment paralyzed by his lack of control over his compulsive overeating, depressed about his rounded body shape, and terrified of his rageful impulses. B. was a large, strong, but soft-spoken man, who said, "I'm big enough to hurt someone. To me food is a drug. I would inject it to stop that feeling." He added, "I learned early in life that I could calm myself down with food. Food is like an injection." Hunger was the only feeling he believed he could control, and he controlled his rageful impulses with food as well. When he arrived home at night, he immediately started eating to settle himself down.

At age 10, he began using food as an escape from what he perceived as humiliations at home and school. He felt that his acne, his clothing, and his blushing were constant problems and caused him pain that only food could stop. He began daily bingeing and vomiting, and from then on was plagued by a lifelong weight problem.

Beginning before age 5 and continuing for over 10 years, B. was physically abused by both of his parents on a daily basis. They used belts and clothes hangers to beat him, sometimes so badly that he could not go to school. His persistent memory of childhood was believing that he was going to die, and he felt tortured when he was spanked "until he would stop crying."

B.'s father had been overseas in the military service for the first 3 years of B.'s life. When he returned home, (he was a traveling salesman, away for weeks at a time), B. said, "He never did anything for me—just beat me up and threatened me." As a child, his fantasy was of being a kid 1 inch tall so that he could get into the woodwork and live there, where he could see his parents but they couldn't see him.

He recalled that when he was 11, a man fondled his penis, but his mother didn't believe his story. He also told about an incident in the gym when some boys wanted to have oral sex with him. He acknowledged that he felt comfortable about his sexual feelings toward men and would not mind being a submissive partner in a homosexual act.

He left home at an early age and married his girlfriend after impregnating her. They had two children. She had casual sex with anyone who was around, and on one occasion when he confronted her about her extramarital sex, she fled to a distant state with their two children. That breakup led to a period of extreme self-starvation, and B. eventually gave up his successful professional training to follow his wife. The marriage ended when his wife decided she was gay.

B. spent the next 7 years alone, during which time his weight stabilized and he stopped bingeing and vomiting. Eventually he remarried and had one more child. Immediately after the remarriage, his bingeing and vomiting returned. He became enraged with his wife during arguments, and felt he was being treated unfairly. When he reached the point of explosion, he threw everything he could at the windows. "I got so pissed off I could have taken a two-by-four and broke it over my leg." Afterward, he felt sorry, apologized, and cleaned up the mess.

B. feared his wife would find out something bad about him, and would criticize or humiliate him. He acknowledged that he feared his wife, and that he did not feel "manly" when talking about this weakness.

My understanding of B. was that he suffered from boundary disturbances resulting from severe physical abuse. His father was absent during the first years of his life, and when B. attempted to identify with him in a move away from his mother, he was met by physical assault. Unable to return to the mother because she was also abusive, he turned to compulsive overeating to soothe himself. Self-induced vomiting was less prominent for B. He doubted his worth as a man, felt easily humiliated by women, and feared losing control of his rage. On the other hand, he used his rage to clearly define his separateness from women and his identification with his father.

B. had become irrevocably male. His problems existed in the content and meaning of masculinity. He ate in order to avoid hurting someone, and in order to undo or reverse his identification with an aggressive and hostile father. He ate to get away from his father and take in his mother. He felt "weak" when he talked about "feelings," and equated manliness with his father's violence. He felt that he could not demonstrate his masculinity because it would be aggressive. He kept himself round and feminine to avoid becoming violent like his father, but in the process he felt threatened that he was losing his masculinity. He ate when angry, trying not to be like his father; at the same time, he worried that he was becoming feminine—a constant doing and undoing.

Case 4: Mr. L.—Vomiting to Refuse What Mother Gave Him

Mr. L. was a 44-year-old, extremely obese, bulimic, married man. He came to treatment because of his wife's urgings and because of his own health concerns.

Until L. was 4, his father was away in the military. "When he first came home, I ran away from him. I didn't know who he was." His paternal grandmother lived with L. and his mother. "Whenever I would cry, although I had just eaten, my grandmother would come and give me another bottle to calm me down, so I was never really allowed to be anxious. . . . When I had a full diaper my mother and grandmother shoved a bottle in my mouth instead of changing me." When he was 18 months of age, L. and his mother moved to a military post in a remote part of the country to live with his father. However, L. developed a near-fatal case of dysentery, so his mother used this as an opportunity to move back home immediately.

When he was 5 years old, his mother told him he had had a stillborn twin brother. As his mother put it, "You probably ate him, since you seem to be eating everything else." During his childhood, his overweight mother force-fed him and then took him with her to her diet doctors to get shots and pills for "their" weight problem. These visits were made against the wishes of his father and kept secret from him. L. heard his father tell his mother, "Don't you dare take him to a diet doctor," and wondered if his father, who was thin, didn't want L. to be like him. The mother gave L. food and other things and would warn him not to tell his father. L.'s compulsive eating became a major issue when, at age 11, his mother developed cancer and was hospitalized in a distant city, causing a 11-week separation between mother and son.

L.'s father's absence and his primary involvement with his mother took their toll on L.'s relationship with other boys. When L. was 6, he went to summer camp and recalls, "I got real scared. Kids were playing this game called baseball. I didn't know if I was left- or right-handed, or how to use a bat and ball. When my father visited me, I asked him to buy me a glove. So he bought me a glove, but it was a left-hand glove instead of a right-hand glove."

L. was a very bright student, but cut so many classes he didn't graduate from high school, and was eventually kicked out and sent to a military school.

L.'s remembrances of his time with his father were few— conversations in which his father talked to him constantly about time, money, and success, and disciplining accompanied with physical punishment. "I got so scared that I couldn't be successful." Otherwise, L.'s father was emotionally absent from L. He was away for months at a time on vacations with his brother, and L. felt relieved during these times because "I didn't have to put up with him and I could get my mother to do anything I wanted." In fact, she did his homework for him when he was upset. L. said, "Maybe if I'm powerful I'll become a real prick. My father was a prick. My mother was a nice guy, but more covert about how she did things."

My understanding of L. was that he had problems in the early identification process. His father was effectively absent during his growing up. He always felt inadequate as a man and identified with his mother through food. His mother identified him with his lost twin, and he was the object used to reduce her own guilt about the infant's death. She had attempted to resolve her feelings by developing a symbiotic relationship with her son—one that involved overfeeding and overindulgence. He, in turn, handled his anxiety by eating, becoming fat, and identifying with her.

At the time of his prepubescence, L.'s mother began to encourage him to diet and lose weight; he experienced this as a plea to become more masculine. During this time, he starved himself and/or vomited to gain control, or perhaps to reject his mother's projection onto him, while he developed a masculine exterior, ridding himself of the fat associated with his feminine identity. He fought a losing battle to maintain his masculinity, and eventually gave in to his mother and became extremely obese.

Case 5: Mr. K.—Creating an Internal World with Food

Mr. K., 42 years old, came to treatment with desperate fears of losing his girlfriend. In the first consultations, he whined, complained, and demanded that I do something to save their relationship.

He was thin, and had a history of multiple hospitalizations for bingeing and vomiting—a pattern occurring from 30 to 40 times a day, beginning when he was 15. His first hospitalization was at age 20, precipitated by his moving away from home to college. He slept only 2 hours a night, had a chronic potassium deficiency, and had only 25% of his teeth. He did not want to let a meal stay inside him for fear that he would feel something.

Because of his chronic condition, he stated that he could sense his potassium level by his physical and affective experience. He found this terrifying, because it signified that he was losing himself, becoming nonexistent. He indicated that when he ate, he felt the heat rise from the warmth of his blood flowing through his veins; the rest of the time he kept himself ice cold. He acted as if his internal world did not exist unless it was fed.

K.'s father owned a business in another state; he was rarely home when K. was a young child, and when he did return, he was too busy to spend time with his son. K. remembered the few times they did spend together as "great." When K. was 7, his father died of colon cancer. He had been ill for 2 years before he died, slowly withering away. Once K. sneaked in to see his sick father, despite his mother's warning against entering his room, and was appalled by his father's emaciated appearance. When his father died, he felt it was "absolutely the cruelest thing in the world; people are down to nothing before they die.

His mother played a powerful role in keeping K. from his father, and he perceived her as one of the few people who didn't love his father. After his father's death, he idealized him and went on a "crusade" to discover his father by visiting relatives in other states. K. developed fantasies to supplement the father he felt he didn't have. His mother continued to be his "greatest friend in the world," but he felt betrayed by her when she told him that the father he held so dear was in fact a "worthless, no-good liar." K. felt doubly betrayed when she remarried, after telling K. that there would be just the 2 of them. His mother allowed her second husband to abuse K.

In high school, K. became attached to a skating teacher who was "real anorexic—thin." K. wanted to skate and look exactly like him. Because he was out of the house and consumed with his new interests for long hours, his mother stopped holding meals for him. Formerly, from childhood on, meals had been an important part of their relationship. For

2 years he ate only cereal (Wheaties—the "Breakfast of Champions") in order to lose weight. Skating became his life. "I feel I've lost my identity, but out on the ice, I'm in touch with the real me."

My understanding of K. was that his food rituals served both to bring his mother to life in a merged fashion, and to create a father. His purposely maintained low potassium level (resulting in dizziness and loss of drive) and his constant bingeing and purging kept him helpless. These patterns were primitive attempts to deal with his desperate feelings; in order to function, he needed to fill himself up with his mother's love.

His incessant binge–purge rituals were attempts to create a masculine identity, which he felt had been withheld from him. The natural father he remembered was so pathetic, so cachectic, that it was terrifying to think of becoming like him. When he felt thin, he was frightened of becoming this appalling, no-good, skinny, dying father. When he filled himself up, he was frightened of merging with his mother.

K. felt hopelessly lost in his binge-purge ritual. "What I do to myself is really cruel. If I were to look at my body as another person, I'd be really angry at myself. It's not a person, it's a thing—a living thing. A life form like that is really cruel."

Case 6: Mr. D.—Attempting to Capture Masculinity

Mr. D., a 26-year-old homosexual male, came to treatment because he was depressed and unable to control his bingeing and vomiting. His weight was normal at the time but had fluctuated greatly for the past 16 years; at one point it was up to 305 pounds. He was ambivalent about his sexual identity and was concerned that, being gay, he would never father or raise children.

Even when he didn't feel hungry, he felt driven to eat. He attributed this to fears of getting close to somebody, because he didn't feel good about his physical appearance. With food he felt in control, but in other aspects of his life he felt "less than a whole person."

Early in treatment, D. binged and vomited before coming to a session and described the experience as being like orgasm—a sexual release. At other times, following a binge, his associations led to thoughts of passively pleasing others. "I'm pleased to give to someone else sexually. I'm in control. I usually don't come, not allowing good things to come in or stay in. I prefer to go home and masturbate by myself." He collected a large number of partners—lots of experiences where he had control and did not reach orgasm. For him, real sexuality took place away from people. This was similar to his bingeing and vomiting, and had to do with "control of sad and happy feelings. Food [was] an alternative to feelings."

His mother was a diabetic housewife, and his father an overweight, "humongous" truck driver who was on the road much of the time. D. felt that he could not please his parents, and that he was unlovable.

The case of D. contained problems in all three of Tyson's (1982) types of gender development. Although he talked a great deal about his homosexuality and seemed somewhat conflicted about it, his core gender identity confusion was the more significant issue. There was a close connection between D.'s sexuality and his bulimic symptoms—trying to be in control of whom he took in sexually, in an effort to acquire the masculinity he desired. Sex and his eating disorder were enactments of the same dilemma. On the surface, people did with him whatever they wished, but on a less apparent level he turned this into a triumph; he was controlling them.

His dramatic attempts to control the "in" and "out" suggested that his symptoms were connected to early maternal nurturing concerns. He feared that if he did not exert control he would be enslaved by his controlling mother, who displaced her rage toward her husband onto her son. The father failed to protect D. from the mother's physical assaults, such as the time she gave him a bloody lip, or the time she broke a stick over his back. The father showed his own unpredictable anger toward D. and had unrealistic expectations for his son, who already was doing excellent academic work. The father's disappointment began when D. lacked interest in competitive sports as a young boy, and instead chose passive interests. D. belived he must have been unlovable and deserved to be beaten because he was male. The father was not available to balance the picture, and D. felt he had to disavow his maleness, though did not disavow masculinity entirely. Instead, he treated it as something to be attained in a secret way. D.'s multiple sexual partners, like his use of drugs and alcohol, represented futile attempts to capture the maleness from an absent father. His compulsive multiple sexual encounters were efforts to take into himself a strong phallic and masculine presence. His being full of the semen of several men "proved" that he contained masculinity within his body. At the same time, his passive sexual role and his somatic illness were part of a feminine identification with his diabetic mother.

Case 7: Mr. M.—How Will I Know Who I Am?

On the telephone, M.'s voice was hard to place, and I thought "her" name, "Candy Valentine," was a caricature of femininity, not unlike the names some bulimic women have been given. M. told me he wanted help to control his weight and out-of-control bingeing. He had stopped his self-induced vomiting earlier. He was late for his first appointment, and my office door was open when he arrived. I was suprised to see an extremely large man lumbering down the hallway with a cane. He wore dark glasses, a large print dress, and a wig that looked more like a floor mop, with Adidas running shoes and calf-height, Army-issue green socks.

M. told me he had been a very chubby baby, and was overweight between the ages of 5 and 10. From 10 to 13, he was thinner and more active on the playground. He was a good long jumper until the eighth grade. He had wrenched his knee 3 times by age 14, marking the end of his involvement in athletics and the beginning of a period of drinking.

As a child, he preferred to play with girls and dolls. By age 13, he had his first boyfriend. He eventually learned that if he acted tough and played at sports, the kids would not make fun of him for being effeminate. However, as an adolescent, a boy made a pass at him, and he was labelled a "queer."

Throughout this period, M.'s father was abusive, although he said he had not realized this until recently. He was still angry toward his father, indicating this his father, "for all his years of work, is a failure," whereas his mother "had a long job history." M. said, "I was *not* an unwanted child before I got here. He [the father] tried to get her to go for an abortion, but she wouldn't go." His father was away in the military service for the first 3 to 5 years of his life, and although his mother stayed married to her husband, she constantly told M. how terrible his father was and how much she hated him.

His father told him that he was stupid, dumb, and ugly. M. remembered the nicest parts of his life involved going to ice cream parlors with his mother when he was 2 to 3, and also when he was 5 to 6 with his grandfather. Throughout this period he was overweight, and got teased for that. He was physically abused by his father until he was age 14, when he hit him back.

It was after M. lost weight and stopped self-inducing vomiting that he investigated undergoing a gender change. He spent a lot of time in bars with transsexuals, although previously he had not cross-dressed; he was afraid that once he started, he would not want to stop. He went to gay bars, experimented sexually, started drinking, and a year later became convinced that he was not happy being a man. He indicated that this was not a sexual problem, but an identity problem. His mother was very upset when he started becoming a transsexual, telling him, "You killed my son"; his father rejected him completely.

This is a typical pattern for secondary transsexualism, as described by Stoller (1979). M. knew he was anatomically male, and took exhibitionist pleasure in knowing he had a penis, but was "tricking the unsuspecting" by his clothing and mannerisms. However, the clothing and mannerisms were not truly feminine. He dressed in a feminine way to act out his hostile caricature of femininity—perhaps implying that he was, or could become, "a better biological woman than women," having both feminine characteristics and a secret penis.

M. had not been feminine for his whole life. His mother, a very strong woman, married a somewhat passive and distant male who was absent from the family during M.'s infancy and early childhood. The mother was depressed, and maintained a symbiotic relationship with her son. She seemed to have used him as a reason to envy males. In M.'s case, there was some attachment to maleness and masculinity earlier in life. The bulimic symptoms were a compromise solution to his gender identity concerns. When the self-indiced vomiting disappeared, it was replaced by a new and more radical gender identity compromise.

COMMON FEATURES IN THE CASES

Review of these seven cases highlights several important similarities. In general, these men are more disturbed than a random selection of female bulimics. Every one of the seven cases involved a father who was physically absent early in the development of the infant. If the father eventually was physically present, he was nevertheless passive and uninvolved. This in itself does not result in bulimia or gender identity symptomatology, so obviously other factors played a role as well. Of equal importance is the mother's attitude regarding the father in each case, and the potential role of that attitude in shaping the son's view of the father as an appropriate or desirable object of identification. In five of the seven cases, the mother was very critical of the father—sometimes demeaning and hostile. In five of the seven cases fathers, or fathers and mothers, were physically abusive.

Hence problems in developing male gender identity were common to all of these cases—both for those who were homosexual and for those who were heterosexual. There was apparent disturbance in the mother–son relationship, as well as in the father–son relationship. I propose that the reason so many bulimic men are homosexual is because of their disturbance in gender identity. The disturbances in gender identity may have begun during the same period as disturbances in the mother–infant feeding relationship.

Most of the cases described here involved clear evidence of an atypical role of food in the mother–son interaction as far back as early childhood. These seven cases were specifically selected to demonstrate the existence of gender identity disturbances underlying male eating disorders. They are, however, typical of the male bulimics I have treated.

By examining a psychoanalytic developmental theory with case illustrations, I have attempted to explain the apparent link between eating disorders and homosexuality. These theoretical formulations have helped me in my understanding and treatment of male bulimics. My hope is that they will now serve to stimulate new dialogue regarding the role of gender identity issues in male bulimia nervosa.

Acknowledgments. I am grateful to Dr. Charles Fisher and Dr. Thomas Ogden for their helpful comments during the writing of this chapter.

NOTES

1. I use a broad concept of gender identity outlined by Tyson (1982), and influenced by Stoller (1968), which is composed of the following: (1) core gender identity—one's early primitive unconscious and conscious sense of belonging to one sex and not the other (Stoller, 1968, 1976, 1978); (2) gender role identity— one's overt behavior in relationship to other people, including the child seeking "self-like objects" as role models with whom to identify; and (3) sexual partner orientation (Green, 1975), referring to the preferred sex of the love object. Using this comprehensive model allows us to account for the various levels of early relationship difficulties that culminate in confused gender identity.

2. Fairburn and Garner (1986) have this to say on anorexia versus bulimia:

First, approximately 50% of patients with anorexia nervosa manifest the symptoms of bulimia (Casper, Eckert, Halmi, Goldberg, & Davis, 1980; Garfinkel, Moldofsky, & Garner, 1980). Second, it is well-established that many patients move between anorexia nervosa and bulimia nervosa at different points in time (Vandereycken & Meermann, 1984). Third, patients with these disorders have numerous features in common: in particular, "bulimic" anorexia nervosa patients, bulimia nervosa patients with a history of anorexia nervosa, and bulimia nervosa patients with no such history, have been found to be similar on virtually all the clinical and psychometric dimensions that have been measured (Fairburn & Cooper, 1984a, 1984b; Garner, Garfinkel, & O'Shaunessy, 1983, 1985; Garner, Olmsted, & Garfinkel, 1985). While these subgroups of bulimic patients can be distinguished from "restricting" (i.e., non-bulimic) anorexia nervosa patients on some measures of their psychopathology, on most measures all these patients display equivalent levels of disturbance (Garner et al., 1983; Garner, Olmsted, & Garfinkel, 1985). Since anorexia nervosa and bulimia nervosa are so similar, the validity of the diagnostic distinction may be questioned. (pp. 411–412)

3. Of bulimics, from 0.4% (Halmi, Falk, & Schwartz, 1981) to 8.9% (Pyle et al., 1983) are male.

4. Refer to Note 1.

5. Mahler et al. (1975) discuss symbiosis as follows:

The term *symbiosis* . . . is a metaphor. Unlike the biological concept of symbiosis, it does not describe what actually happens in a mutually beneficial relationship between two *separate* individuals of different species. It describes that state of undifferentiation, of fusion with mother, in which the "I" is not yet differentiated from the "not-I" and in which inside and outside are only gradually coming to be sensed as different. (p. 44)

6. Stern (1985) defines attunement as "the predominant way to commune with or indicate sharing of internal states" (p. 142).

7. Erikson (1959) introduced the idea that organ modes—for instance, incorporation for the mouth—generalize to body organs other than the original zone of charged biological activity, leading to the eventual formation of an individual's characteristic behavior and psychic patterns of functioning:

In addition to the overwhelming need for food, a baby is, or soon becomes, receptive in many other respects. As he is willing and able to suck on appropriate objects and to swallow whatever appropriate fluids they emit, he is soon as willing and able to "take in" with his eyes whatever enters his visual field. (1959, p. 57)

This in turn leads to:

Firm establishment of enduring patterns for the balance of basic trust over basic mistrust. . . . [The] amount of trust derived from earliest infantile experience does not seem to depend on absolute quantities of food or demonstrations of love, but rather on the quality of the maternal relationship. (1959, p. 63)

Hence, when the feeling act lacks normal maternal relating, the infant learns a lack of trust.

8. I make the distinction, as does McDougall (1985), between "penis" and "phallus."

If the phallus (as distinct from the penis, in that it is the symbol of unity and fertility that belongs to and joins both sexes) acquires its true significance, the child, boy or girl, finds his or her place and gender identity guaranteed. If instead the penis becomes detached from its symbolic significance, many dramatic scenes arise for both sexes. (1985, p. 44)

REFERENCES

Abelin, E. (1971a). The role of the father in the separation–individuation process. In J. B. McDevitt & C. F. Settlage (Eds.), *Separation individuation: Essays in honor of Margaret S. Mahler*. New York: International Universities Press

Abelin, E. (1971b). *Esquisse d'une theorie etiopathogenique unifée des schizophrenies*. Bern, Switzerland: Huber.

Abelin, E. (1975). Some further observations and comments on the earliest role of the father. *International Journal of Psycho-analysis, 56*, 293–302.

Abelin, E. (1977). The role of the father in core gender identity and in psychosexual differentiation [Abstracted by R. Prall]. *Journal of the American Psychoanalytic Association, 26*, 143–161.

American Psychiatric Association (1987). *Diagnostic and statistical manual of mental disorders* (3rd ed., rev.). Washington, DC: Author.

Barclay, A. G., & Cusumano, D. R. (1967). Testing masculinity in boys without fathers. *Transactions, 5*(2), 33–35.

Blos, P. (1985). *Son and father*. New York: Free Press.

Bruch, H. (1971). Anorexia nervosa in the male. *Psychosomatic Medicine, 33,* 31–47.

Casper, R. C., Eckert, E. D., Halmi, K. A., Goldberg, S. C., & Davis, J. M. (1980). Bulimia: Its incidence and clinical importance in patients with anorexia nervosa. *Archives of General Psychiatry, 37,* 1030–1035.

Chodorow, N. J. (1989). *Feminism and psychoanalytic theory*. New Haven: Yale University Press.

Crisp, A. H. (1967). Anorexia nervosa. *Hospital Medicine, 1,* 713–718.

Crisp, A. H. (1970). Anorexia nervosa, 'feeding disorder', 'nervous malnutrition', or 'weight phobia'? *World Review of Nutrition and Dietetics, 12,* 452–504.

Crisp, A. H. (1983). Some aspects of the psychopathology of anorexia nervosa. In P. L. Carby, P. E. Garfinkel, D. M. Garner, & D. C. Coscina (Eds.), *Anorexia nervosa: Recent developments in research* (pp. 15–28). New York: Alan R. Liss.

Crisp, A. H., & Toms, D. A. (1972). Primary anorexia nervosa, a weight phobia in the male: Report on 13 cases. *British Medical Journal, i,* 334–338.

Dally, P. (1969). *Anorexia nervosa*. London: Heinemann.

Deneux, A., Soms, P., Le Clech, H. G., & Messak, E. (1977). Three cases of mental anorexia in men. *Revue de neuropsychiatrie de l'Ouest, 14,* 83–95.

Diatkine, R. (1966). Aggressivité et fantasmes d'agression. *Revue Français Psychanalytique, 30,* 15–92.

Emde, R. N. (1980). Toward a psychoanalytic theory of affect. In S. I. Greenspan & G. H. Pollock (Eds.), *The course of life: Psychoanalytic contributions toward understanding personality development: Vol. 1. Infancy and early childhood* (pp. 63–112). Rockville, MD: National Institute of Mental Health.

Erikson, E. H. (1959). *Growth and crises of the healthy personality. [Psychological Issues,* Monograph No. 1, Vol. *1*(1), 50–100]. New York: International Universities Press.

Fairburn, C. G., & Cooper, P. J. (1984a). Binge-eating, self-induced vomiting, and laxative abuse: A community study. *Psychological Medicine, 14,* 401–410.

Fairburn, C. G., & Cooper, P. J. (1984b). The clinical features of bulimia nervosa. *British Journal of Psychiatry, 144,* 238–246.

Fairburn, C. G., & Garner, D. M. (1986). The diagnosis of bulimia nervosa. *International Journal of Eating Disorders, 5*(3), 403–419.

Freud, S. (1961). The ego and the id. In J. Strachey (Ed. and Trans.), *The standard edition of the complete psychological works of Sigmund Freud* (Vol. 19, pp. 3–66). London: Hogarth Press. (Original work published 1923)

Garfinkel, P. E., Moldofsky, H., & Garner, D. M. (1980). The heterogeneity of anorexia nervosa: Bulimia as a distinct subgroup. *Archives of General Psychiatry, 37,* 1036–1040.

Garner, D. M., Garfinkel, P. E., & O'Shaughnessy, M. (1983). Clinical and psychometric comparison between bulimia in anorexia nervosa and bulimia in normal-weight women. In *Understanding anorexia nervosa and bulimia:*

Report of the fourth Ross Conference on Medical Research. Columbus, OH: Ross Laboratories.

Garner, D. M., Garfinkel, P. E., & O'Shaughnessy, M. (1985). Validity of the distinction between bulimia with and without anorexia nervosa. *American Journal of Psychiatry, 142,* 581–587.

Garner, D. M., Olmsted, M. P., & Garfinkel, P. E. (1985). Similarities among bulimic groups selected by weight and weight history. *Journal of Psychiatric Research, 19,* 129–134.

Glazer, N., & Moynihan, D. P. (1963). *Beyond the melting pot.* Cambridge, MA: MIT Press.

Green, R. (1975). Sexual identity research stereotypes. *Archives of Sexual Behavior, 4,* 337–352.

Greenacre, P. (1957). The childhood of the artist. *Psychoanalytic Study of the Child, 12,* 47–72.

Greenson, R. (1968). Disidentifying from mother: Its special importance for the boy. *International Journal of Psycho-Analysis, 49,* 370–374.

Gull, W. W. (1874). Anorexia nervosa (apepsia histerica, anorexia hysterica). *Transactions of the Clinical Society* (London) 7, 22–28.

Gwirstman, H., Roy-Byrne, P., Lerner, L., & Yager, J. (1984). Bulimia in men: Report of three cases with neuro-endocrine findings. *Journal of Clinical Psychiatry, 45(2),* 78–81.

Halmi, K., Falk, J., & Schwartz, E. (1981). Binge-eating and vomiting: A survey of a college population. *Psychological Medicine, 11,* 697–706.

Herzog, D., Norman, D., Gordon, C., & Pepose, M. (1984). Sexual conflict and eating disorders in 27 males. *American Journal of Psychiatry, 141,* 989–990.

Herzog, J. M. (1980). Sleep disturbance and father hunger in 18–20 month-old boys. *Psychoanalytic Study of the Child, 35,* 219–233.

Johnson, C., & Connors, M. E. (1987). *The etiology and treatment of bulimia nervosa, a biopsychosocial perspective.* New York: Basic Books.

Korner, A. F. (1973). Sex differences in newborns, with special reference to differences in the organization of oral behavior. *Journal of Child Psychology, 14,* 19–29.

Krystal, H. (1988). *Integration and self healing.* Hillsdale, NJ: Analytic Press.

Lang, J. L. (1958). L'abord psychoanalytique des psychoses chez l'enfant. *Psychoanalysis, 4,* 51–82.

Lebovici, S., & Diatkine, R. (1954). Étude des fantasmes chez l'enfant. *Revue Francais Psychoanalytique, 18,* 108–155.

Leclaire, S. (1958). À propose de l'épisode psychotique que presente "l'homeaux loups." *Psychoanalysis, 4,* 83–110.

Lewin, B. D. (1955). Dream psychology and the analytic situation. *Psychoanalytic Quarterly, 24,* 169–253.

Lichtenstein, H. (1961). Identity and sexuality: A study of their interrelationship in man. *Journal of the American Psychoanalytic Association, 9,* 197–260.

Mack-Brunswick, R. (1940). The preoedipal phase of the libido development. In R. Fleiss (Ed.), *The psychoanalytic reader* (pp. 231–253). New York: International Universities Press.

Mahler, M. S., & Gosliner, B. J. (1955). On symbiotic child psychosis: Genetic, dynamic and restitutive aspects. *Psychoanalytic study of the child, 10*, 195–212. New York: International University Press.

Mahler, M. S., Pine F., & Bergman, A. (1975). *The psychological birth of the human infant*. New York: Basic Books.

McDougall, J. (1974). The psychosoma and the psychoanalytic process. *International Review of Psychoanalysis, 1*, 437–459.

McDougall, J. (1985). *Theatres of the mind: Illusion and truth on the psychoanalytic stage*. New York: Basic Books.

Mischel, W. (1958). Preference for delayed reinforcement: An experimental study of a cultural observation. *Journal of Abnormal Social Psychology, 56*, 57–61.

Mintz, I. L. (1983). Anorexia nervosa and bulimia in males. In C. P. Wilson, C. C. Hogan, & I. L. Mintz (Eds.), *Fear of being fat: The treatment of anorexia nervosa and bulimia* (pp. 263–303). New York: Jason Aronson.

Mitchell, J., & Goff, G. (1984). Bulimia in male patients. *Psychosomatics, 25*, 909–913.

Morton, R. (1694). *Phthisiologia: Or a treatise of consumptions*. London: S. Smith & B. Walford.

Murphy, L. (1962). *The widening world of childhood*. New York: Basic Books.

Neubauer, P. B. (1960). The one-parent child and his oedipal development. *Psychoanalytic Study of the Child, 15*, 286–309.

Ogden, T. (1988). Misrecognitions and the fear of not knowing. *The Psychoanalytic Quarterly, 57*, 643–666.

Ogden, T. (1989). *The primitive edge of experience*. Northvale, NJ: Jason Aronson.

Piaget, J. (1951). *Play, dreams, and imitation in childhood*. New York: Norton. (Original work published 1945)

Piaget, J. (1954). *The construction of reality in the child*. New York: Basic Books. (Original work published 1937)

Pope, H., Hudson, J., & Jonas, J. (1986). Bulimia in men: A series of fifteen cases. *Journal of Nervous and Mental Disease, 174*, 117–119.

Pyle, R. L., Mitchell, J. E., Eckert, E. D., Halvorson, P. A., Newman, P. A., & Goff, G. M. (1983). The incidence of bulimia in freshman college students. *International Journal of Eating Disorders, 2*, 75–85.

Ritvo, S. (1985). Mothers, daughters, and eating disorders. In H. P. Blum, Y. Kramer, A. K. Richards, & A. D. Richards (Eds.), *Fantasy, myth and reality*. New York: International Universities Press.

Russell, G. (1979). Bulimia nervosa: An ominous variant of anorexia nervosa. *Psychological Medicine, 9*, 429–448.

Schafer, R. (1968). *Aspects of internalization*. New York: International Universities Press.

Schaffer, H. R., & Emerson, P. E. (1964). The development of social attachments in infancy. *Social Research and Child Development*, Monograph 94(29), 3. Lafayette, IN: Child Development Publications.

Schneider, J. A., & Agras, W. S. (1987). Bulimia in males: A matched comparison with females. *International Journal of Eating Disorders, 6(2)*, 235–242.

Schneider, J. A., O'Leary, A., & Jenkins, S. (1990). *Sexual object choice, gender and eating disorders*. Unpublished manuscript.

Segal, H. (1957). Notes on symbol formation. *International Journal of Psycho-Analysis, 38,* 391–397.

Selvini, M. P. (1965). Interpretation of mental anorexia. In J. E. Meyer & H. Feldman (Eds.), *Anorexia nervosa: Symposium am 24/25 April 1965 in Gottingen.* Stuttgart: Thieme.

Sours, J. (1980). *Starving to death in a sea of objects.* New York: Jason Aronson.

Sperling, M. (1978). Anorexia nervosa (Part 4). In D. Sperling (Ed.), *Psychosomatic disorders in childhood* (pp. 129–173). New York: Jason Aronson.

Sperling, M. (1983). A reevaluation of classification, concepts, and treatment. In C. P. Wilson, C. Hogan, & I. L. Mintz (Eds.), *Fear of being fat: The treatment of anorexia nervosa and bulimia* (pp. 51–82). New York: Jason Aronson.

Stern, D. N. (1985). *The interpersonal world of the infant.* New York: Basic Books.

Stoller, R. (1968). *Sex and gender* (Vol. 1). New York: Science House.

Stoller, R. (1975). *Sex and gender* (Vol. 2). New York: Jason Aronson.

Stoller, R. (1976). Primary femininity. *Journal of the Amreican Psychoanalytic Association, 24*(5), 59–78.

Stoller, R. (1978). Boyhood gender aberrations: Treatment issues. *Journal of the Amreican Psychoanalytic Association, 26,* 541–558.

Stoller, R. (1979). Fathers of transsexual children. *Journal of the American Psychoanalytic Association, 27*(4), 837–866.

Sugarman, A., & Kurash, C. (1982). The body as a transitional object in bulimia. *International Journal of Eating Disorders, 1*(4), 57–66.

Sugarman, A., Quinlan, D., & Devenis, L. (1981). Anorexia nervosa as a defense against anaelitic depression. *International Journal of Eating Disorders, 1*(1), 44–61.

Taipale, V., Larkio-Miettinen, K., Valanne, E. H., Moren, R., & Aukee, M. (1972). Anorexia nervosa in boys. *Psychosomatics, 13,* 236–240.

Tyson, P. (1982). A developmental line of gender identity, gender role, and choice of love object. *Journal of the American Psychoanalytic Association, 30,* 61–86.

Vandereycken, W., & Meermann, R. (1984). *Anorexia nervosa: A clinician's guide to treatment.* West Berlin: de Gruyter.

Winnicott, D. W. (1956). Primary maternal preoccupation. In *Collected papers: Through paediatrics to psycho-analysis* (pp. 300–305). New York: Basic Books.

Yager, J., Kurtzman, F., Landsverk, J., & Wiesmeier, E. (1988). Behaviors and attitudes related to eating disorders in homosexual male college students. *American Journal of Psychiatry, 145*(4), 495–497.

Yarrow, L. J. (1964). Separation from parents during early childhood. In M. H. Hoffman & I. W. Hoffman (Eds.), *Review of child development research,* (Vol. 1, pp. 89–136). New York: Russell Sage Foundation.

III

FEMINIST PSYCHODYNAMIC PERSPECTIVES

·. *10*·.

New Maps of Development, New Models of Therapy: The Psychology of Women and the Treatment of Eating Disorders

CATHERINE STEINER-ADAIR
*The Project on the Psychology of Women and
the Development of Girls, Harvard University
and Middlesex Family Associates, Lexington, Massachusetts*

The high incidence of women with eating disorders challenges psychotherapists to integrate the current research on the psychology of women and apply it to traditional models of therapy in order to be able to work more effectively with eating-disordered women.

The extreme reality of eating-disordered patients, who corporally express their emotional starvation and their difficulty in digesting interpersonal nourishment, forces us as therapists to examine how we are present in the therapy relationships, what we feel for and with our patients, and what constitutes a therapeutic and healing relationship. Through their tortured preoccupation with food and their bodies, women with eating disorders highlight difficult questions for us as therapists about what is a genuinely nourishing relationship in the context of therapy. As we help these patients make their terrifying journey from their objectified bodies to connecting to their selves, they reveal to us the necessity of expanding our practice in individual psychotherapy from the traditional model—which highlights distance and objectivity—to a model that integrates connection.

REVISING THE SEPARATION–INDIVIDUATION MODEL

The traditional separation–individuation approach to eating disorders, as written about by Bruch (1978), Crisp (1980), Selvini-Palazzoli (1974), and others, casts eating disorders as a failure to separate and attain autonomy. An eating disorder is seen as an attempt to forestall maturation to adulthood, which is equated with independence. However, this approach requires critical analysis, given that current research by Gilligan (1977, 1982, 1986a,) Chodorow and colleagues (Chodorow, Lamphere, & Rosaldo, 1974; Chodorow, 1978), and Marcia (1980) on female adolescent development challenges the validity and applicability of this development map for females (see also Steiner-Adair, 1986, 1989). Furthermore, longitudinal research on girls' psychological development suggests that a model for therapy based on separation–individuation theory risks recreating the development crisis experienced by girls at adolescence.

Gilligan (1982) has demonstrated that the language of separation and individuation can have different meaning for males and females. When Gilligan asked males and females to speak about dependence and its opposite, she got different answers. From males, Gilligan (1982) heard the same perspective as that embedded in separation–individuation theory—that is, one of dependence as something negatively connoted, to be outgrown for independence, which was its positively connoted opposite.

In contrast to males, the females interviewed by Gilligan talked about dependence as something of value; they defined it as active engagement and, at its highest form, life-sustaining. When asked what the opposite of dependence was, many females said "Isolation," and thus associated independence with the danger of detachment. From this perspective, a different map of development appears—one of movement from an unequal dependent relationship (where a child is more dependent on a parent) to one of mature dependency (where the parent and the now adult child depend on each other in different ways) or interdependence, involving mutual engagement and reciprocity (Gilligan, 1982).

Within this different developmental map, there appears a different developmental crisis—what Gilligan (1990) calls a "crisis of connection." Longitudinal cross-sectional research on girls of diverse ages, races, and social classes, begun in 1981 at the Project on the Psychology of Women and the Development of Girls (Harvard University), identifies a developmental experience of confusion for girls: They must adapt to psychologically debilitating sex-role stereotypes and androcentric cultural norms, which unrealistically idealize nurturing and actually promote individualism and autonomy.

In "Narratives of Relationship: The Development of a Care Voice in Girls Ages 7 to 16," Brown (1989) observes in her nonclinical longitudinal sample "a pattern of losses and vulnerabilities girls face as they grow up . . . a nonlinear pattern which simply does not fit very well with hierarchical stage descriptions of development" (p. 131). Furthermore, Brown hears "a loss of voice and a struggle over issues of authorization that can result in confusion, uncertainty and self-doubt" (p. 131), for some girls in eating disorders (Steiner-Adair, 1986). Briefly summarized, Brown's (1989) mapping of female development looks like this: Up until age 11, girls are relatively confident and articulate about the full range of emotions experienced in relationships; girls at 11 see relationships in a realistic, nonidealized way, as places where people grow in the experience of joy and pain. Around 11 or 12, as girls look outward to the culture, they begin to perceive cultural norms in which relationships are idealized, and women are valued and accepted to the extent that they are on the one hand "all-caring" and on the other hand "independent." By age 15 or 16, girls are far less confident and articulate; they withdraw and go "underground" (Gilligan, 1988), and become silent as they struggle to hold on to their nonidealized knowledge about relationships in a culture that expects and rewards the "nice" and "perfect" girl.

In the process of maturation, we hear in girls' language a progression that is also a regression—from, the 10-year-old's resounding "I think . . . ," to the 12-year-old's doubting "I don't know," to the 16-year-old's loss of her own voice. The self-involving personal pronoun "I" is replaced with the externalization of authority or "you know"; in this pattern of development, adaption signifies the loss of self-authorization.

Thus, for girls, the developmental "crisis of connection" centers around the loss of the relational world as they come of age in a culture that does not value or acknowledge relationships as the girls have known them to be—that is, experiences of growth in the context of connection to others, in which anger and conflicts, love and connection, can be voiced and valued (Brown 1989). Instead, for girls at age 11 or 12 in the current culture, which both idealizes and devalues care in women, the "tyranny of kind and nice" sets in as girls are expected to be "polite" and avoid "mean" and "hurtful" treatment of others (Brown, 1989, p. 208). When girls reach early adolescence, they are confronted with a developmental double bind (Steiner-Adair, 1986), in which the cultural expectations and norms for adult womanhood direct girls to disqualify the complex world of relationships and replace it with an idealized and superficial version of nurturance and care in women. At the same time, the culture directs girls to replace their previously held value for the relational world with the cultural bias for autonomy (Rothchild, 1979), which also exists in our psychological theories.

These cultural norms are embodied in the ideal image of the "Superwoman," who is "independent," "has a husband but doesn't need one," "earns $50,000 in a high-status professional career," has "a successful marriage and perfect children," and is "thin and beautiful" (Steiner-Adair, 1986, p. 104). By the middle teens, the image of the "perfectly nice girl" is joined with an expectation of independence (which is perceived to mean not needing or depending on others) and self-sufficiency. Furthermore, as girls perceive messages from adults not to call attention to relational inequities, unfairness, and detachment, the world of relationships no longer is safe because it is not real.

It is at this point in their development that girls cease to be confident. Instead, they become silent in their struggle with androcentric cultural norms, which present an unreal view of (1) females as all-caring; (2) relationships as all-inclusive; and (3) adulthood as a kind of individualism, autonomy, and independence that does not include interdependence. It is also at this point that girls begin to wish for the "perfect relationship" in which no one gets hurt, and try to be the perfect girl who "doesn't have a mean bone in her body"—a strategy for relationships that is destined to fail (Gilligan, 1988). From this perspective, the type of behavior in teenage girls that is often described as "cliquey" or "catty" can be seen not as behavior inherent to females, but as the by-product of a culture that encourages falsification of relationships and suppresses direct acknowledgment of nonidealized emotions.

Perhaps most critically, it is at this point that girls' solution to this dilemma is to turn what is initially an issue of political resistance (i.e., the refusal of 10-year-old girls to deny the truth about relationships) into an experience of psychological resistance (Gilligan, 1988). That is, girls at this point show an unwillingness or inability to know what they already know, as seen in the painful loss of self-confidence and the onset of psychological distress that can lead to behaviors related to eating diorders (Steiner-Adair, 1986). Brown (1989) has found that by 10th grade, although girls sometimes doubt and criticize the culture, they far more frequently doubt and criticize themselves. As a result of this, Brown concludes "that what can be known at one age can be lost or buried in self-doubt and confusion at another, and that there is no simple relationship between maturation, social-cognitive complexity or social adaptability, and psychological health" (p. 221).

In light of this research, I think it becomes very important to think about what it means to say to a teenager with anorexia that the goal of therapy is to "separate." I think in the worst case, you risk recapitulating the young girl's worst fear—that growing up means isolation and that the goal of therapy is no longer to need anybody. Furthermore, a therapist who practices a model of psychotherapy in which he or she remains personally distant and never speaks of his or her reactions and experience in the relationship further risks reinforcing a presentation of phony or false relationships: The therapist practices a professional version of "the tyranny of kind and nice" by remaining distant behind "neutrality" or objectivity."

Longitudinal research on girls' development points to the enormous impact on girls of their observations of adults, particularly adult women, silencing themselves in relationships, especially in the face of relational inequities. How can a therapist expect a young female with an eating disorder to reinhabit her body if there is no "I" or self that speaks directly from within the body of her therapist, and the girl must struggle alone with the dilemma? If the therapist is not present as a real person, he or she risks recreating the cultural image of perfection, "niceness," and social acceptability that requires the truth of one's feelings and beliefs to live underground. In other words, longitudinal data indicate that girls at 15 struggle with the dilemma of "How can I be fully present and authentic if my observations and feelings are unacceptable in the cultural ideal image for women?" This raises serious questions for therapists about what kind of solution to the dilemma to model. "Much of what is known by psychologists is also known by adolescent girls. But as girls themselves say clearly, they will speak only when they feel that someone will listen and will not leave in the face of conflict or disagreement" (Gilligan, 1988, p. 23). The challenge of working with teenage girls with eating disorders raises useful questions to therapists about who is the someone who "stays" and "listens" in the context of psychotherapy.

REFRAMING THE GOALS OF THERAPY

New research on women's development (Brown, 1989; Gilligan, 1982; Miller, 1976) offers a different paradigm for identity development, and therefore a different model for therapy. In contrast to the emphasis on separation and autonomy, the psychology of women focuses on self in relation to others and on the reciprocal meaning that individuals have for each other. This model, which holds interdependence as the goal of adulthood, suggests that therapy hinges on both the patient's and the therapist's ability to experience themselves in a mutual relationship that acknowledges both individual's sense of self—in a way that includes both individuals' need to care for and to be cared for. The developmental paradigm provided by Gilligan (1980) is one of self-differentiation within the context of relationships; thus, therapist and patient are two separate people who are also reciprocally connected to each other.

The psychology of women offers a new way of thinking about a real relationship—as an experience in interdependence and connectedness, where one is able to move and be moved by another, to influence and be influenced. In false relationships, people are either not affected by the other, or they hide the fact that they are. Women with eating disorders have a particular area of expertise: They are experts in false relationships. Although they do not arrive at therapy aware of their knowledge about false relationships, they have vast experiences of what it is like to be in a relationship that has the outward form of connection but is lifeless or dead at the center, in which the other is emotionally absent and therefore cannot be directly engaged. Much of the work of therapy—and in this chapter I am referring specifically to individual psychotherapy with patients who are well enough to be seen on an outpatient basis—is to make conscious and valid eating-disordered women's perceptions of previous false relationships, which have blunted their hope, desire, and ability for true relationships.

Because this paradigm involves reciprocity in relationships, it eliminates status in the realm of interpersonal connection and posits a mutual (albeit asymmetrical) relationship by acknowledging that both patient and therapist are actively engaged in a real relationship that has unique dynamics due to position and role, commonly called "transference" and "countertransference." The asymmetry is ever present in that only one person's experience is the focus of the work, money is exchanged for expertise, and so forth. However, instead of focusing on separation or individuation, this model holds a tension between self-differentiation and connection, and tensions arise around issues of separateness and connectedness in different ways for both patient and therapist. In the language and paradigm of this new theory, I have come to view the central dynamics of individual psychotherapy with women who have anorexia and bulimia in the way I describe (in highly condensed and summarized form) below. I talk generally about women with anorexia and bulimia, and assume that readers will adjust my comments with respect for significant differences along the mild-to-severe continuum; I also assume that readers will hear overlapping themes between the two syndromes from theories of normal female identity development.

PROBLEMS IN RELATEDNESS IN WOMEN WITH EATING DISORDERS

Females who have anorexia nervosa exhibit a seeming lack of relatedness, which is based on an underlying starvation for an experience of closeness that is not fusion, and separateness that is not detachment. Anorexics confuse engagement with enmeshment; they fear connection because it represents the loss of a separate sense of self. At worst, they fear that to connect is to lose oneself in a malevolent, overwhelming presence—and to admit a need for connection is to put themselves at jeopardy in an annihilating, dependent position—from which to separate is to destroy self and others and incur great wrath. The false relationship looks like this: The only way to relate is to be connected without separateness—a theme of selflessness that resonates throughout the psychology of women. Their stance in therapy is "I'm not going to need you, because if I need you I lose me—because you want and need me too much." My stance as therapist is "You do and can need me, and still not lose your separateness. Our relationship can survive the intensity of your need without either of us being destroyed, and I'm not going to harm you." Because anorexics believe that their need for others is dangerous, their struggle originates not in a struggle to control the therapist as much as a struggle to control themselves, their desire to connect to the therapist.

At the more pathological extreme, for an anorexic to acknowledge her need for others feels like a suicidal loss of self. At the less pathological end of the continuum, when a female is restricting a little, the behavior becomes a scoring system that says, "As long as I'm denying myself a little, it's OK to receive; as long as I keep some part of myself out, I can try to be in." At either end, therapy works toward integrating connection, and the therapist holds and makes safe the tension between separateness and connection. When the work is going well with a patient who has anorexia, it feels good because she is inviting you in.

In contrast to the tension of integrating closeness with anorexics, the core tension in work with bulimic women focuses on integrating differentiation. Rather than being afraid of the therapist's involvement, women with bulimia want the therapist to do all the work because they struggle with connection in fear of separation and they struggle with separation in fear of fragmentation and abandonment. Their overt message is "I do need you," but their convert message is "I don't need you"; it is a cybernetic cycle that feeds on itself. It sounds like this: "I really need you, but I don't want you to know how much, because although I look as if I have my act together, you'll be destroyed by my neediness." Separation is more dangerous than connection, and bulimics are extremely involved with the therapist's perceptions of them (which they distort with paranoia and humiliation). They don't trust the "we," so they grab on to the connection and try to control both the therapist and themselves, and bring the relationship down in fear that differentiation and individuation will destroy connection. For them, differentiation is toxic, and their need for both closeness and separateness is dangerous. The tension in the relationship here is more difficult, because it has to do with inclusion and exclusion, separateness and connection.

NEW NORMS FOR RELATEDNESS
AMONG THERAPISTS

We hear in the psychology of women a shift in language from detachment, depersonalization, and objectivity to a language of emotional directness and personal reference, in the service of learning. (See also Rogers & Gilligan, 1988.)

The language from the psychology of women attempts to create an interactive phenomenology (Gilligan, Brown, & Rogers, 1988) that more accurately describes the therapist's experience of himself or herself in the therapy relationship. This requires that the therapist think about how to use himself or herself more directly in the relationship. When I talk about the therapist's experience of using self in the real relationship, I am not talking about fusion, induction, smothering, or inappropriate revealing of the therapist's self. Nor am I talking about an absence of boundaries, but rather a different vision of boundary—a boundary not in the traditional "walled-up" definition of self as a distinct entity, but a boundary modeled from women's development. That is, I see this boundary as a permeable membrane that allows the relationship to flow back and forth.

From recent research on female psychological development that locates the process of identity formation in a mutual relationship, the central metaphor for therapy becomes dialogue rather than mirroring: The self is defined through the gaining of perspective, which is discovered through the experience of engagement with the therapist. This perspective is quite similar to the research on therapy efficacy (LeBerie & Sturnillo, 1988) in which patients are reported to experience self-involving statements by the therapist (which are defined differently from self-disclosing statements) as positive and helpful. (See also Stiver, 1985.)

Self psychologists (Kohut, 1971; Kernberg, 1976) are looking at a separate narcissistic line of development of the self, in which the therapist is a self-object. The relational line of development as described by Surrey (1985) is seen as an irreducible and continuous line of development, in which relationships with self and others are seen as continuous and developing through life—an approach that is consistent with Daniel Stern's (1985) research on infants and mothers. In this model, the therapist's self does not remain distant in the presence of the patient. In self psychology, empathy implies an identification of feelings: The patient looks into a mirror of the therapist, and sees the same feelings; self and other feel the same. This different definition of empathy, or "cofeelings," as described by Gilligan and Wiggins (1987), implies an ability to participate in another's feelings, signifying an attitude of engagement rather than observation. Miller (1984) and Jordan (1984) write about the importance of the approach toward empathy in which one person is using his or her own experiences to try to understand the other. This in no way implies an absence of difference or a failure to distinguish between self and others; rather, it gives rise to an awareness of two individuals who affect each other in an interactive process.

REFRAMING COUNTERTRANSFERENCE

From this perspective, I have found it useful to look at countertransference as thoughts and feelings that take the therapist out of connection with the patient. This is just the opposite approach to what is traditionally meant by countertransference—that is, those thoughts and feelings that interfere with objectivity and distance. Here I am talking about feelings that interfere with responsiveness and connection, so countertransference problems are problems of disengagement and of failures in a relationship.

Like the traditional defintion of countertransference, this perspective also questions breaks in empathy and overidentification, or moving too far so as to fuse with the patient, which extinguishes the patient as a separate person. However, this perspective does not hold suspect feelings (conscious or unconscious) of connectedness—love, caring, sorrow, pity, envy, joy, anger, frustration—and it stresses the importance and usefulness of appropriately articulating these feelings directly in the therapy relationship in the here and now. I do not want to be misunderstood as saying that therapists should randomly be telling their patients that they love them and hate them. I am talking about a model of therapy that offers different guidelines for using the therapist's feelings about the patient and the relationship—a model that is grounded in theories of the psychological development of women.

Like patients with eating disorders, who are unable to find a way to speak directly about the quality of their connection to important people in their lives, I experience a real bind as a therapist when I try to speak in the language of traditional psychoanalytic theory directly about my experiences of caring about my patients, and what I feel in relationship to patients. Psychoanalytic theory tends to cast my sense of myself as a real and separate person with strong feelings about my patients, especially compassionate feelings, in a pathological light of either fusion or gratification or seduction. As Stiver (1985) says, "It's not that therapists don't care about their patients, but that the caring goes on behind closed doors and is hard to speak about, both in training and in therapy."

In her paper, "The Conquistador and the Dark Continent: Reflections on the Psychology of Love," Gilligan (1984) traces the limits of psychodynamic language for talking directly about the therapist's experience in the therapy relationship to the difficulties in psychoanalytic theory in talking about love. She writes, "By using Freud's terminology of 'objects[,]' which carries with it the premise of separation by casting the 'other' always in the image of self-gratification, [psychoanalytic theory] creates a landscape of love [and, I would add, an image of the therapy relationship] unparalleled in its depersonalization" (pp. 90–91). In this world, where the therapist is an object and the relationship a holding environment designated to facilitate separation, it is truly difficult to discuss real experiences of closeness. Furthermore, when the therapist's caring for the patient is associated only with mothering, which in itself is cast in a regressive light—as in Winnicott's description (see "The Conquistador . . .", p. 90) of the "good enough mother," who in her "primary maternal preoccupation" (i.e., motherly love) withdraws from herself and sinks into a "withdrawn state" resembling a "disassociated" or "schizoid episode"—it is difficult to feel proud of one's feelings as a therapist (or a mother). Gilligan (1984) notes that "this language of borders and boundaries, splitting and fusion, creates an imagery of love and connection that is undistinguishable from the imagery of war" (p. 90). Indeed, one hears in the classical definition of countertransference a theme that associates intimacy with danger. This is just the opposite of the association found in women's psychological development, which associates detachment with danger.

It strikes me that in listening to eating-disordered women's fears about their desire for closeness and connection, I hear the same fear as that expressed in some of the traditional definitions of countertransference and models of it. That is, if the therapist reinforces his or her own feelings or expresses care about the patient by saying something like "I'm sorry that happened to you," this is seen as dangerous, gratifying, or seductive. Any desire on the part of the therapist to refer to or include himself or herself in the dialogue is not legitimate. (For example, a supervisor might tell a trainee that he or she should have said "How did you feel about that?" instead of using the pronoun "I.") This sounds like a mirror image of the patient with an eating disorder who believes that her own desire for closeness is toxic and that in order to stay connected in the relationship, she must hide or tightly control this part of herself. At the most extreme, the therapist's feelings for the patient are generally kept out of the therapy relationship (either hidden in the mind of the therapist or discussed in supervision, which is a different relationship), and we get a picture of a therapist who relates to the patient much as the woman with anorexia appears to relate to her starving body—in a detached, dispassionate, and purely objective manner.

The model of therapy being proposed here suggests that therapists look at how they feel distance and frustration toward their patients and how they use those feelings, but that they look also at how they feel care and compassion toward their patients and how they directly use these feelings. The therapy focuses on experiences of both patient and therapist—of separateness and connection, distance and closeness, as well as self. The goal is for therapist and patient both to be watchful and aware of the nature of the rational bond in the present (what Surrey [1983] calls being "vigilant" in the relationship), and countertransference feelings are used to inform the therapist's watchfulness.

In this context, there are particular times when direct expressions of the therapist's reactions of being moved with compassion, which demonstrate that the therapist cares about and is affected by what he or she is hearing, are not fusion or seduction and are not blocks to good therapy; rather, they constitute a necessary foundation in the creation of a real relationship, or what is commonly called the "therapeutic alliance" (again, this term carries echoes of the language of war "allies"). Responses like "I'm so sorry that happened to you," or "I'm so happy for you," are simple yet potentially powerful examples of what might precede the inquiry "How did you feel about that?" It is not surprising to me that work with eating-disordered patients is clarifying this dimension of therapy, because Gilligan's (1982) work on the morality of care, as revealed by the study of female moral reasoning, defines moral failures in relationships as failures to acknowledge, claim, and respond to attachment. This failure to acknowledge and respond to connection is the "unfairness" that our patients with eating disorders often speak of.

Perhaps if the field of psychotherapy dealt more directly with the "problem of love in psychotherapy" (Gilligan, 1984), there would be significantly less acting out on the part of therapists in the sexual exploitation of patients. With respect for the seriousness of the ways in which a therapist can abuse the notion of care and connection for the patient, the fear of expressing caring feelings in traditional models is not unlike the eating-disordered patient's fear that to say who she is would be to destroy the connection or alliance. Clearly, these are complex interactions requiring theoretical guidelines that must include evaluating the risks, such as pushing the patient into a false position of compliance. The brevity of this chapter does not allow a comprehensive clinical discussion of the application of this model. The intent here is to introduce the issue of direct expression of feelings of connection that is highlighted in the psychology of women. In a way, this is nothing new. We hear repeatedly that the quality of the therapy relationship is what makes therapy effective. What is new is that the map of female development provides a model and language for therapists that can elucidate and elaborate this aspect of therapy.

Epstein and Feiner (1979), in the book *Countertransference*, list the following reasons why it is important to express feelings of anger and hate to patients—in some appropriate expression of frustration. Why shouldn't the same reasons hold true for expressing feelings of love and compassion, which, just like anger, are often expressions of caring?

1. To not show that you are angry with your patient is to keep her in the position of an infant who cannot understand what she owes to her parents.
2. The subjectivity of anger/hating feelings needs to be recognized to teach relational skills.
3. If the patient experiences the therapist as a real person, the effect is to open the relationship up and move toward further activity.
4. The therapist reveals that she too is human, and it is normal to feel angry.
5. To restrain intense feelings of anger may give the patient the message that these feelings are only allowed to children or patients; which could reinforce their fear that to grow up and get better is to lead a life of endless battle of control and to hide the depth of one's feelings. (p. 229)

These issues are central to female identity development and are ever present in work with eating-disordered women (Steiner-Adair, 1986, 1987, 1989). Because she has lived in false relationships, a female with an eating disorder feels that her needs and desires to be taken care of are bad and that her ability to care successfully for others is quite inadequate. She comes to equate care with self-sacrifice and believes that she must empty herself of all need for closeness in order to connect. Her self-esteem is tied to her capacity to give to others what she cannot get for herself. All of these internalized messages have individual, family, and cultural determinants.

A therapist's telling a patient that he or she cares about her feels real to both of them, because it makes emotional sense and speaks to the truth of their presence in each other's lives, which the patient needs to hear directly. Since, as a female, her self-esteem is closely tied to her sense of interpersonal efficacy (Kagan, 1964), she needs to hear that she has a place in the therapist's life. Also, as a female, she develops her identity by comparing herself to others (Rosenbaum, 1979). To hear that the therapist has caring feelings as well as feelings of frustration helps her achieve a more tolerable distribution of badness, to the extent that she feels her love is bad. What Epstein (1979) says about anger is also true about love: The therapist rescues the patient from the maddening and symptom-syntonic position that she is all bad for caring and the therapist all good for controlling and hiding his or her caring.

Women with eating disorders are terrified that their need for love and connection will devour or destroy others. By responding to mutual feelings of care, the therapist protects the patient from her terrible fear of the consequences of her love; moreover, the therapist, by talking about his or her feelings as well as the patient's, shows that caring feelings will not destroy either of them or the relationship. Furthermore, working with eating-disordered patients forces us to challenge the assumption that growth and change can only occur if a therapist does *not* gratify the patient by telling her that he or she cares about her—a perspective that requires the therapist to be objective, distant, and neutral. I do not think any of us can be neutral about a teenager starving herself to death—or question the usefulness of telling a bulimic woman that she deserves to hold inside her food and emotional sustenance, that she needn't expel from herself her desire for love in order to be loved.

THE NEED FOR AN INTERACTIVE LANGUAGE

This theory calls for the therapist to create a highly interactive relationship with a patient who is terrified of relatedness. Females with anorexia and bulimia have difficulty believing that they can be separate and connected to the therapist and that it is possible to be attached to someone in a relationship where self, other, and "we" are all equally recognized. The reassurance must be directly heard—body language and posture are not enough. Their distortions and fears lead to incredibly complex and difficult relational dynamics, and their controlling behavior often appears as an expression of hopelessness about the possibility of integrating these two modes of relatedness. The challenge of engaging with the therapist hinges on their increasing willingness to be vulnerable with the therapist—that is, to be willing to experience an unprotected softness that allows for real and spontaneous contact (R. Berezin, personal conversation, 1987). The same vulnerability in a different way is required of the therapist.

What follows are some more brief examples of how this can be applied. Application hinges on personal reference on the part of the therapist; the use of the pronoun "I" and directly addressing the "we" of the relationship; and an acknowledgment that dynamics flow back and forth. Conceptually, this is similar to Schaeffer's writing about the need for an action language. There are situations in which I'll say something simple like "I'm sorry you felt that way for so long," or "Hearing you say this makes me feel so good," or "I see how important this is to you." The communication is "What you are telling me moves me," and then "How does it affect, move, and influence [consciously and unconsciously] you?"

Examples of things I've said that speak to the relationship dynamics when someone is struggling with distance are as follows:

"There's something about the way you're telling me this that makes it really hard for me to feel with you. . . . I wonder why?"

"There's something about the way you're telling me this that makes me feel like you're pushing me away from you."

"One of the things we both know is that when you talk *at* me like this, rather than *with* me, you're usually scared." I might add something like this:

". . . scared that I won't understand or accept you," or

". . . scared about something related, but deeper. What's going on for you right now? How are you feeling as you talk?" or

". . . scared about being close to me or known by me. Do you feel too vulnerable?"

My experience is that instead of interfering with or blocking the analytic work, such acknowledgments deepen the therapeutic process and allow necessary exploration to proceed. When someone is projecting and distancing, I'll say, "What just happened? Who did I just become for you? There was a sudden shift in your tone of voice." If someone has just told me about something about which she feels enormous shame or embarrassment, I might ask something like "How does it feel to you to have me know about this?" or "How do you imagine that my knowing this affects how I see you?" One woman with whom I've worked for several years will still jokingly say, "OK, now *this* will be the thing I say that will convince you that I'm a stupid fool" (a favorite statement of her father's for her). Her saying this has become a shorthand for us, a brief communication about the way in which she can feel extremely exposed and frightened about revealing herself. In this model, which emphasizes teaching relational skills, teaching the process of projection directly and early in the therapy is seen as helpful. At the same time, if I've made a mistake, I'll claim it with something like this: "I think I missed something important you were trying to tell me. I'm sorry."

Searles (1975) has said that the therapist's ability to see the real relationship will guide the work of the therapy. I agree, and I think that therapeutic impasses often occur when the therapist pulls out of the relationship. Females with eating disorders are highly attuned to and easily discouraged by people distancing from them. They have spent years locked in an isolated, lonely, and secret world of desperately trying to make sense of relational dynamics, and sometimes they will use their symptomatic behavior in a way that looks like resistance, regression, or manipulation to indicate to the therapist that he or she is too far away and therefore no longer feels real.

CULTURAL COUNTERTRANSFERENCE

Because eating disorders are so closely tied to cultural images of perfection in women, the extent to which any therapist is embedded
in the cultural ideal will clearly affect the therapeutic process and the
therapist's vulnerability. Research on the development of girls highlights
the necessity of (1) helping female adolescents recognize developmentally disabling norms and the reality of the cultural context in which
they live and to which they are connected, and (2) helping female adolescents hold on to their early adolescent voice of resistance and cultivate
an ability to take a stand apart from disabling norms. From a feminist
perspective, it is essential to address the sociocultural context in therapy.

The dilemma of resistance in adolescent girls raises questions of
resistance for therapists. I have observed two countertransference reactions that indicate contrasting vulnerabilities in therapists working
with women who have eating disorders. On the one hand, I have often
heard therapists, primarily those following a traditional psychoanalytic
model, state that any time a patient refers to sociocultural images, she
is "resisting deeper work." Although there are times when this may
be true, the unilateral dismissal of the validity of a sociocultural perspective is illustrative of a process in which the healthy attempt of
the patient to identify and resist disabling cultural norms is resisted by
the voice of authority and relegated to the underground of psychopathology. In my observations, when a therapist responds inaccurately with
this interpretation, a regression may occur. At this point one must
ask this question: In response to whose resistance is the regression occurring?

On the other hand, if a therapist introduces cultural values in a way
or at a time that leaves the patient behind, and in so doing pulls himself
or herself out of the relationship, at that moment I think the therapist experiences a cultural countertransference. What I have often seen
as a supervisor is that in these moments, the therapist gets mad at the
culture; the patient gets confused and thinks that the therapist is
mad at her, which can lead to confusion, distance, or resistance in
the patient.

THE THERAPIST AS THE PERFECT,
ALL-CARING MOTHER

Another danger I see for therapists working with eating-disordered
women is that a therapist may present himself or herself as the perfect
mother. This is doubly dangerous, for it reinforces two cultural values

that are disabling to female development. The first is that it reinforces the notion that women (or caretakers) are in direct competition with each other in all aspects of their lives (perfect mothers, perfect lovers, etc.)—a message that males have long received and women are now the beneficiaries of. As a supervisor, I see this played out in therapy when a therapist sets himself or herself up as the ideal or perfect mother, in opposition to the patient's mother, and the therapist becomes invested in maintaining this position. Unfortunately, this position reinforces the treacherous model of the all-caring caretaker, or the "tyranny of kind and nice." This is not to be confused with carrying an idealizing transference, which originates within the patient. Nor am I in any way suggesting that therapists deny their patients anger at their mothers. Rather, research on the psychology of women suggests that in order for women to feel whole, they need to be able to identify with their mothers in some way (if only from a multigenerational perspective), and be able to understand their mothers' context. "Failure to know your mother, that is your position and its attendant traditions, history, and place in the scheme of things, is failure to remember your significance, your reality. . . . it's the same thing as being lost or isolated, self-estranged and alienated from your own life" (Allen, 1988, p. 15).

At times I have heard therapists get stuck in a competition with their patients' mothers. It is important in thinking about this to recall that there are still few legitimate ways for women to get angry in our culture. If they are angry at men, they become angry at their mothers; they get cheered on by the androcentric culture and by many of our psychological theories, and their anger is legitimized. A lot of attention is paid to helping women with eating disorders express their anger, especially at their mothers. Certainly identifying and expressing one's anger (as well as one's love) and understanding one's family are integral parts of recovery. However, it is also extremely important that therapists help their patients understand their mothers' struggles and social context as well. Any therapy that stops without this, and sets up an unacknowledged competition between an all-nurturing therapist and an awful mother, colludes with an unfortunate history in the field of psychotherapy of isolating and blaming mothers.

IS THE THERAPEUTIC RELATIONSHIP A RELATIONSHIP?

Women with eating disorders have highlighted to us a question that has been most difficult and problematic for therapists: "Is the therapy relationship a true or false relationship?" Women with eating disorders call our attention to the dilemma of connection versus difference between therapists and patients, which is a real dilemma in the context of therapy. By this I mean the following: How do we as therapists conceptualize ourselves in the therapy relationship as different from our patients, yet simultaneously connected to them and involved in a real relationship? On the one hand, conceptualizing the relationship merely in terms of transference and countertransference puts undue emphasis on differences. On the other hand, idealizing the relationship as a perfect, equal union ignores the asymmetrical factors of money being exchanged, unequal self-disclosure, a limited time construct, training and position, and so on. Both are constructs of false relationships: It is impossible to talk about connection without acknowledging differences or separateness, and vice versa. The question of how to connect in the presence of difference, and how to differentiate in the context of a relationship, is not only central to women with eating disorders; it is central to psychotherapy and also a central human dilemma (between individuals, families, sexes, races, classes, and nations).

If we listen to Freud's observation that symptoms have meaning and are a way of speaking, recent research on the psychology of women can help us better understand how to respond to what is being indirectly said, so that the symptom may be replaced by direct communication. If we look at eating disorders as expressions of a body politic rather than a body pathological, the symptoms become a statement about the enormous difficulty of growing up female in the current culture, which casts out that which is central to female development and human nature (Steiner-Adair, 1986). From this perspective, the challenge of therapy is to transform that which initially appears as psychological resistance into political resistance—that is, a refusal not to know what one knows with regard to corrupt presentation of truth in the public world. The map of female development highlights a process of self-discovery and authorization in the context of real relationships, and moral failures are often identified as failures to claim and respond to attachment. Recent research on the psychology of women suggests that if therapy is to be an experience in which the loss of the complex relational world may be reclaimed, and the body reinhabited, then therapists must find a way to acknowledge and claim the truth of a real relationship in the context of therapy, if healing is to occur.

Acknowledgments. This chapter was presented at the 1986 conference of the Center for the Study of Anorexia and Bulimia, New York. I would like to acknowledge my research colleagues at the Project on the Psychology of Women and the Development of Girls, Harvard University.

REFERENCES

Allen, P. G. (1988). Who is your mother? Red roots of white feminism. In R. Simonson & S. Walker (Eds.), *Multi-cultural literacy: The Greywolf annual five* (pp. 13–28). St. Paul, MN: Greywolf Press.

Brown, L. (1989). *Narratives of relationship: The development of a care voice in girls ages 7 to 16* (Monograph No. 8). Cambridge, MA: Harvard University, The Study Center.

Bruch, H. (1978). *The golden cage: The enigma of anorexia nervosa.* Cambridge, MA: Harvard University Press.

Chodorow, N. (1978). *The reproduction of mothering.* Berkeley: University of California Press.

Chodorow, N., Lamphere, L., & Rosaldo, R. (Eds.). (1974). *Women: Culture and society.* Stanford, CA: Stanford University Press.

Crisp, A. H. (1980). *Anorexia nervosa: Let me be.* New York: Academic Press.

Epstein, L., & Feiner, A. (1979). The therapeutic function of hate. In L. Epstein & A. Feiner (Eds.), *Countertransference* (pp. 213–224). New York: Jason Aronson.

Gilligan, C. (1977). In a different voice: Women's conceptions of the self and of morality. *Harvard Education Review, 47,* 481–517.

Gilligan, C. (1982). *In a different voice.* Cambridge, MA: Harvard University Press.

Gilligan, C. (1984). The conquistador and the dark continent: Reflections on the psychology of love. *Daedalus: Journal of the American Academy of Arts and Sciences, 113,* 75–95.

Gilligan, C. (1986a). Remapping the moral domain: New images of the self in relationships. In T. Heller, M. Sosna, & P. Wallenberg (Eds.), *Reconstructing individualism* (pp. 237–252). Stanford, CA: Stanford University Press.

Gilligan, C. (1986b). Exit voice dilemmas in adolescent development. In A. Foxley, M. McPherson, & G. O'Donnell (Eds.), *Development, democracy, and the art of trespassing: Essays in honor of Albert O. Hirschman* (pp. 283–300). Notre Dame, IN: University of Notre Dame Press.

Gilligan, C. (1990). Teaching Shakespeare's sisters: Notes from the underground of female adolescence. In C. Gilligan, N. Lyons, & T. Hamner (Eds.), *Making connections* (pp. 1–29). Cambridge, MA: Harvard University Press.

Gilligan, C., Brown, L., & Rogers, A. (1988). *Translating the language of adolescent girls: Themes of moral voice and ego development* (Monograph No. 6). Cambridge, MA: Harvard Graduate School of Education, Center for the Study of Gender, Education & Human Development.

Gilligan, C., & Wiggins, G. (1987). The origins of morality in early childhood relationships. In J. Kagan & S. Lamb (Eds.), *The emergence of morality in early childhood* (pp. 277–305). Chicago: University of Chicago Press.

Jordan, J. (1984). *Empathy and self boundaries* (Work in Progress Paper No. 16). Wellesley, MA: Wellesley College, Stone Center.

Kagan, J. (1964). Acquisition and significance of sex typing and sex role identity. In M. Hoffman & L. Hoffman (Eds.), *Review of child development research* (Vol. 1, pp. 137–167). New York: Russell Sage Foundation.

Kernberg, O. (1976). *Object relations theory and clinical psychoanalysis*. New York: Jason Aronson.

Kohut, H. (1971). *The analysis of the self*. New York: International Universities Press.

La Berie, G., & Sturniolo, F. (1987). *Effects of self-involving statements on the counseling relationship*. Paper presented at the annual meeting of the American Psychological Association, New York.

Marcia, J. (1980). Identity in adolescence. In J. Adelson (Ed.), *Handbook of adolescent psychology* (pp. 1–99). New York: Wiley.

Miller, J. B. (1976). *Toward a new psychology of women*. Boston: Beacon Press.

Miller, J. B. (1984). *The development of women's sense of self* (Work in Progress Paper No. 12). Wellesley, MA: Wellesley College, Stone Center.

Rogers, A., & Gilligan, C. (1988). *Translating the language of adolescent girls: Themes of moral voice and ego development* (Monograph No. 6). Cambridge, MA: Harvard University, The Study Center.

Rosenbaum, M. (1979). The changing body image of the adolescent girl. In M. Sugar (Ed.), *Female adolescent development* (pp. 234–296). New York: Brunner/Mazel.

Rothchild, E. (1979). Female power: Lines to development of autonomy. In M. Sugar (Ed.), *Female adolescent development*. New York: Brunner/Mazel.

Searles, H. (1975). The patient as therapist to his analyst. In P. Giovacchini (Ed.), *Tactics and techniques in psychoanalytic therapy: Countertransference* (Vol. 1). New York: Jason Aronson.

Selvini-Palazzoli, M. (1974). *Self-starvation*. London: Chaucer.

Steiner-Adair, C. (1986). The body politic: Normal female adolescent development and development of eating disorders. *Journal of the American Academy of Psychoanalysis, 14*, 95–114.

Steiner-Adair, C. (1987). *Weightism: The politics of primary prevention in the treatment of eating disorders*. Keynote address to the Fourth National Conference on Eating Disorders, Columbus, OH.

Steiner-Adair, C. (1989). Educating the voice of the wise woman: College students and bulimia. In L. Whitalier & W. Davis (Eds.), *The bulimic college student: Evaluation, treatment, and prevention* (pp. 151–169). New York: Haworth Press.

Stern, D. (1985). *The interpersonal world of the infant*. New York: Basic Books.

Stiver, I. (1985). *The meaning of care: Reframing treatment models* (Work in Progress Paper No. 20). Wellesley, MA: Wellesley College, Stone Center.

Surrey, J. (1983). The relational self in women: Clinical implications. In J. Surrey, J. Stiver, A. Kaplan, & J. Jordan (Eds.), *Women and empathy* (Work in Progress No. 13).

Surrey, J. (1985). *The "self-in-relation": A theory of women's development* (Work in Progress No. 14). Wellesley, MA: Wellesley College, Stone Center.

Wooley, O., & Wooley, S. C. (1982). The Beverly Hills eating disorder: The mass marketing of anorexia nervosa. *International Journal of Eating Disorders, 1*, 57–60.

Wooley, O., Wooley, S. C., & Dyrenforth, S. (1979). Obesity and women: II. A neglected feminist topic. *Woman Studies International Quarterly, 2*, 81–92.

Wooley, S. C., & Wooley, O. (1980). Eating disorders, obesity, and anorexia. In A. Brodsky & R. Hare-Mustin (Eds.), *Women and psychotherapy* (pp. 135–159). New York: Guilford Press.

Wooley, S. C., & Wooley, O. (1984). Intensive outpatient and residential treatment for bulimia. In D. M. Garner & P. E. Garfinkel (Eds.), *Handbook of psychotherapy for anorexia nervosa and bulimia nervosa* (pp. 391–430). New York: Guilford Press.

∴ *11* ∴

Uses of Countertransference in the Treatment of Eating Disorders: A Gender Perspective

SUSAN C. WOOLEY
University of Cincinnati College of Medicine

Countertransference is a topic that makes most therapists uneasy. Embedded in its history are the worrisome notions of unconscious expressions of one's own faulty development or character structure, the likelihood of therapeutic failure, and the possibility of unwanted self-exposure. Indeed, Freud's early discussions of countertransference suggested that the occurrence of any inner state other than neutral attentiveness was a serious problem requiring a return to analysis. Whether or not Freud really meant to make suspect all human feeling in therapists, his legacy has been one of fear that several decades of renewed interest in countertransference has failed fully to remove. This is particularly unfortunate, since the therapist's emotional experience is often the best—some might argue the only—tool for comprehending the inner life of the patient and the transactions of the therapeutic relationship.

A strong dichotomy between the intellectual and emotional was, of course, a prominent feature of the culture in which Freud worked. Objective, rational thinking, associated with males, stood in stark contrast to the hysterical, irrational style attributed to females. It was but a few years before Freud began his work that the prominent American neurologist S. Weir Mitchell had warned Charlotte Perkins Gilman of the great dangers to her health involved in any further attempts by her to think, read, or write—a prescription immortalized in the classic feminist short story "The Yellow Wallpaper," in which the heroine's futile attack on the walls of her gendered prison propels her into madness. Differential encouragement of emotional responsiveness and intellectual objectivity remains at the heart of male and female socialization, and must be recognized as the source of differing experiences of male and female therapists.

Eating disorders, perhaps more than any other contemporary psychological disorders, have as a central feature difficulties in the successful integration of the traditionally feminine and masculine poles of personality organization. They are undeniably gendered disorders. In restricting anorexia,[1] the rejection of female nurturance and disavowal of needs reaches its ultimate expression. In bulimia, conflict between the expression and disavowal of needs leads to oscillations in behavior, typified in the doing and undoing of the binge–purge ritual. In some bulimics impulsivity predominates in the basic character structure, while in others compulsivity predominates; however, in either case bulimic symptoms signal the existence of an inner war, which usually carries many layers of symbolic meaning.

Because this inner war is, to some extent, a part of the psychological experience of all men and women socialized in confining gender roles and undergoing changes in relevant aspects of their value systems as they progress through adult life, there is an inevitable resonance between patients' and therapists' issues. This struggle is mirrored again in the therapist's decisions about the management of countertransference reactions: whether to acknowledge them, whether to attend to them, whether to act on them, and whether to disclose them. These resonances hold the potential for a uniquely rich therapeutic encounter in which the therapist's own behavior is dense in meaning for the patient—telling her what it is to be a man, to be a woman, to struggle with dissonant parts of the self, and to be in a relationship.

The years since Freud's contributions have brought many revisions in the concept of countertransference. Despite continuing anxiety about the dangers of therapists' emotional responsiveness, there has been a progressive effort to admit a fuller range of therapists' feelings into consideration, to identify the ways in which therapist–patient interactions generate feelings in the therapist, and to elaborate on the therapeutic uses of more broadly defined countertransference phenomena.

This chapter briefly addresses the topics so far alluded to: female development, the evolving concept of countertransference, and the issues typically presented by patients with eating disorders. It examines countertransference issues, especially as they are experienced by male and female therapists and in the treatment of anorexic, bulimic, sexually abused, and borderline patients. Therapeutic uses of countertransference are discussed, as well as the revelatory potential of experiential techniques that permit participants, including therapists, to step out of their narrow roles and "act out" responses in defined and safe ways.

EMOTION, OBJECTIVITY, AND GENDER SOCIALIZATION

A summary of the differences in male and female socialization in our culture might go as follows. In the course of their development, boys are encouraged to ignore and transcend the currents of emotion that comprise the shared consciousness of family and community life. The development of immunity to these emotional forces is believed, undoubtedly with some justification, to permit the development of a level of objectivity that informs our most cherished social institutions, and that, by freeing males of excessive concern for the emotional needs of others, maximizes their intellectual and physical achievements. To be able to transcend feelings is largely what is meant by "being a man."

Girls, by contrast, are encouraged to be attuned to the feelings of others, to feel responsible for meeting others' emotional needs, and to create and sustain human relationships. Although a girl may be encouraged to achieve, her experience leads her to feel that an accomplishment won at the expense of others is a hollow victory. Through most of history, emotional responsiveness has been the defining characteristic of a "good woman." If the imperative to attend has created a unique set of burdens and problems for girls and women, the imperative to ignore, not to know, has created a parallel set of burdens and problems for boys and men. If females are often enslaved by interpersonal relationships, men are often excluded from them. If women are often blocked from achieving, men are often blocked from doing anything else.

Although there is enormous cultural continuity in these socialization processes, it is difficult to know to what forces they should be attributed. A feminist analysis would invoke the historically powerful influences of patriarchal society in which women were not people but property, banned from the pursuit of autonomy and charged with the care of men and children. A biological analysis would emphasize probable differences in the drive states of boys and girls. Boys, this argument might go, have a more formidable task in the mastery of aggression and sexuality, requiring a socialization that emphasizes the transcendence of feeling states, in contrast to girls, whose affiliative and nurturing instincts do not require cultural suppression.

Freud located what he saw as essential differences in males and females in their different anatomies. Women—lacking a penis, and therefore spared castration anxiety—were not impelled to achieve the clear-cut oedipal resolution necessary to full superego development. Women's superego was never, in Freud's (1925/1961) view, "so inexorable, so impersonal, as independent of its emotional origins as we require it to be in men" (p. 257).

To many, important male–female differences are attributable to the fact that girls are usually nurtured by someone of the same sex and boys by someone of the opposite sex. Chodorow (1978) argues that the formation of male identity requires a greater firming of ego boundaries than is the case for girls. This developmental necessity, a consequence of the almost exclusive nurturing of children by females, diminishes the capacity of males for empathy and causes intimacy to represent a threatening regression to preoedipal relational modes. Female identity, by contrast, involves a sense of continuity with and relatedness to the external object world, which is threatened by individuation. These forces in early development equip females for the later nurturing of children, thus reproducing sex roles.

> Women, as mothers, produce daughters with mothering capacities and the desire to mother. These capacities and needs are built into and grow out of the mother–daughter relationship itself. By contrast, women as mothers (and men as not-mothers) produce sons whose nurturant capacities and needs have been systematically curtailed and repressed. (Chodorow, 1978, p. 7)

Dinnerstein (1976) also emphasizes how our construction of women is irrevocably conditioned by their mothering role, calling attention to the enduring ambivalence so created:

> So long as the first parent is a woman, then, woman will inevitably be pressed into the dual role of indispensable quasi-human supporter and deadly quasi-human enemy of the human self. She will be seen . . . as the being so peculiarly needed to confirm other people's worth, power, significance that if she fails to render them this service she is a monster. . . . And at the same time she will also be seen as the one who will not let other people be, the one who beckons her loved ones back from selfhood . . . to engulf, dissolve, drown, suffocate. (Dinnerstein, 1976, pp. 111–112)

Predisposed, in Chodorow's (1978) view, by her biological sameness to experience a greater degree of merger with her mother, the way and degree to which a girl achieves separateness and self-definition become of particular interest. Chodorow argues that the development of identity requires that a girl turn to her father, who becomes for her "a symbol of freedom from dependence and merging" (p. 121). Miller (1984) has questioned whether maternal care indeed implies merger, arguing instead that the infant's sense of self is, from the outset, a self-in-relation, which is augmented throughout girls' development but discouraged in boys' development.

> The very notion of true caretaking precludes anything that would lead the infant to feel submerged, fused or merged with the other. These are words which may describe some of the phenomena observed after *distortions* in caretaking, but they are unlikely to characterize the infant's prototypic sense of self. (Miller, 1984, p. 4)

And Miller, like most theorists of female development, questions the role of separation in the development of self:

> Development of the self presumably is attained via a series of painful crises by which the individual accomplishes a sequence of allegedly essential separations from others and thereby achieves an inner sense of separated individuation. . . . Almost every modern psychiatrist who has tried to fit women into the prevalent models has had . . . obvious difficulty . . . (Miller, 1984, p. 2)

The apparent dilution of the girl's bond with her mother during the "oedipal period" and her increased interest in her father have been an enduring subject of controversy. At the heart of this debate is the concept of "penis envy," said by Freud to constitute the basis for girls' angry rejection of "deficient" mothers and attraction to their fathers. Revisions of this view have argued, variously, that penis envy stems more from envy of male prerogatives than of male anatomy; from envy of the anatomical differences that facilitate the boy's separation from the mother; and, finally, from envy of the male's greater attractiveness to the mother. A more fundamental question is whether girls do in fact reject their mothers at this time.

Implying that all of these processes occur, but that they do not involve a severing of the mother–daughter bond, Chodorow summarizes the events of the oedipal period for girls as follows:

> The [girl's] turn to the father . . . is embedded in a girl's external relationship to her mother and in her relation to her mother as an internal object. It expresses hostility to her mother; it results from an attempt to win her mother's love; it is a reaction to powerlessness vis-à-vis maternal omnipotence and to primary identification. Every step of the way . . . a girl develops her relationship to her father while looking back at her mother. (Chodorow, 1978, p. 126)

Thus, in the oedipal phase, a boy experiences a relatively clear-cut separation from the mother and an identification with a father who has, from the outset, been experienced as a separate person with his own interests. A girl continues her relationship and identification with her mother. Particularly in traditional families, she is dependent on her father to introduce her to the outside world and to help her feel a part of it. His emotional absence may stunt her sense of self and cause her to experience her relationship with her mother as suffocating. But however present he may be, awareness of the bodily differences between herself and her father makes ambiguous for the girl the extent to which the world her father shows to her can someday be her own.

Adrienne Rich gives a firsthand account of these feelings in *Of Woman Born:*

> I don't remember when it was that my mother's feminine sensuousness, the reality of her body, began to give way for me to the charisma of my father's assertive mind and temperament; perhaps when my sister was just born and he began teaching me to read. . . . But the early pleasure and reassurance I found in my mother's body was, I believe, an imprinting never to be wholly erased, even in those years when, as my father's daughter, I suffered the obscure bodily self-hatred peculiar to women who view themselves through the eyes of men. (Rich, 1976, pp. 219–220)

For boys, physical differences appear to make the process of self-differentiation less complicated, contributing to a sense of autonomy and "difference from" that characterizes their interpersonal relationships in much the same way that the girl's sameness provides a lifelong basis for connection and empathy. To a degree, this assures females greater lifelong access to the kinds of emotional experiences associated with early nurturing—neediness, attachment, and softening of interpersonal boundaries. But the girl is also learning that to be female is more to give nurturing than it is to get it. Taking becomes colored with guilt—not so much the shame that males feel when neediness threatens to undermine their identity, but concern that taking will be at the expense of others.

> The boy's restitutive urges toward the early mother—as echoed in later relationships with her and with other females—are less tinged than the girl's with fellow-feeling. For him, the mother . . . [is] a natural resource that has been assaulted and must now be restored lest it cease to provide. . . . For the girl, too . . . but she is also—more vividly than for the boy—a creature who suffered injury just as one can suffer it oneself, and who needs to be soothed and protected just as one needs her to soothe and protect one's vulnerable self. (Dinnerstein, 1976, p. 103)

It is at puberty, when a girl's bodily changes threaten to transform her into her mother, that the meaning of being female is perhaps most forcefully brought home to her. She may begin to anticipate the sacrifice of selfhood associated with the female role. She may feel abandoned by a father whose presence in her life has previously suggested other choices and provided a needed dilution in her relationship with her mother. She may equate the development of a woman's body with the interruption of a trajectory of achievement that up to that point may not have differed much from, or may even have exceeded, that of male peers. She senses the difference in the full permission given to boys to achieve and to meet their own needs and in the qualified permission given to girls. Her responses to this knowledge may include acceptance, depression, confusion, or rebellion and a surge of ambivalent anger toward her mother. The greater the constriction and sacrifice of her mother's life, the more painfully the daughter will experience her growing similarity to her:

> The most notable fact that culture imprints on women is the sense of our limits. . . . As daughters we need mothers who want their own freedom and ours. We need not to be the vessels of another's woman self-denial and frustration. The quality of a mother's life . . . is her primary bequest to her daughter. (Rich, 1976, pp. 246–247)

As Gilligan (1982) has demonstrated, the differences between boys and girls, evident even in early childhood play, eventuate in profound differences in the later sense of responsibility for others. While boys subordinate relationships to the game and depersonalize the players, girls subordinate the game to relationships and practice roletaking. Later, while males build right and wrong around concepts of impartiality and fairness, females construct theirs around the personal and the need to care.

> [M]ale and female voices typically speak of the power of different truths, the former of the role of separation as it defines and empowers the self, the latter of the ongoing process of attachment that creates and sustains the human community. (Gilligan, 1982, p. 156)

Confronted in adolescence with increasingly painful choices between their own aspirations and others' needs, girls become confused. Those least able to identify and begin working through conflicts between their girlhood values and new constructions of female "success" become particularly susceptible to eating disorders (Steiner-Adair, 1986). For the separate developmental paths of boys and girls are not equally respected. Females must struggle with the cultural devaluation of even their most pronounced successes as those of a woman. It is the external achievements of males that are celebrated, not the interpersonal ones of females. Even more problematic, the emotional and relational style of men—detached, impartial, independent—is viewed as superior to women's more personal, emotionally attuned, and interdependent style. Thus many females are caught between guilt if they assume the right to autonomy taken for granted by males and shame if they forgo it.

Gilligan (1982) argues that in successful female development, ways to balance the conflicting needs of self and others are eventually achieved. The young woman accepts responsibility to herself as well as to others. She recognizes that connection is diminished and responsibility obscured when people shrink from the need to be honest about their own wants and needs. Basing morality on a foundation of responsibility, "women begin to see their understanding of human relationships as a source of moral strength" (Gilligan, 1982, p. 149). "The conflict between self and other . . . constitutes the central moral problem for women, posing a dilemma whose resolution requires a reconciliation between femininity and adulthood" (Gilligan, 1982, p. 71).

To prevent her connection to others from obliterating her sense of self, a woman must learn to express the full range of human feelings, trusting the reparative force of truth. This is a sophisticated lesson—one that cannot be comprehended in a family in which feelings are concealed and in which conflict is avoided or never resolved. Eating disorders typically develop at a time when, lacking this understanding, females experience the greatest conflict between selflessness and self-interest, the most confusion about the meaning of being female. Gaining this understanding is the heart of therapy.

As male or female therapists, entering our patients' lives at different stages in our own development, we bring to the therapeutic encounter vastly different constructions of the world. Though these constructions are brought into some degree of concordance by our training and experience as therapists, they are nonetheless profoundly influenced by our gender. An examination of therapeutic relationships must always take the gender of the patient and the therapist into account.

THE EVOLUTION OF COUNTERTRANSFERENCE THEORY

It is evident that Freud's definition of the therapeutic mission relied on models drawn from male development. The point is not so much that his theory did a better job of elucidating male than female development (although it did) as that the therapeutic stance in psychoanalysis was modeled after the goals of male development. The analyst was, in a sense, the ultimate expression of successful male socialization—freed completely of inappropriate and nonfunctional emotion, impersonal in his response to the patient, totally objective in his understanding. His goal was to help the patient be as much as possible like him. The "blank screen" required to adequately encourage transference resembled the vision of "blind justice" that has informed our legal system—each made effective by virtue of its nonresponsiveness:

> I cannot advise my colleagues too urgently to model themselves during psychoanalytic treatment on the surgeon, who puts aside all his feelings, even his human sympathy, and concentrates his mental forces on the single aim of performing the operation as skillfully as possible. . . . The justification for requiring this emotional coldness is that it creates the most advantageous conditions for both parties: for the doctor a desirable protection for his own emotional life and for the patient the largest amount of help we can give him today. (Freud, 1912/1958, p. 115)

Such a view of the therapeutic relationship is profoundly alienating to women, who can locate in it little, if anything, resembling their own experience or aspirations. If men have trouble, as we must certainly imagine they do, achieving the state of objectivity dictated by Freud, they at least have experience in striving for it; it is a recognizable goal. Trying to explain why this tenet went so long unchallenged, Racker (1957) cited the "infantile idealization" of training analysts by trainees—a process that undoubtedly owed much of its power to the repetition of form and content from the trainees' relationships with their fathers.

Tracing the history of shifts in views of countertransference, Tansey and Burke (1989) note that it took nearly 40 years for it to be widely acknowledged that "a therapist often responds with powerful emotions to his work with given patients and that this reaction does not necessarily indicate a pathological impingement from the therapist on the therapeutic process" (p. 5). It is perhaps not entirely coincidental that the first tentative challenge of the long-prevailing view came from a woman, Deutsch, writing in 1926. Deutsch (1926/1953) rejected the classical view, which restricts the meaning of countertransferance to the therapist's unconscious reactions stemming from unresolved conflict. Instead, she anticipated the totalists by arguing that countertransference includes unconscious identification with the patient through the revival of the therapist's memory (the basis of "intuitive empathy"), as well as identification with the patient's early objects that can occur when the patient responds to the therapist as if to a past relationship.

Although the term "projective identification" was first introduced by Melanie Klein (1946), it has acquired a different meaning than that which she originally gave to it: the projection by an infant of unacceptable aggressive impulses onto an internal object. Coming to represent the projection of both self-representations and object representations onto others in actual relationships, projective identification is now a major organizing concept for countertransference, describing the process by

which the therapist is brought into the patient's most central and enduring relational modes.

In 1950 Heimann, in a decidedly female voice, made what Tansey
and Burke (1989) describe as the "landmark statement" of the totalist
perspective, arguing that countertransference should refer to all the
therapist's feelings toward the patient, since the distinction between
"realistic" and "distorted" ones is so difficult to make. She also challenged
the view that regarded countertransference as an unwanted, if inevitable,
intrusion in the therapy process:

> I have been struck by the widespread belief amongst candidates that the
> countertransference is nothing but a source of trouble. . . . [M]y thesis is
> that the analyst's emotional response to his patient . . . represents one of
> the most important tools for his work. . . . [O]ften the emotions roused
> in him are much nearer to the heart of the matter than his reasoning . . .
> (Heimann, 1950, pp. 81–82)

Heimann further argued that it is the task of the analyst "to sustain
the feelings which are stirred in him as opposed to discharging them (as
the patient does) in order to subordinate them to the analytic task." Thus,
the therapist's feelings, rather than being eliminated, must be tightly
held. The "containing" metaphor has been given many meanings in
therapy, but probably none is more important than the therapist's ability
to keep alive feelings that the patient must be helped to reclaim.

Little (1951) and Tower (1956) similarly argued for greater acceptance and use of countertransference phenomena and for a decrease in the
"rigidity and prohibitiveness" passed from one generation of analysts to
the next. Little called upon analysts to adopt a less "paranoid" or "phobic"
attitude toward countertransference. Although she retained a definition
of countertransference based solely on past experience, she argued for the
benefits, even the necessity, of discussing countertransference in the
therapy:

> In my view a time comes in the course of every analysis when it is
> essential for the patient to recognize the existence not only of the
> analyst's objective or justified feelings, but also of the analyst's sub-
> jective feelings. . . . The very real fear of being flooded with feeling . . .
> leads to an unconscious avoidance or denial. Honest recognition of such
> feeling is essential to the analytic process, and the analysand is naturally
> sensitive to any insincerity in his analyst and will inevitably respond to it
> with hostility. (Little, 1951, pp. 37–38)

But it was Racker (1957) who best consolidated these ideas. He
argued that the analyst can make either of two mistakes, adopting an
"obsessive ideal of objectivity" leading to repression and blocking of

subjectivity, or, at the other extreme, "drowning" in countertransference. He defined countertransference broadly to include the analyst's transference responses to the patient, concordant identification with the patient's psychic structures, and complementary identifications with the patient's internal objects. Incomplete awareness of these responses, he maintained, leads the analyst into destructive repetitions from the patient's and/or analyst's past.

Tansey and Burke (1989) refer to the years since 1970 as the "specifist" period in countertransference theory, and describe efforts to classify countertransference responses along various dimensions. Although expressive of continuing interest and of the need to refine observation and theory, this era of "list making" probably also reflects some anxiety over the growing recognition of the importance and inevitability of therapists' feelings. Although this was a time in which the totalist view gained wider acceptance, the classical view nonetheless retained many proponents.

This chapter is written using a totalist definition of countertransference. "Countertransference" refers to all the therapist's responses to the patient, occurring at varying levels of awareness, to all of the patient's verbal and nonverbal communications. These include (1) what Winnicott (1949) called "objective countertransference," reactions with a basis in reality that would be shared by most people; (2) responses common to groups of people with some basis for a common outlook (e.g., gender, age, nationality); (3) idiosyncratic "transference" responses occasioned by one's unique developmental history; and, most important, (4) responses attributable, in Tansey and Burke's (1989) phrase, to "interactional pressure"—that is, to the patient's unconscious effort to direct the therapist into an experience of feeling as the patient does or feeling toward the patient as important people in the past have done. These include "concordant projective identification," in which the therapist temporarily shares the patient's experience (this is usually called "empathy"), and "complementary projective identification," reflecting the complementarity of the patient's internalized representations of important relationships. Complementary identifications can have two forms, one in which the patient plays his or her original historical role and another in which the roles are reversed.

Thus, in response to a male patient's bullying tone, I might be irritated, as would most people. I might, along with many other women, feel a pull to protect myself through ingratiation and to protect him from emotional discomfort, responses reflecting gender training. Unconsciously associating him with my father, I might feel affection and might try even harder to please him, an idiosyncratic response. I might, if receptive, begin to experience some of the agitation this man felt when, in childhood, he had been bullied by his own father. And at moments when the patient dropped his toughness, revealing a vulnerable side, I might discover a bully in myself, prepared to take advantage of his weakness. My own gender training, his projection onto me of a role filled by females, and my projection onto him of a male transference figure to whom I respond as I have in the past all work in concert to cause me to have a strongly "gendered" response.

The existence of multiple concurrent feelings, while confusing, is typical of much experience. Usually one feeling predominates; however, given adequate time and receptivity, all of the important unresolved relationships in the patient's past are likely to emerge in the interactional experience of the therapy. Except in extreme situations, some choice is possible as to which to attend to and amplify. Feelings may be tested for their probable significance and therapeutic usefulness. Since it is the unexpected feeling that carries the gift of unexpected insight, it should be kept alive by the therapist until it is fully understood. Control over feelings is limited, and since the therapeutic encounter can at times elicit overwhelmingly powerful emotions, it is helpful to maintain awareness of and reflection upon feelings, in preparation for moments in which reflection is made difficult by the intensity of affect.

The task of discussing countertransference in the treatment of eating disorders requires generalization and must inevitably result in the sacrifice of particulars. Despite a body of knowledge indicating that anorexia and bulimia are each associated with relatively characteristic early experiences and personality traits, clinicians have seen instances of each associated with nearly every imaginable background and character structure and have experienced nearly every form of countertransference. And yet some generalization is possible.

In many cases countertransference responses have been examined as a function of therapist gender. Conceptualizing eating disorders as a legacy of centuries of gender role stereotyping, it is disturbing to me to engage in gender stereotyping in discussing therapy. And yet gender is almost certainly the single strongest organizing force in our experience of others. We have difficulty evaluating any fact about a person unless we know that person's gender. Without this information we feel at a total loss, deprived of a crucial context for understanding.

Training as a therapist might be regarded as a process of "degenderization": Men learn to be more attuned to feelings and relationships; women learn to be less indsicriminately caretaking, more thoughtful and deliberate in their responses. Perhaps at some level of experience, distinctions between male and female responses begin to disappear. However, this process is never complete. Moreover, countertransference represents the recruitment of the therapist into the patient's most primitive construction of male and female. Therapists are drawn into almost archetypal roles that inevitably color their experience. It is my hope that readers will be able to apply what fits their experience, ignore the rest, and transcend the inevitable irritation elicited by overgeneralization.

COUNTERTRANSFERENCE AND ANOREXIA

As bulimia began to emerge as a defined clinical syndrome in the late 1970s and 1980s, it was inevitable that it would be compared to anorexia nervosa, from which it often evolves and to which it often reverts. At first glance, anorexia and bulimia seemed to be opposites—the one involving total self-denial, the other total self-indulgence. And yet, on closer examination, it became obvious that anorexics and bulimics share many characteristics: Both feel fat, both fear fat, and both aspire to an asceticism marked by food rejection and torturous regimens of physical work. Bulimics are, in a sense, failed anorexics, unable to control not only the impulse to eat but often the impulse to shoplift, to use drugs or alcohol, and to engage in so-called "casual" sex.

There soon developed a sort of debate within the field as to which group is more disturbed, reflected in studies that counted symptoms and compared such indices as social adjustment and rate of recovery. Therapists held opinions that seemed to them so self-evident that they were hard pressed to understand a differing response. Thus, some saw the bulimic binge as an obvious manifestation of a life force missing in anorexics, whereas others saw it as evidence of faltering ego control. To some, the fact that bulimia often occurs as a later stage in anorexia suggested that it falls on the route to recovery, while to others this suggested that it falls on the route to chronicity. To some, the empty perfection of the anorexic's life was horrifying; to others, the overflowing mess of the bulimic's was to be abhorred. These opinions were, for the most part, refractory to data, having little to do really with the course of the illness or recovery rate, but rather with subjective responses to the syndromes that were divided to some extent along gender lines. It has seemed to me that males are often more comfortable with anorexia, females with bulimia.

Gender Differences in Countertransference

To the extent that there indeed exists a gender difference in response to these syndromes, it is easy to see why this might be so. For anorexics display a severe arrest with respect to the goals of female development, while often keeping pace (or nearly so) with the goals of male development. The opposite is true of bulimics. The anorexic girl, far from moving toward a more sophisticated concept of interdependence, has rejected it altogether. She neither receives nor gives nurturance and is withdrawn from and seemingly uninterested in relationships. At the same time, she is fiercely motivated toward autonomy and achievement. In wrenching her body from dependence on anything, even nourishment, and bending it to her astonishing will, she is symbolically expressing traditional male "strength" in caricatured form.

Female therapists, in my experience, react with a much deeper horror to the curtailment of relational growth in anorexics than do males. I generally find "classical" restricting anorexics the hardest of any diagnostic group to work with. No matter how well prepared I may be, I am often baffled and stung by the rejection of my care and offended by the anorexic patient's lack of concern with others. Viewed solely by the standards of female development, she is a monster. And I know that there will be moments when I will recoil from her—when I will seek out people, food, and intense feeling as though I were starving myself—just as she will recoil from the monster she sees in me and in the bodily changes that threaten to make her like me.

Men do not, it seems to me, react with the same disapproval of anorexics that women do, and may even find traits to admire. For, threatened with a loss of selfhood, the anorexic girl has brought the force of an army to her battle against the flesh. In male therapists' attempts to treat her, she will not be rejecting the parts of themselves males hold most dear; in fact, men often put to good use their capacities to rationally assess, to teach, and to manage, escaping the devaluation of their "mothering" abilities.

Treatment may progress extremely well under the *Pygmalion* model, in which Henry Higgins firmly but gently tutors his young charge, ignoring her irrationality, successfully managing not to "personalize" her rejection, and laying out a developmental agenda as well thought out as Higgins's phonetic teaching method. If the treatment goes well, he will at some point have to endure his pupil's rejection of his definition of the relationship and respond to her demand for a more personal connection in which he shares feelings held in abeyance through the tutelage. If, like Higgins, he denies that such feelings exist or, if they do, that they are relevant or important, he will, like Higgins, squander much of the bond so painstakingly built.

Of course, the responses of male and female therapists to anorexics are colored by the responses of anorexics to male and female therapists. For most anorexic women, the onset of illness represents a retreat from relationships that threaten to overwhelm an already precarious sense of self, and this threat is embodied more by women than by men. There are some exceptions to this generalization. The violation of boundaries through incestuous emotional appeals or frank sexual abuse appears to trigger anorexia in a substantial minority of instances. If, as is usually the case, the perpetrator is male, then men will be more feared than women. Unmanageable losses may also cause a defensive regression. But in most cases, anorexia emerges in the context of increased pressures for relational growth attendant upon puberty, and against a family background in which she has long felt at risk of having her life co-opted by others.

Perhaps she is not valued for the unexpected gift of her never-before self, but is encouraged to conform to the limiting expectations of parents who do not value the unexpected in themselves, who are profoundly constricted, and whose own lives are shaped by the need to please. Perhaps she has felt tyrannized by parent(s) with a driven need to control. Following the theories of Selvini-Palazzoli, Johnson, and Connors (1987) argue that anorexia is the result of parental intrusiveness, which depending on whether it is "benign" or "malevolent," produces either a false self or borderline personality organization. Writing from a self-psychological perspective, Goodsitt (1984) contends that in anorexia the child's needs have been so consistently subordinated to those of the parents that vital self-functions have failed to develop. And probably in many instances parental overinvolvement is responsive to subtle deficits manifested early in the anorexic's childhood, which have prevented her from developing gratifying peer relationships. In this situation, mother and daughter may feel trapped in a relationship that they do not choose but cannot escape.

As the primary caretaker in most families, the mother is most often implicated in the problems noted above: the model and instructor of conformity, the intrusive parent who fails to maintain an appropriate boundary, or the parent who steps in to fill the gap in an isolated child's life. The father's contribution to the problem is usually excessive distance, robbing both the mother and the child of a connection that could attenuate the demands they place on each other. Detached, depressed, or unexpressive fathers intensify rather than compensate for maternal overinvolvement.

Treatment by Female Therapists

Confronted with a warm, interested female therapist, an anorexic patient is likely to feel alarmed. She fears being taken over by yet another woman, and may be ambivalent about even much-wanted progress, expecting that the therapist will take it as her own accomplishment. Identifying with an intrusive mother, the female therapist is likely to feel unwanted, thwarted, and anxious about how the patient's failure to thrive reflects on her. At the same time, she may be hard pressed to find traits and actions to encourage and admire, and, as noted earlier, she may be privately appalled by the anorexic's failure to embody values dear to her.

This is one instance in which countertransference disclosure is almost certainly destructive. The anorexic will hear any discussion of the therapist's response as criticism that she is not performing well enough or as a complaint about not being given enough power. Indeed, a female therapist is in a real dilemma. The expression, intentional or accidental, of her most honest feelings is likely to be understood not as an attempt to allow both therapist and patient to be more real and spontaneous, but as her attempt to force herself upon the patient and to gain control. In my experience, the way a female therapist can be most useful to an anorexic in the early stages of therapy is to accept her anger and rejection without retaliation or withdrawal. At this stage, even interpretations are apt to be heard as manipulative. But each time the patient criticizes or ignores the therapist, only to find that the relationship is still intact, she is learning something she needs to know: that a relationship can accommodate her painful search for self.

The female therapist will at times experience an identification with the patient's emptiness, her dearth of energy. In putting into words what she senses the patient feels, she gives the patient the experience of being genuinely understood. Even this the anorexic girl is likely to experience with ambivalence: To be understood is to be vulnerable to control. Moreover, what the therapist articulates is a source of despair in the anorexic's life, evidence of the tragic limitations of her attempted self-organization. For these reasons her reaction is not likely to be one of pleasure deriving from connection; indeed, she may pale even more.

Anorexics can feel to their female therapists like emotional black holes, absorbing seemingly infinite amounts of energy with no remaining trace. Women who have had adolescent girls may have an easier time with countertransference reactions, having experienced in a normal relationship the uniquely confounding combination of dependency and repudiation that requires a mother always to be concerned but never to care too much. Postmenopausal women, past some of the performance anxiety inherent in child rearing, may have an easier time still. However, it is never easy.

The successful treatment of anorexics by females often involves a paradoxical twist. Constrained in the early phases of treatment to relinquish as much control as can safely be done and to absorb hostility, the female therapist reaches a point at which confrontation and the assertion of her feelings are vital to the successful completion of the therapy. For as much as she is occupied with defusing the power of the mother vis-à-vis her daughter, she also symbolizes the mother's, and by extension the daughter's, power vis-à-vis the world. Often the daughter has tolerated her mother's having power over her because she senses her mother's vulnerability and the impoverishment of her other relationships. Now her mother, held at ransom by her daughter's illness, is reduced to utter powerlessness in even this relationship. To be able to reinvest in being female, the anorexic needs an opportunity to identify with a strong woman.

At first, confrontation by the therapist is best addressed not to what the patient has done or is doing to her, but to how she is cheating herself and others by her lack of engagement. The therapist's behavior must say, "I have wanted you to have the freedom you needed in our relationship, but I am not afraid of you. And when I need to, I can be very powerful." The patient's experience of a woman who is at once in favor of individuality, insistent upon responsibility in relationships, and powerful in conflict carries a crucial message about being female. Eventually the female therapist must include herself as a person with needs, giving her patient permission to do the same.

It can be helpful for an anorexic to see her female therapist in a group or in settings other than her own individual therapy where, in the therapist's responses to a variety of people and situations, she exhibits differing capacities. Although the anorexic is not likely to say so for a long time, she watches her female therapist carefully. Assessing the therapist's integrity in relationships, the patient decides how much to trust her. Watching the therapist's freedom to express herself and to take risks, the patient begins to revise her view of her own potential to communicate directly rather than through her body. Having made her relationship to her body the almost sole focus of her often considerable intelligence, she is attentive to her therapist's comfort or discomfort with her own body.

I have found it useful to talk to anorexic patients about my own body and body image, but with a few cautions. To do so too early deprives the patient of the opportunity to have her own reaction and to reflect upon it. Also, premature discussion is apt to be seen as propaganda. The therapist who does open this topic must be honest, for insincerity will be readily apprehended. Female therapists will have a difficult time working with anorexics if their own weight or appearance is an area of appreciable conflict for them. They may be unable to successfully contain the patients' anxiety and may unwittingly communicate envy, enhancing the patients' already intense sense of competition with, fear of control by, or guilt in relation to their mothers and sisters.

As important as the model a female therapist provides is the help given an anorexic's mother to live in a way that both meets her own needs and reassures her daughter. Whatever problems she may have had before her daughter's illness are almost surely intensified as her daughter's failure to thrive fills her with fear and casts suspicion upon her mothering ability. If the anorexia preserves the mother–daughter bond by arresting the daughter's development, it also makes a mockery of it. A "cure" that helps the daughter while ignoring the mother is likely not to be a cure at all. If the mother can be empowered with respect to her own needs and goals, this is the surest way to encourage her daughter to grow.

The injunction not to replace a parent unless truly necessary is more easily followed with anorexics than with bulimics, because mothering them is not so gratifying. Nevertheless, this can be a problem. The countertransference joy that a female therapist feels when an anorexic patient finally lets her in, combined with a tendency to overidentify with anger at the mother, often causes the therapist to place herself between mother and daughter rather than furthering their relationship. A persistent lack of interest in involving family members is, in my opinion, a countertransference problem in which the therapist is inducted into the patient's belief that improved relationships with family members are either unimportant or unattainable. Instead, the therapist supports the patient in trying to achieve an inappropriate and unrealistic agenda of self-sufficiency and autonomy.

Treatment by Male Therapists

A male therapist is apt to be experienced by anorexics with more curiosity and interest than a female one. Representing, as he probably does, a disengaged father whose unavailability has led to idealization, the male therapist's presence will be more welcome. His management of the anorexic's care (e.g., his instructions on eating, hospitalization, and weight restoration), though met with some resistance, may be experienced positively as an indication of involvement and concern, and as an opportunity for a wanted rather than a feared identification. The male therapist's generally less emotional style will probably make the patient feel safer, and, especially in the early stages of treatment, the relationship is likely to be smoother than with a woman. For the absent father is usually seen as valuable and desirable, and a wish to please him may yet exist in a girl who wants only to frustrate her mother. He is the "lost object" regained. My sense of male therapists' experience of therapy during this stage is that, for the most part, they feel relatively important and competent. Although males, like females, are subject to identification with patients' emptiness, this is less prominent, perhaps because their very presence alleviates it.

However, the patient's responses to her male therapist are certain to vacillate. The more she is pleased by his attention, the more she will feel disloyal to her mother, forcing her at times to withdraw. The more he attempts to understand her, the less he will please her, reminding her then not of her father but her mother. Any positive identification she feels with him will be tempered by the realization that she cannot become like him, but must instead remain a girl or become a woman.

Although the anorexic's idealizing transference to her male therapist provides an opportunity for her own sense of self to flourish in its reflected glow, she can as easily wither if he unwittingly mirrors her belief in the superiority of men. She may already distrust his affections, projecting onto him the devaluation of women implied in her father's detachment. The dynamics of the relationship will be as much those of courtship and defense against rejection, as of the control struggle and defense against merger experienced with a female therapist.

A crucial juncture in therapy comes when the patient, now attached to the male therapist, demands a glimpse into his feelings both as evidence that she is special to him and as proof that to have and express such personal feelings is not an aspect of female inferiority. The male therapist is apt to resist this subtle or overt request because of its seeming irrelevance, because of its impropriety, and because of the simple discomfort involved. But he can help her best by responding to this need. Strober and Yager (1984) suggest that therapists treating anorexics do well to have a sense of humor and flair for the dramatic. And it may be at moments just such as these that the therapist's expressive abilities provide anorexics with the much-needed lesson that everyone has a life of the heart.

Case Examples

The following examples illustrate a range of countertransference responses to anorexic patients whose overt behavior provided little obvious reason for the very different reactions elicited in the therapists. In each instance, the reactions became understandable with additional information about the patient's past. The first example concerns a fairly typical "empty" anorexic with onset of illness in adolescence.

Example 1

Lynette was asked by her college to seek residential treatment when, in her first year, her weight dropped to 80 pounds. She had little insight into her situation, able only to identify lifelong awkwardness with peers, which had lessened temporarily when she received positive attention for weight loss. Despite attributing her problem to peer rejection, she showed little interest in the women in the group and appeared immune to their increasing irritation with her failure to eat. Listening to her in groups, I would again and again drift into an abyss, becoming anxious as I realized that I had lost track of what she had said and had no idea how to respond.

During the multifamily session, our first impression of her father was of a man from a Western movie, jaw set firm and without a trace of visible emotion. Her mother, relocated from her own to another small Southern town because of her husband's work, seemed terribly anxious, self-doubting, and eager to please. She echoed Lynette's anxiety about peer acceptance as she talked about her social isolation, the impossibility of "breaking into" the town, and her eventual escape into work as a teacher. The father made a few stiff comments on request but otherwise remained silent. Her older brother, once socially backward and the identified family problem, seemed reluctant to get involved.

Lynette was petulant and irritable. Aware that she was not progressing and wishing to give the parents something to which they could respond, the therapists pointed out that Lynette was not doing well; she had, if anything, lost weight since entering the program. At this, her father became very angry. Showing feeling for the first time, he confronted her passionately about manipulating them and lying to them throughout her past treatments. Filled with emotion, he fought back tears as he described his fears for her.

Her mother then stepped in, supporting what her husband had said, but also telling him how angry she was about his usual lack of emotion and involvement. He acknowledged that she was right to be angry. Her voice began to sound less doubting. Lynette, now in tears, said that she had lied to them in the past but she was making a solemn promise to get better. And on that day she began eating voluntarily.

The heart of the countertransference to Lynette was an identification with her gaping emptiness. Growing up in a town in which they were forever strangers, their mother lonely and inhibited, their father irretrievably disengaged, she and her brother had both had difficulty relating to anyone. Neither had experienced themselves as people who could bring joy or stir passionate feelings in others. Lynette's flat recitation of her difficulties with peers was but a rote and hollow imitation of her mother's words, and did not reflect any real interest on her part in developing outside relationships. Indeed, it was when she left home and lost the bond of shared isolation with her mother that her anorexia had worsened. When her father became angry in the family session, she experienced, possibly more vividly than she ever had in her life, a sense of importance and possibility implied in his unexpected aliveness. This was enhanced by her mother's expression of anger at her father, which broke a pattern of silence, providing a model of real feeling and indirectly giving her permission to take care of herself.

Example 2

The next example illustrates a very extreme reaction of female therapists (myself and a colleague) to a young anorexic woman, an apparent result of projective identification.

Karalee was as remote an anorexic as I had ever seen and evoked an almost immediate distaste in me. Sitting motionless in groups, Karalee never spoke unless spoken to. Then an expression of annoyance fluttered across her face, as though she were tired of being interrupted. She seemed especially to resent the need to explain herself, and although she rejected as incorrect any guesses as to what she might be feeling, she never volunteered any clarification. Whatever moving event might occur in group, Karalee remained unmoved. Her individual therapist, also a woman, felt no connection to her and admitted that she had been disappointed when, after preliminary meetings, Karalee had decided to come into the program.

Her mother told us that at ages 3 and 4 Karalee had gone into trance-like states during which she masturbated, and that in grade school she had had an imaginary companion whom she blamed for anything bad she did. Karalee had had several hospitalizations, followed each time by renewed weight loss; her younger sister had also been anorexic, though less severely so.

During the multifamily session, concerns began to mount as Karalee passed up first one chance and then another to talk, saying wearily that she didn't feel anything. We came to a point where we had finished helping another family express their feelings to their dead mother, represented by a makeshift "corpse," and commented that the image of death must be one with which Karalee's parents lived all the time. It was decided that Karalee should lie in the place of the corpse so they could show her what they would feel if she were to die. Crying, her father expressed both sorrow and anger; her mother said that, after much therapy, she knew that whatever happened her life would go on. But her feisty sister, Emily, the carrier of life in the family, seemed the most genuine.

Asked what she had felt, Karalee said as usual, "I didn't feel anything," but added, "until Emily talked. Then I felt sad." This reminded me that she described crying when she looked at pictures of them together as children. Their relationship had ruptured in early adolescence when the family's absorption in Karalee's swim meets and the attention paid to Karaleee by Emily's male friends had caused Emily to withdraw in resentment. Karalee's illness began shortly thereafter.

We suggested that she and Emily spend the evening together. Both seemed excited when we asked Emily to bring down some of their old stuffed animals and "sleep over." I remembered that one of Karalee's few initiatives in the group had been to ask that the group have a pillow fight. As the group moved out of the circle for a break, Karalee waited for Emily and caught her hand. She said later that she was a little scared to spend the night with Emily because afterwards she might miss her even more. Watching her talk to Emily, I felt a tug of genuine affection for Karalee.

In this example, our response of uninterest and discouragement was responsive to the patient's projection of an irrelevant intrusion. At an early age, Karalee was observed to be different from other children. Her relationship with her sister was her most important one, vital to her sense of self and to her psychological stability. Her difficulty in relating to peers was compensated for during childhood by her bond with her sister, her accomplishments, and the extra attention she received from her parents. But this deficit placed her under greatly increased stress at puberty. Perhaps sensitive to her escalating vulnerability, her parents further increased their attention to her. This, combined with greater attention from peers, contributed to the rupture of her bond with her sister and her subsequent food refusal, the concrete manifestation of her inability to survive alone. Further anxious attention by parents and therapists only exacerbated the problem. Attempting to save her, her sister had followed her, becoming anorexic herself; however, being less dependent on the relationship, Emily had recovered. Karaleee could see in her "helpers" only useless obstacles to her real but unarticulated needs.

Example 3

In the final example, a very different reaction to a restricting anorexic signaled a different etiology and dynamic.

At 70 lbs., 42-year-old Mattie had the wizened face of an ancient medicine woman. Her frightened, childlike voice and gestures therefore came as a surprise. In our first group meeting, we asked each patient to tell us what she understood about her eating disorder. Waiting until last, Mattie professed bewilderment. Weight-preoccupied since adolescence, she had begun a diet 2 years ago. The weight loss had escalated into anorexia when her husband and daughter were in a near-fatal car accident. She had herself come close to death during several ensuing hospitalizations. Mattie made no connections among these events. She seemed barely to know what was going on in the room. I found myself wishing that I were sitting closer to her, feeling interested in and protective of her.

In a seminar preparatory to family meetings, the patients drew genograms. They were asked to indicate with blue arrows the direction of any physical, sexual, or emotional abuse by family members. "I can't talk about this," said Mattie. Then, shaking uncontrollably, she described 10 years of daily sexual abuse by her father, a violent man who had met her sister's dates in the driveway with a gun. She had also been abused by her older brother.

This time I was sitting beside her as she talked. I put one hand firmly against her back, another on her shoulder. When she finished talking I reached over to hold her. Sobbing in jerky gasps, her bony frame shaking, she clung to me for many minutes. Looking around, I saw the other women in the group, eyes overflowing, eager to come over and hug her, to tell her what her disclosure had meant to them.

The therapist's positive countertransference stemmed from a sense of being wanted and needed. Severely traumatized in childhood, Mattie had found refuge in a marriage to a gentle man and in her devotion to her daughter. When this was threatened by the accident, she could no longer maintain herself. Although fearful of rejection by her mother and sisters, she longed for their love and care. Therapists, too, were seen as valuable, with the potential to meet her needs.

COUNTERTRANSFERENCE AND BULIMIA

If anorexia represents abandonment of the normal female developmental line, bulimia represents an intense and seemingly unresolvable struggle with its core task: balancing the needs of self and others. Usually victims of some form of neglect, abuse, or trauma, bulimics are needy, emotionally labile, scared, and angry. Although binge-eating may be one of the few ways in which the bulimic woman permits the expression of her needs, the binge embodies for her, in the most frightening terms, what she regards as inappropriate, immature, and insatiable appetites—a source of both terror and shame. She fears exposure and rejection, and she fears uncontrollable regression and disintegration of her ability to cope and to stave off depression and self-destruction. She is also fearful for others, having usually seen at too close range the vulnerability of people she depended on.

In response to these fears, she has developed a defensive counterself who furiously disavows needs and directs her energies to caring for and pleasing others. More than an interpersonal strategy, this is an active opposition to her truer self, a striving to be wholly free of needs. In childhood, justifiably worried about the care available to her, she learned to take care of her caretakers. Now she gives to others what she needs herself, and tries to need nothing. She tries not to need food, but she fails, purging to reinstate the counterself following its collapse in binges. Like the anorexic, she strives for self-discipline, autonomy, and high levels of performance; however, unlike the anorexic, her needs are stronger than her resolve and may begin to be expressed not only in eating but in stealing, substance abuse, or other impulsive behaviors. Intimate relationships, while offering the hope that some of her needs might be met, are also a threat to her attempted self-organization, tempting her to expose unacceptable feelings and stimulating unacceptable dependency longings. Frequently she retreats from relationships, becoming perilously isolated.

Treatment by Male Therapists

It seems to me that, in general, male therapists have more problematic countertransference reactions to bulimics than do female therapists. They are more apt to feel unnerved or disgusted by the bulimic's collapse of self-control, and less apt to understand the relentless pressure of her concern for others. The male therapist is confronted with the bulimic's failure to achieve the goals of male socialization, and is further confused by her ambivalent endorsement of them—for if she finds needs unaccept-able in herself, she is unable to ignore the same needs in others. Failing in her attempts to be like a man, she is also the most frightening kind of woman, most like the male's representation of the mother from whom he felt such a powerful need to separate: caregiving, care-needing, emo-tionally larger than life.

It is perhaps for these reasons that many of the therapies developed for bulimia are therapies of "containment"—therapies designed to help the woman "manage," "cope with," "redefine" in more moderate terms, suppress, or "master" her needs. Discussion of the care of bulimic women by men is often riddled with distancing language ("these people") and military terminology ("attack symptoms," "monitor," "strategize," "devel-op a battle plan") not heard so often with respect to other problems. Bulimic women, I think, make men nervous, and men make bulimic women nervous in return, for bulimic women are exquisitely sensitive to signs of revulsion to their neediness. Male therapists, raised to deny such needs in themselves and to be critical of their expression by other men, may be tempted to encourage a male adaptation, which they believe to be more conducive to "success." Alternatively, male therapists may differen-tiate themselves from females by encouraging their female patients to show their emotions, while covertly feeling and perhaps conveying dis-approval.

Women in general, and bulimic women in particular, are so sensitive to this response by men that they are apt to curtail their expression of feelings before a male therapist has an opportunity even to become aware of his developing feelings, or of the fact that he is in any way communicat-ing them. The result is that unless his bulimic patient is unable to conceal her feelings, the male therapist may feel very little. He is being suc-cessfully "managed" by someone very good at it, and will be permitted to give advice or make interpretations with no hint of the rage these may be instilling in the patient or her sense of utter fraudulence in the relationship.

Bulimics, for their part, tend to bring to therapy more distrust of men than of women—the opposite of the pattern that occurs in anorexia. A fairly large minority of bulimics are exceptions to this rule; these are cases in which the daughter has received most of her nurturing from her father or, in an attempt to escape the plight of her mother, is strongly identified with him. But in most instances, the bulimic woman has a primary loyalty to her mother, having experienced her father as indifferent, abusive, or (most commonly) out ot touch. None of these transferences predispose her to experience a male therapist as receptive or understanding, and she may, at the worst, take some pleasure in keeping him excluded, rendering him stupid and contemptible by concealing from him the most important facts of her life.

Even in those instances where the father has been the nurturant parent, he has rarely been a true confidant, and she knows she has to relate to him at a level that does not strain his capacity for personal disclosure. Asked whether she is close to her father, such a woman will say, "Oh, yes. He would do anything for me." Asked, "Do you talk to him about your feelings?", she will reply in surprise, "Oh, no. I wouldn't do that." Thus, apart from (or in concert with) their fears of male disapproval, bulimic women have low expectations for men in terms of psychological-mindedness and tend to shut them out. When this is going on, male therapists may feel confused, and, when working in a team, aware of being excluded. How they react to this depends on how ego-syntonic this role is for them. Some will find it relatively normal; others may feel hurt and faintly paranoid.

The male therapist must work hard not to play out the bulimic patient's projections onto him. He must help her to express feelings in the face of her distrust of his capacity to understand or accept them. He must hold in check signs of approval for composure, self-control, or the apparent lessening of need, despite her attempts to elicit such approval from him. For he does her a disservice if he allows himself to be cast as a stereotypical father figure, or if he uses the relationship to prop up her crumbling defenses against legitimate needs. He must help her to hear his questions about her feelings for what they are, rather than as part of his assessment of her. She can all too easily elude him, responding to his questions with many facts but no meaning.

Countertransference disclosure can be immensely helpful in moving the relationship past this arid repetition of past interactional failures. If the male therapist can identify and articulate his sense of being shut out of a real relationship by the patient's silence, ingratiation, or editing of her feelings, he immediately changes the relationship. No longer can she project onto him indifference, detachment, or insensitivity; he is telling her that he sees beneath the surface of their interaction, that he too has feelings, that he is able and willing to talk about them, and that he is concerned about the quality of the relationship. This is likely to be so different from what the patient has come to expect from men that at first she may not know how to respond. But with repetition the male therapist's insistence on an authentic connection forces her to recognize the assumptions she has brought to their encounter and to move beyond them. When she does begin to open up, he needs to be explicit about his reactions to what she says, encouraging her to ask him any questions she has about what he is feeling. This is necessary to counter her projection of disgust or disapproval, which, if not contradicted, can again silence or slow down further disclosure.

What makes this process so difficult for male therapists is this: The projection is one so commonly made by females onto males that it may not produce any distinctive affect that can signal to the therapist his induction into a pathological process. As will be discussed later, female therapists are often unaware of their entry into a "depleted mother" identification because the associated feelings of worry, fatigue, and even victimization by others' emotional demands so often overlap with their "normal" state. Similarly, male therapists may be accustomed to interacting with women who are concealing the real intensity of their feelings, protecting them, or seeking their approval, and so may feel no special discomfort or altered self-experience when inducted into a patient's "detached father" projection. But if the male therapist attends closely to his experience of the interaction, he can uncover and modify his patient's limiting constructions of men. If he does so successfully, he may confer a special gift, encouraging her to settle for no less in her future relationships with men.

Treatment by Female Therapists

The female therapist faces an entirely different set of issues stemming from the similarity of values and conflicts. I find bulimic patients to be among the easiest to work with. I do not disapprove of their impulsivity nearly as much as I approve of their concern for others. Sensitive and caring, they are "good women" who I feel deserve help. I understand their needs and their worries, and, for the most part, they learn to trust me and gratefully accept my nurturance. I think that many women share this attitude, although as I look back I realize that I have not always felt this way.

Initially, treating bulimics made me anxious. I think that I readily identified with their conflict and felt tremendous pressure to help them "get control over things," but, like them, had no idea what this meant or how to do it. Experience has since taught me not to take a patient's worries about faltering control so seriously; I have come to realize that control will subside as an issue as her real needs and feelings are addressed. Later, as I was building my own career, I overidentified with bulimic patients' ambition, wanting them to "suceed," to "break free" of their "inadequate" families. Eventually, I felt compelled neither to "fix," "improve," nor "launch" bulimic women. I began to see that what they really needed from me and from their families were relationships in which they could safely express their pain. And I now saw their family members as victims of similar unmet needs, capable, like the bulimics themselves, of insight and change.

Over the years I have also become more comfortable with being frankly nurturing. For if female patients feel shame over expressing their needs, female therapists often feel shame over meeting them. In the context of female development, giving and getting are part of the same process, and it is one that is held suspect, especially by women working in predominantly male-defined systems. Both the need for and the willingness to provide mothering may be perceived as aspects of female inferiority. My sense is that many women therapists have long been nurturant to patients but have been reluctant to talk about it. Comparing her feelings and behavior to the therapeutic stance first described by Freud, and little changed since, the female therapist can hardly avoid feeling like a fraud.

Even if she knows that her patients get better, she may be haunted by a feeling that the process represents a second-rate shortcut. And, certainly, nurturing may at times be an inappropriate shortcut—one that blocks the patient's expressions of anger or other strong feeling, ignores or denies important tensions in the relationship, and ingratiates or infantilizes the patient. But surely women, raised to be experts in the art of real support, artists in the application of love and restraint, should trust their instincts in these matters, learning from mistakes.

It is perhaps for these reasons that many women therapists have moved away from the perceived confines of psychoanalytic theory; they have turned to theories of female development that include rather than omit, value rather than cast suspicion upon, their experience in therapy. In her discussion of these issues elsewhere in this volume, Steiner-Adair explains:

> I experience a real bind as a therapist when I try to speak in the language of traditional psychoanalytic theory . . . about my experiences of caring about my patients. . . . [It is a theory that]tends to cast my sense of myself as a real and separate person with strong feelings about my patients, especially compassionate feelings, in a pathological light

of either fusion or gratification or seduction. (Steiner-Adair, Chapter 10, this volume)

I do not think any examination of these issues can avoid asking how much the neutral stance advocated by most theories owes its existence to the needs and problems of men conducting therapy. The methods of therapy overlap with male skills, and the goals of therapy overlap with the goals of male development. And there are real problems in men trying to do therapy like women, more worrisome even than the problems of women trying to do therapy like men. For while women can, in most cases, safely nurture and touch female patients, when men do this there is a greater risk of sexualization of the relationship.

Tender feelings can slide unexpectedly into sexual ones. And men experiencing the same nurturing impulses that a woman might are justifiably wary of touching or holding a female patient. To do so is to stress a boundary that is imperfect in the best of us and whose integrity the patient may interpret differently than the therapist. Thus, touch experienced by a therapist as supportive and paternal may feel romantic or sexual to a patient. If, as is often the case with bulimic women, there is an undisclosed history of sexual abuse by a male in authority, touch by a male therapist can be particularly destructive.

This may reflect an advantage for women therapists, which, however unfair, cannot be denied and which constitutes an argument for their involvement in the treatment of abused and neglected women. Although Johnson (1989) has argued that, in treating bulimics, therapists should depart from technical neutrality and "err in the direction of being human," this is a harder task for the male than for the female therapist to negotiate, and one he must find difficult to talk about, given taboos against feelings in general and sexual feelings in particular. In treating male patients, I am acutely aware of the potential for sexual feelings to emerge and feel more constrained in my use of touch, even when it might facilitate mourning. The higher rates of sexual involvement with patients by male therapists may, in part at least, reflect the fact that in a society in which the majority of therapists are heterosexual and the majority of patients are female, men are more frequently exposed to temptation.

And yet female therapists have their share of difficult countertransference problems in treating bulimia. The bulimic woman typically projects onto the therapy relationship her relationship with her mother— usually one of neglect, born of the pressures of conflicting demands, inadequate support, and the continuing effects of her own unmet needs for mothering. Although the patient's deprivation and need may be great, so is her empathy. And so, in her relationship with her therapist as in her relationship with her mother, she is as likely to subtly provide care as to make demands, so that the transference is a relatively "silent" one. This projection, containing as it does the issues of many women, may very well "alloy" with the therapist's own introjective configuration such that she settles easily into her assigned role, reinforcing the patient's definition of the relationship by her own history as a daughter whose needs felt too great and later as a mother and therapist whose capacities for care felt too meager.

Because this identification can be so powerful, the female therapist must be watchful that she is not taken care of in ever more subtle ways by a patient always willing to ignore, deny, postpone, or readjust her needs to what she thinks can be given, expressing them only in the private fury of the binge. She must constantly question the patient's seeming contentment, asking always what else the patient feels, what hurts she is still concealing, what doubts about the work she is holding in reserve, in what ways (even within a seemingly positive relationship) the therapist is disappointing her. The therapist must not encourage her to continue taking care of others at her own expense by recoiling from the necessity to help her patient confront the perpetrators of past abuse, express the pain of her neglect, or make clear what she can no longer give. She must watch that she does not use kindness to suppress her patient's feelings, by offering sympathy when she needs to encourage her to go deeper and further. Therapists who work regularly with bulimics may not realize how dependent they have become on their ingratiating style until an experience with an entitled or hostile patient brings this to awareness.

As important as it is for the female therapist to help her patient be authentic in the relationship, it is equally important that she do the same, requiring both to transcend the limits of their history. This is the critical task in female development and the critical task in the treatment of bulimia. To ask the patient to be real by herself—to conduct an honest relationship all alone—is absurd at many levels. There is no authentic context within which to respond. She is asked to relate to her therapist in an artificial situation in which, by definition, her feelings will always turn out to be wrong: to be feelings more properly addressed to her mother or her father or anyone other than the therapist, who disavows all but neutral interest. The experience of being honest with a person who shows no responses is nontransferable to a world inhabited by people with real feelings.

In disclaiming her responsibility for an honest relationship in the guise of maintaining neutrality, the female therapist abandons the patient. She models nothing of value; instead, she mirrors her patient's problem, saying by her actions that a helping stance defined by an absence or transcendence of personal feelings is the best way to be. Female therapists find it far easier to deal in an honest way with their positive feelings than their negative ones. For as Adrienne Rich says, "Mother-love is supposed to be continuous, unconditional. Love and anger cannot co-exist. Female anger threatens the institution of mother-hood" (Rich, 1976, p. 46).

It is imperative that as women therapists we show our female patients the place of integrity in relationships. It is not enough to tell them that there are no "secrets"—that feelings, though unexpressed, are always betrayed. It is not enough to tell them that the anger they do not claim will nonetheless find its target. It is not enough to say that anger is as much a part of love as caring. We must show them that we mean these things by acting on them in this relationship. For as they struggle to free themselves from the necessity to ignore their own feelings while attending to others, bulimic women consciously or unconsciously test their female therapists' ability to do the same.

Case Examples

Example 1

The first example shows how a therapist's identification with a neglectful parent can be acted out in therapy. This is probably one of the most recurrent problems in the treatment of bulimia, and is often difficult to recognize. The therapist and her patient may engage in effortless repetition of parent–child interactions in which the child, having long ago learned that her needs cannot be met at an acceptable expense to others, now skillfully conceals them.

Jenny was in training to be a therapist. Avoiding the obvious pitfall of setting herself apart, Jenny was a good group member who made herself emotionally available. When her parents had divorced many years ago, only she of all the children had maintained a relationship with her father as well as her mother—a stance that had at times led to angry rejection by her siblings. Her father gave very little emotionally, refusing to initiate contacts with his children and controlling them through money.

The family session was the first time the parents and children had been together in years. On behalf of herself and her siblings, Jenny challenged her father's unavailability and extreme emotional detachment. Alternatively defending his stance and then seeming to "come around," he kept himself the focus of most of the interactions. Nonetheless, the children were able to discover similarities in their feelings, which had been obscured by past differences in alignment in the parental triangle. If, in the end, Jenny suspected that she had lost her father, she also felt that she had found her brothers.

The following week the body image group began dealing with sexuality. There were many difficult issues within the group: incest, rape, molestation, abortion, bodily shame so intense that one woman found it hard to bathe. Jenny said that she had no real issues. One morning, concerned about dividing the time, we asked group members to position themselves in relation to the center of the room to represent their readiness to work. To my surprise, Jenny went to the center. We had decided to have each member explain the issues they wanted to address and let the group decide which would be most beneficial to them. Jenny described fear of abandonment by men, and was selected by the group to work.

I was stunned by the group's decision. How could they have chosen an issue so clearly less important? Was this a popularity vote? Unfortunately, I stifled these feelings, and my cotherapist and I began a bloodless attempt to bring the issues to life in psychodrama—an attempt that, needless to say, failed. By the end of the group, all were convinced that Jenny was blocking the feelings connected with her father's abandonment of her. As the group was ending, I said that perhaps in focusing on her father, we were missing some issues with her mother. Jenny then told us that her mother, whom she had so far portrayed in positive terms, had not spoken to her for a year after a fight following the divorce. Jenny had learned to dress herself at 3, while the other children had continued to be cared for.

When I discussed the group with my cotherapist (who was also Jenny's individual therapist), we found that we had both been immensely irritated when Jenny had asked for help, "denying" her siblings what they needed and placing an unexpected burden on us. As the first girl, her mother had probably counted on her to suppress her needs and to help out. In their next session, her therapist offered this interpretation. Jenny intellectualized the problem, analyzing it from many sides. But when, as the session neared an end, the therapist responded to the impulse to put an arm around her, Jenny erupted in sobs, crying in her arms until the session was over.

In this example the other female therapist and I, initially eager to help, both made a concordant identification with the patient's neglectful mother. Eventually we so took for granted the patient's ability to deny her needs that we were enraged by her unexpected demand for help and acted out our anger before examining it. When we did, we discovered an even more important issue than the patient's abandonment by her father, to which we had been attending. The patient's pain was released not by words, of which she had probably had a surfeit, but by a touch that spoke directly to her emotional deprivation.

Example 2

The second example deals with an unexpected moment of truth in therapy. Confronted by the patients' inability to own and express their feelings, the therapist (myself) was brought to a choice point about whether to express her own.

This group was one unusual for its predominance of distant and conflicted relationships between the patients and their mothers. Only Leslie could count on her mother, but she felt trapped in the relationship. She sculpted an image of herself with no arms or legs; when I tried to explore the meaning, she hit me "by accident" in the head with a ball of clay.

During the multifamily therapy, each woman made some efforts to repair her relationship with her mother. The success of these efforts was mixed and when the family work was over, many of the women drew into themselves, seeming to be processing what had taken place.

Over the next few days, Leslie and the other patients became increasingly passive–aggressive, showing less and less initiative, "forgetting" assignments, tuning out the therapists. Arriving in the room one day to find them lying on the couch and reluctant to rise, I told them that I felt a surge of anger because they were using my energy without putting in any of their own. I ended a frustrating group session with a similar comment.

The following day, I opened the group room to a surprising scene. All the lights were off. A candle was lit, a radio was playing softly, and all but one patient (who arrived with me) were stretched out as though sound asleep, with covers over them. "Oh, you guys," I murmured in appreciation of their parody of my feelings the day before.

Like sleepy children, they gradually rose, yawning and stretching, stumbling to their places in our circle. "That was wonderful," I said. "I know a picture is worth a thousand words, but do any of you want to put some words to that?" They looked at me blankly. "I thought it was a reference to my having gotten on you yesterday for lying around when I came in." Speaking for the group, Leslie denied any meaning, deflecting the topic with maddening non sequiturs: "Is there any psychological significance to which side you sleep on?"

"That makes me feel so alienated that I don't know what to say. To do that in response to what happened yesterday, and then for all of you to disown that it had any communication value makes me feel like you just walked up and slapped me." Still no one responded. At last, I said, "I'm so angry I don't know what to do. I feel like leaving." My cotherapist asked, "Do you need to leave for a while?" "Maybe so," I said, and walked out into the hall. I immediately hurried back into the room.

"I shouldn't have left," I said, "that was a huge mistake. That's probably what made you afraid to say what you feel in the first place—the fear that you would be left." One of them said, "I felt you didn't really mean it; you were just trying to get a reaction, but you weren't really upset."

"Well, I was upset," I continued with obvious feeling. "I don't know what it takes to get through to you guys that I really do feel things and that I'm in here struggling with you as human beings and I'm sick of this shit. . . . I want more for you. And you should too. You're cheating everyone who's ever going to come in contact with you. This is not the way you fight. You fight with courage, you don't do it in this incredibly underhanded and dirty way. You face stuff. I was very wrong to leave the room."

"It makes me so sad for you," I began anew, "because I do understand that it's hard for you to trust—at some level all of you have been betrayed." I began to cry. "I'm so sorry that happened, but you have to trust again." I looked up to see their eyes filling with tears and I stopped talking. They began to talk.

In this example the origins of the countertransference response were perhaps less important than what to do about it. Clearly many of the patients had distrusted my sincerity and interest—a fact that became evident in further discussion. Many feared that this was "just a job" for me and expressed pain over such incidents as seeing me in the hall between sessions and having me simply say "hello" and pass by. Behind the anger was great need for a mother who really did care. Leslie, whose relationship with her mother was secure if oppressive, became the provocative "spokesperson" for the group's anger and led them to act out what was, in effect, an escalating test of the sincerity of my relationship with them. Together we created an event that could reassure them of their importance to me. This settled, they were freed up to risk more honest relationships with one another.

Interpretation might never have resolved this impasse. "If you want us to be real," they seemed to say, "you do it first." As they well knew, I had much less to lose. My response was not, however, one planned and chosen with these considerations in mind. The target of intense interactional pressure in my relationships with them, I found myself with sudden and strong feelings I could barely hide. The only choices were to be honest, hoping that my feelings contained more than irrelevant residues of my own past, or to irrevocably distance myself from them with a series of covering lies.

The best argument for countertransference disclosure is that honesty nourishes and sustains human connection. The second best argument is that there is often no acceptable alternative. Our feelings toward our patients are determined, more than by anything else within our control, by whether or not we express them. The relationship comes to consist either of the infinite compounding of unventilated feelings or the fresh occurrence of new ones. Countertransference disclosure almost always gives both patient and therapist the opportunity to experience one another newly. A therapist I know said often that no therapeutic error is serious unless it is repeated; any mistake that is caught can be fixed. In the spirit of her remark, I feel we do best to trust and use our strong feelings—prepared, if necessary, to correct mistakes, but not to let relationships die of malnutrition.

COUNTERTRANSFERENCE AND SEXUAL ABUSE

Because so many eating-disordered women have been victims of sexual abuse, it seems important to give some attention to the countertransference issues in their treatment. In our setting, 59% of a series of women coming for intensive residential treatment of bulimia were found to be victims of incest, childhood molestation, or rape (Kearney-Cooke, 1988). The issues of sexually abused women overlap markedly with the issues of bulimic women, and it is not surprising that bulimia is one way in which abuse victims' pain is often expressed.

Sexual abuse instills or intensifies body shame, creating in many women a drive for "purification" that may be served by self-starvation or purging. Like bulimics, sexual abuse victims are often parentified children who habitually deny their own needs. Indeed, human contact is apt to feel dangerous. And like the bulimic, the victim of childhood abuse has been neglected, her need for protection having gone unmet. In most cases of incest, the nonabusing family members have been unavailable to her. Similarly, the rape or molestation victim suffers more serious consequences when she feels she cannot turn to her family to assist her in recovery. Finally, a history of abuse, like bulimia, constitutes a shameful secret that creates social and emotional isolation.

Countertransference Horror

Therapists are often shocked and sickened by revelations of abuse, and understandably so. The inability to overcome this aversion might be considered a countertranference manifestation that has contributed to the suppression of abuse disclosure, beginning with Freud's recasting of reported abuse as patient fantasy and continuing in attenuated form to the present. To protect ourselves, we have apparently sent powerful messages to our patients not to burden us with such disturbing information. There are a few similar examples in which a "rare" problem is suddenly found to be common because a change in therapists' awareness facilitates disclosure. Indeed, female therapists' reports of high abuse rates among their eating disorder patients have at times been held suspect by male therapists who did not "see" this phenomenon.

In some instances men seem to feel an even deeper horror in

response to revelations of abuse than do females. Perhaps this stems from a greater tendency to identify with the perpetrator; perhaps it stems from their greater sense of responsibility to protect women; perhaps it arises from the fact that identification with the victim's experience of boundary violation represents a threat to identity as well as to safety. Also, women often carry some small measure of immunity to abuse, gained from inoculations in their own history. In withholding information on abuse from their male therapists, patients may be protecting them. Within our staff, however disturbed the female therapists were by the details of abuse, the males were more so. In other cases, patients who withhold disclosure of abuse from male therapists may be protecting themselves, anticipating disbelief or blame. Obviously, many males in our society have an ability to distance themselves from the horror of abuse; this is inevitably true of some male therapists, though it is hardly the rule.

Experience in working with abuse tends to correct the problem of initial horror, but therapists who have achieved tolerance may still at times be unexpectedly overwhelmed by the details of some event. It is not harmful for a patient to see her therapist's response, provided that the therapist makes it clear at all times that it is the perpetrator's and not the victim's behavior that is shocking. It *is* harmful for the therapist to emotionally pull away at such times. Abuse victims are usually very sensitive to even subtle manifestations of distancing and require continuing encouragement to complete the necessary description of details. As "countertransference horror" subsides, other problems take its place. Two kinds of complementary identification are common: identification with "unseeing" parent(s) and identification with the abuser.

Complementary Identifications

Identification with the "unseeing" parent is a remarkably powerful dynamic with potentially destructive consequences. It is not synonymous with the suppression of disclosure discussed above, but occurs in therapists who have had much experience working with abuse. In essence, the patient engages the therapist in a re-enactment of parental inaction, in which even disclosed abuse is repeatedly forgotten, ignored, or minimized. Therapists experiencing this form of countertransference may feel the reported details of the abuse slipping away like fragments of a dream as they struggle in vain to hold onto them. Or they may find themselves numb, even bored. When this happens, it seems to me that countertransference disclosure is essential to repair the damage. The therapist must acknowledge what the patient knows—that the therapist has neglected the patient's vital and legitimate needs. The two must then struggle to understand how this happened and what it means.

If, in ignoring the patient, the therapist replicates parental indifference, in acknowledging and trying to understand the neglect the
therapist is doing something the patient's parents have not done: admitting and taking responsibility for inappropriate behavior. The patient is
not only reassured to know that others can be concerned enough about
her to scrutinize themselves, but often learns something about how she
helps to perpetuate nonresponsiveness—not only with respect to abuse,
but with respect to other needs and problems as well. The problem of
forgetting what has been said is so common that therapists who work with
abuse do well to routinely take notes or to audiotape or videotape sessions
so that information can be retrieved.

The second common countertransference phenomenon is complementary identification with the abuser. These feelings are so unacceptable to therapists that they almost always come in disguised form, in
which contempt for the victim masquerades as something else. This often
takes the form of a rapidly growing impatience with the victim's "inability" to feel or express anger toward the perpetrator. The therapist's
frustration with the patient for her defense of the perpetrator may es-
calate into near-rage. This is, of course, in part an identification with the
patient's unexpressed feelings, and therapists are certainly more comfortable seeing it as such. But self-examination will usually reveal a telling
element of sadism, particularly toward women who have been the victims
of rape or other violent abuse.

This countertransference response carries a great deal of energy and
in groups is often shared by a number of people. Ignored, it may lead
group members to unconsciously reject the victim, allowing her to embody unworthiness and weakness. In my opinion it must, at some point,
be discussed, since it is inevitably felt by the patient and may otherwise
leave her feeling diminished and afraid of the therapist and other
patients. However, it may be used in various ways. A common dilemma
in treatment is that even after much work that honors the complexity of
the patient's feelings, she may indeed experience a block in reclaiming
dissociated anger, which leaves her vulnerable to further abuse. She may
work through the dangers associated with feeling to re-experience the
terror; she may work through her loyalty to the perpetrator to know that
he or she is guilty; and yet she may still be unable to feel or assert the
anger that would signal that she claims the right to protect herself.

Sometimes by accident and sometimes by design, the expression of
countertransference anger by therapists or fellow patients becomes the
experience-near arena in which anger is mobilized. In telling them to get
off her back, the victim of abuse is speaking to her abuser. Because of its
ability to re-empower, a therapist may choose to let this countertransference be acted out, to be followed by an analysis of what occurred. In such

situations, other patients feeling the anger may need help to understand their responses as much as the victim does. The shared experience of the dynamics of abuse gives group members a powerful and useful insight into the way in which the helpless rage of victimhood is transformed into the heady power of abusiveness, particularly when a suitable "victim" is made available.

Case Examples

Example 1

The following example illustrates the power of the hear-no-evil, see-no-evil phenomenon within a treatment team drawn into identification with unseeing parents.

Jane announced by her words and demeanor in the first group the likelihood that she would "blow-off" treatment. She matter-of-factly listed past failures, described her family's frustration, and announced that she had brought her computer and planned to do a lot of studying while here. I commented that she seemed to have a plan already in mind to sabotage her treatment. She agreed. The therapist and group members were soon frustrated by Jane's intellectualizing. Sculptures and pictures of herself depicted a disembodied head. I liked her but became reluctant to do work focused on her, knowing I would get nowhere.

On the first morning of the multifamily session, each family constructs a genogram, using a color code to identify traits of individuals. The patients have already done this before their families come, but now the family must try to achieve consensus. Afterwards each patient presents her genogram, along with comments on what she sees in it, to the larger group. After this, families are divided up for a half hour or so while mothers meet together, as do fathers, siblings, husbands, and children.

I was meeting with the bulimic women. One of them had noticed Jane's name on the genogram circled in yellow, indicating a sexual issue, and asked about it. Jane shook her head furiously, hands held up in front of her, saying "Oh, no." The group eventually persuaded her to reveal a violent rape. She had told her sister about it. Although she realized that her parents had been told by her sister, it had never been discussed. When we urged her to bring it up with her family, she adamantly refused; however, I was confident that we could help her do this, as we often had with others in the past.

When the staff met that noon, I shared Jane's disclosure. No one ever thought of it again until 3 days after the family therapy had ended, *after* Jane again brought it up. At this point the therapist who had helped the group construct the first set of genograms remembered that even in that session Jane had circled herself in yellow. "I went around and asked everyone about every yellow circle, but I completely forgot to ask her."

The next day in group I told Jane that I felt we had let her down badly, ignoring the problem just as her family had. When she was unable to describe the rape, I suggested that she enact each person in her family, articulating their unwillingness to hear about the rape. She eventually asserted her need to talk about it, said that the exercise had been helpful, and in a later group vented some of her anger.

Still, she refused our suggestion that the family be brought back and became increasingly agitated. Two days later Jane arrived at her individual session with a note saying that at 13, on a combined family fishing trip, her uncle had molested her. He had succeeded in disrobing both of them and there had been a violent struggle. When she had told her parents they had dismissed it, saying he was just being affectionate.

In this example, every member of our staff with experience in treating sexual abuse responded to the patient's interactional pressure to ignore her abuse. The repetition of parental indifference required that we be repeatedly informed of the abuse and then suppress the information. Jane was forever caught in a leap between two cliffs, unable to go forward and unable to go back. Her need to have her experience known and her fear of the consequences constituted a classic approach–avoidance conflict. The intensity of her conflict was matched by the consistency with which we failed to deal constructively with her situation. When this was recognized and acknowledged, she was able to move forward in small steps.

Example 2

The following example illustrates complementary identification by therapists and fellow patients with the perpetrator of abuse. The countertransference response was used within the group to further the patient's work.

Toby was an extreme people pleaser. With a long history of bulimia, alcoholism, and cocaine abuse, she certainly had her troubles, but she always smiled and had something positive to say. She was living with a man who had terminal cancer, unable to leave him. Each day, Toby heaped praise on the program, saying how much it had already helped her. We saw no progress. Her large family was unresponsive to her— dismissive, defensive, and tired of her promises. Although she had felt enormous pain over neglect by her mother, she could not express her anger to her.

In the third week of treatment, Toby revealed a series of abusive incidents including a date rape. In a courageous enactment of this, Toby relived hurt and terror. But as we tried to empower her to push away the perpetrator, she could not speak without smiling, could not mobilize her body. Sensing the group's growing agitation and anger, I invited them to parade past Toby voicing their disgust or frustration. "There is an abuser in each of us at times," I said. "If you feel abusive, consider expressing your feeling and seeing what you learn." Several group members did so, as did I. Toby stopped smiling; her face settled into stony anger. She answered the charges directed at her. The women who had criticized her began to feel sickened. I said that while abusers are fully responsible for their own behavior, by playing the part of a victim Toby had elicited our sadistic feelings, allowing us to escape our own feelings of vulnerability.

The next day Toby told us how angry we had made her. For the first time since I had known her, she spoke with authority and congruence. She looked and sounded angry. The group continued to struggle with their feelings about becoming perpetrators, but Toby said she was glad it had happened, because it allowed her to see how she let other people push her around. She continued to seem more real in her interactions.

The ease with which we were able to identify with the abuser was due in part to Toby's projection and in part to our own prior experience in situations containing some of the same elements. Virtually everyone has at some time felt victimized or victimizing even though their experiences may have been far less traumatic than Toby's. The allure of the victimizer stance lies in its ability to free an individual of uncomfortable identification with the victim: to allow another to take on all of one's own vulnerability and to experience power. Toby got angry because this process in essence replicated the original abuse in which another person's sense of power was won at the cost of her own intimidation and terrorization. It is often difficult for a woman to mobilize anger against her real life abuser not only because she senses that it is dangerous but also because her empathy for the abuser's underlying vulnerability is so great. By comparison, the anger may be readily mobilized by lesser expressions of sadism, which pose no actual physical threat and which are used by the individuals involved to reduce relatively minor psychological discomfort.

COUNTERTRANSFERENCE AND BORDERLINE PATIENTS

No discussion of countertransference in the treatment of eating disorders is complete without acknowledging the special problems experienced with certain borderline patients. Borderline personality is a problematic diagnosis, one that sometimes operates as a marginalizing term for women, obscuring rather than calling attention to a history of abuse and neglect and justifying an unwarranted lowering of therapeutic goals. My aim is not to further stigmatize these women but to examine the interactional problems that occur in working with a subgroup whose difficulties might, in my opinion, be better termed interpersonal chaos syndrome than borderline personality disorder. These are women in whom a particular combination of trauma, inadequate parental support, and, perhaps, an enhanced biological susceptibility to intense affective states has led to continuing inner turmoil. Their rapidly shifting projections onto others create emotional havoc, with the result that few relationships endure long enough to provide them with the stability and care that they need in order to heal. The treatment of these patients can involve countertransference reactions so disruptive and disturbing that, without help in processing them, some therapists refuse ever to see such a patient again. For their treatment can arouse an excruciating combination of dread, anger, and the sensation of being gradually but profoundly compromised.

I once told a young colleague that she would know she had seen such a borderline patient if she left the first session feeling slightly sick to her stomach. She would, if she let herself think about it, realize that in response to the patient's pull she had done something that now made her inexplicably uncomfortable. Unless she attended rapidly to these feelings, she would begin a series of attempts to set things right that would leave her feeling ever more wrong. Afraid not to honor what seemed to be an implicit promise already made to go another mile down the river, but to build a fortress there, she would look up to find herself 50 miles downstream and committed to another outing tomorrow. At some point she would be too ashamed of what she suspected were breaches of professionalism to ask for help.

Borderlines and their therapists seem to become trapped in a reverberating circuit of anxiety. The therapist's inability to contain the patient's unmanageable feelings and to set limits on the patient's subtle threats, overt aggression, or seduction creates in the patient an escalating anxiety, triggering more attempts to test or punish the therapist. I have learned over the years that when I can break this cycle by speaking honestly of my own experience, the patient relaxes, feeling a renewed trust in me and in the therapy. This process will have to be repeated many times, but it is a necessary one. In some cases, when the patient must be interrupted in the expression of very strong feelings relevant to abuse, limit setting may produce an initial rage response. But reassurance that her anger will not be ignored and that she will be helped to express it in nondestructive ways allows her to accept the limit.

The histories of all the very poorly integrated borderline patients whom I have treated have combined severe early abuse and an inability on the part of the parents to protect the child from extremes in her own behavior. It is as though the early tantrum in which a tormented and exhausted child begins to fling herself against walls, kick and thrash at those around her, and scream for help has been retained in a modified form in the adult personality. To the extent that we, as therapists, identify with the failing parent, we feel helpless and out of control, alarmed by the readiness with which we have relinquished responsibility to a patient obviously unable to assume it alone. If we become identified with the abusing parent, we feel hardened, cold, even sadistic. Therapists accustomed to feelings of warmth and nurturance toward their patients are astonished and ashamed to find themselves harboring feelings that are sometimes most honestly characterized as hatred. If we identify with such a patient's feelings, we feel cranked up to the breaking point, unable to put whatever feelings we have aside, frantic for someone to help us—in short, on the verge of a tantrum ourselves. These feelings can lead to withdrawal, panic, anger, despair, and heroic but ill-conceived efforts to rescue the patient and salvage ourselves.

Female therapists appear to experience more distress in their countertransference to borderline patients than do males. This may be just "appearance." It may be that men simply deal with the feelings stirred in them differently, maintaining a degree of detachment that protects them from extremes of feelings. If not carried too far, this may serve the patient well. But there is a risk that excessive detachment will leave the patient feeling emotionally abandoned, her suffering "objectified" beyond recognition. Females are, in general, less likely to detach and more inclined to solve problems in relationships by giving more. In contrast to the many situations in which this instinct may be useful, it can exacerbate the tensions of a patient who is already losing control. For while she needs to feel that her therapist is emotionally connected to her, she also needs a competent "parent" who is able to interrupt a "tantrum" without ignoring, rejecting, or punishing the overstimulated and frayed child whose behavior is as chaotic as her inner life.

Often the father or mother of a borderline patient will tell us about his or her abdication of the parental role, stating that the child's moods and behaviors were inexplicably and uncontrollably extreme. In some cases this represents a highly pathological denial or minimization of the known stresses on the child. For example, one mother, herself a victim of severe abuse, complained about how her daughter had "overreacted" to sexual abuse and to seeing her mother beaten. But sometimes the parent is simply inadequate to the task of managing problems that he or she does not understand. Thus, for example, the child may be acting out in response to undisclosed sexual abuse. Problems may be intensified by inborn aspects of the child's temperament. And sometimes family members are just indescribably depleted, becoming helpless in the face of one more demand.

The following dream, told by the mother of a borderline woman named Portia, illustrates her sense of helplessness with respect to the demands made upon her. She told this dream after a session the night before in which two of her daughters had unleashed seemingly limitless rage upon their brother and father for past abuse. The following day, we gave each family member 10 minutes to talk without interruption. There evolved a story of singular loss and tragedy across the generations. Her mother chose to use her time to describe a dream she had had shortly after Portia had asked her to come the more than 2,000 miles to this session.

> I was at home . . . and there were a couple of strange young women in the far end of the room. One came up to me and I realized that she was blind, that they were all blind. She said, "I guess I'll go to bed," and I said, "Oh, don't do that. Sit here with me while I wash dishes and then we'll go for a ride." . . . And then Portia appeared . . . and she said, "I have to go to the library." "You'll enjoy the new one," I told her, and she said, "Well, I've got to have the car."
>
> So, the next thing I know, I had the keys and I was taking off out the door. And then I was on a strange road—a four-lane road—but it was a strange road and I felt like I was maybe 4 miles from home and I said to myself, "What are you doing here? Portia has to have the car." So I thought, "Well, I'll go up to the top of this hill and then I'll get turned around and headed back."
>
> Well, I got there and there was a train across the road and . . . I was boxed in. [T]here was . . . a warehouse there that had accommodations. I apparently stayed the night and in the morning . . . I asked the price and they said it was $92. Well, I was appalled by that. And I wrote them a check . . . and that was when I woke up. So I got the feeling that if we didn't help Portia that it would cost us more in the long run than making this trip would.

The dream seemed to address the difficulties experienced by Portia's mother in responding to the often conflicting needs within her impaired family, represented by the blind children. Surprising even herself, she made a choice not to give in to Portia's demands, but then she turned back. In the end, she perceived that she had been punished for not giving Portia her way in the first place. While her decision to come to the family meeting was, I believe, a good one, the dream revealed a difficulty in setting limits that appeared to have been long-standing. In choosing to tell the dream, she seemed to be trying to tell us something about her relationship to Portia that she could not otherwise articulate.

As an adult, the acting-out borderline patient is frightened when her manipulative or destructive behavior goes unchecked. Seeking temporary refuge in anything that can make her feel better, she still hopes to find a relationship that will heal her, but knows that she drives others away. She is highly sensitive to signs of incongruence in a therapist who is afraid to be honest, and she understands that in winning—in successfully wielding excessive power over her therapist—she is losing again. It is in the extent of her ability to push her therapist into extremes of discomfort that she tests the therapist's ability to contain her destructive assults on the relationship. At times it is necessary for the therapist to set clear limits on the patient's behavior. But the therapist conveys an equally important message each time he or she responds with candor, resisting the pressure to meet a patient's apparent need at the expense of her greater need for an honest relationship.

Case Example

The following example concerns a borderline woman with a history of some fairly extreme acting out in her previous treatments. Caught off guard by her behavior, the therapist (again, myself) rapidly became dishonest. It was a dishonesty more of omission than commission, but caused me to dread contact with the patient until, by owning up to my feelings, I began to establish a therapeutic relationship.

Julia noticed everything and sent signals of approval and disapproval that were hard to ignore, Explaining in a group that each member should do what she needed to do to feel safe, I saw Julia register this message with satisfaction. Later, when I confronted another member's manipulativeness, Julia fairly glowed with approval. But the following day, when we did a long and successful piece of work with that patient, Julia conspicuously removed herself from the group. It no longer, she explained, felt safe. I doubted the sincerity of this response, but I lacked any real evidence.

The next day Julia told us that she had overdosed on laxatives the night before and was experiencing an impulse to harm herself. As the group was nearly over, I asked, "Is there anything we can do to help you now?" "Yes," she said, looking at me with an expression of vulnerability, "I would like to be held." Caught off guard, I prepared to embrace her. She made no move in my direction. "Who would you like?" I then asked. Savoring her power, she looked slowly about the room, circling it with her eyes several times, and then named my cotherapist.

I was embarrassed, but watching the other therapist, I was relieved that I was not the one now locked in an interminable embrace. I remembered her individual therapist reporting that Julia had asked her to hold her during their last session. I remembered a statement on her application for treatment that one of her referring therapists often held her. How could I have forgotten these things? I felt a little sick, but I couldn't think of any useful way to discuss my feelings.

The next day we asked who wanted to work. "I would like to do some work," said Julia. Stalling for time, I asked, "Anybody else?" Another patient mentioned how helpful her work the day before had been. "I'm curious," I said in evasion of Julia's request, "there's a lot more you could do. I wonder if it's hard for you to ask for more." For several minutes my cotherapist assisted me in evasion, broadening the issue to women's trouble in asking for help.

At last I faced what I was doing and said to Julia, "I will admit that when you said, 'I want to work,' my heart sank—that I was hoping it would be somebody else. Because I feel that in working with you, I'm set up for failure. No matter what I do, it won't be good enough and I'll get a very harsh response. As though you were a rattler softly rattling in the bushes and you will strike me at some point. And I say this not to avoid our work—I think it's the heart of our work."

I continued, "As a therapist my job is to help you, and there's a part of me that cares, but there's also a big part of me that doesn't want to be abused. You said you wanted me to be blunt with you and I need to be, because otherwise I will be simulating warmth I don't feel. And you'd pick up on it in a second. I think that may be the way you test people—to see how much they'll act incongruently with what they're feeling."

"Yes," Julia agreed. "But I do need you and other people to be direct with me because people are fearful of me and not direct with me, probably because I can strike out—and sometimes in a real nonverbal way."

I replied, "My sympathy for abuse victims ends at the point where they become abusers. So I think you need to stop it for other people's sake, but also for your own, because I believe you engender much more anxiety and backing off in other people than you're aware of."

Later I mentioned that in interacting with her I felt I had some sense of the fear she felt growing up, as though it was now built into her. "There's an abuse that's perpetuated internally by you and you spread it around."

"It's in my muscles," Julia said, a tear rolling down her cheek.

"What is the tear for?" one of us asked.

She began crying. "I feel like my whole body is a thermometer and a lot of the things I respond to don't even come through my head. And the anger that can come up is like some part of my body has just been touched."

"Where's the pain in that for you?"

She cried harder. "That I'm not in control."

My feeling of dread in this example stemmed from several features of the interaction. First was my sense of Julia's duplicity and my inability to get hold of it so I could talk about it. This left me feeling dishonest and incapable. Next was the incongruence between Julia's presence as a patient (her requests for help, for nurturance) and Julia's subtle assumption of a one-up position in which she became the judge of my cotherapist and me, conferring approval or disapproval on our interventions, relishing the power to choose who would hold her. Finally, there was Julia's maddening presentation of herself as our victim, a projection expressed in her statement that the group was "unsafe," at the same time that her alarmingly sudden mood shifts portended a capacity for unfettered rage.

I was, in part, responding to Julia's rapidly shifting projections of an abusing parent and an incompetent parent. One minute Julia was the frightened victim and I was the abusing and indifferent parent. The next minute Julia was the wily, manipulative child and I was the defeated parent. Because I could not locate the target of my mounting anger—the innocent victim or the provocateur—I could not locate myself and became confused, paralyzed by conflicting inner directives to give more and to give less. Beginning to doubt my competency, I dreaded any interaction with the patient that would further expose me. But Julia, unable at times to control rapid shifts in her experience of others, was compelled to engage them in interactions that provided her with vitally needed information: how the other would respond if she allowed herself to get close, and, as an almost inevitable consequence, subjected the other to her extremes of feeling.

When I expressed my dread, however imperfectly, I was giving Julia her first reason to trust me. Julia saw to her relief, that she could not bully me into silent helplessness. She saw that I could be angry without becoming abusive, an experience missing in critical earlier relationships. She saw that we could be honest with each other. Reassured, she was able to begin talking about her most important problem—the intense feelings that welled up in her, outside her control.

Julia put us to a test before each new piece of work in the group, berating us, rejecting our help, or walking out. In some instances, we simply proceeded with the group's agenda, explaining the choice that was being made. In other cases, when any further postponement would have been to Julia's detriment, a firm insistence that she continue with her work allowed her to resume. Patients such as Julia, more than any others, stir up in therapists the sense of vulnerability associated with intense emotional states. Such patients need their therapists to be able to make an empathic connection: to remember or to grasp the terrible sensation of passing an emotional point of no return. They need their therapists to understand this feeling but not to let them repeatedly act on it to their own lasting detriment. The borderline woman's awareness of her own inability to manage destructive impulses in important relationships is, in the end, her most terrible secret of all.

REVELATION AND COUNTERREVELATION IN EXPERIENTIAL THERAPIES

It has been an article of conventional wisdom that both transference and countertransference most often develop within the context of a long-term relationship between a patient and a single therapist doing individual therapy. It might be more accurate to say that transference and counter-transference become most intransigent within this context. Other forms of therapy—especially experiential ones that involve role taking by patients and therapists—may actually enhance the potential for experi-ence and expression of transference and countertransference, by provid-ing a safer and more evocative format in which the "interactional pres-sure" of projective identification may exert its effects. At the same time, by providing a clear division between the "as-if" or enacted interchange and the return to "real selves" that occurs at the end of such experiences and during their processing, it allows patient and therapist to experience strong feelings toward each other that are less likely to become an enduring part of the relationship. Knowing that there will be an end, and that it is only "pretend," makes it feel safer to both parties to take risks.

These therapies offer the potential of important revelation as patients become aware of the intense and unexpected feelings engendered in them, as therapists do the same, and as both allow a narrative to develop by freely responding to unconscious cues from each other. This is best done in groups for many reasons. More players are available to complete the psychological tableau under construction. The presence of a second therapist makes it possible for the first to enter a role relationship that may temporarily make her or him less useful to the patient as a coach, supporter, or link to reality. Any role can be played by multiple people, in sequence or simultaneously, permitting opportunities to validate the feelings engendered in the role by comparing responses with others. In my experience, projective identification often takes place rapidly and intensely, and the introjective identification may be experienced by several people at once.

A simple example of such an experience might begin by having a patient speak to her mother, played by a member of the group whom the patient selects and instructs in the role. Most patients quickly develop a much stronger affective response than might have been expected by their description of the issues. Other patients may be invited to join in as alter egos, speaking for the patient or the mother.

A therapist, observing without pressure to perform, is likely to develop a sense of the pivotal issues and can then move in to play the mother, voicing the covert message that she believes to be so distressing to the patient. She might, for example, say, "You cannot leave me. I've done everything for you. My life is nothing. I get nothing from your father. You are everything to me." If the "interpretation" is wrong, the patient will say, "No—she wouldn't say that." But if it is correct, her increased emotional response will be immediately apparent. In this example, the therapist, still in the role, might further intensify the interchange by physically grabbing the patient and touching off a struggle in which the patient fights for her freedom.

The evolution of this small drama will usually be revealing. The patient may, despite much greater physical strength than the therapist, struggle ineptly, never getting free. The reasons for her failure will evolve. She may, for example, ignore or turn away needed help from peers. She may become panicky about hurting her mother. One patient gave up, fell into my lap, let out a long sigh of relief and contentedly settled in with her head on my shoulder for the rest of the group. It became obvious to us both that behind the apparent need for autonomy was a far stronger need for closeness. Her fear of rejection, not her fear of entrapment, was the source of her provocative battles with her mother.

In the role of the mother, I may develop a sense of her attitude. I may feel determined and relentless; I may feel sad and depleted; I may become aware that the patient's escape would be a relief to me, because I feel as trapped in the relationship as she does. By allowing the experience to unfold freely, I may make an unexpected discovery. The following is an unusually dramatic example of such a process.

Jessica seemed frightened all the time and stayed at the periphery of the group. She had voiced no complaints about her mother, but feared that her father was having an affair and felt distant from him. One day when we were enacting a dialogue between a patient and her 10-year-old son, Jessica surprised me by volunteering to step into the role of the son, articulating what the mother's illness was doing to him.

Eager to explore this further, I stepped into the role of the mother and grabbed Jessica's arms, saying, "Help me." Jessica responded with alarm. The drama, which began around the common theme of parental dependency, took a curious turn as I found myself becoming increasingly abrupt and beginning to engage in peculiar and frightening behaviors. I began to enact striking her (without, of course, actually doing so) and ended up on the floor wrapped in lengths of cloth and moaning between bursts of angry kicks.

When we stopped to discuss it, Jessica revealed that during her childhood her mother had been violent and abusive, going through what appeared to have been intermittent psychotic episodes. These were never spoken of and, to Jessica's knowledge, she had never received treatment. An interesting detail of Jessica's memory was seeing her mother lying on the bedroom floor wrapped in blankets and moaning.

An episode like this speaks to the power of unconscious communication. Jessica's affect was an unconscious cue made clearer by her contribution to the earlier dialogue. During this experience she shaped the progression of my behavior by dozens of subtle reinforcements to which I was intensely attentive. Together we recreated what she could not talk about. My guess is that if I had seen Jessica in individual therapy, I would eventually have experienced a milder version of these feelings. The regression, recklessness, and unpredictable rage that came and went so quickly and clearly in a 20-minute enactment might have taken the more obscure and perhaps ultimately destructive form of a slowly growing visceral anger and difficulty in maintaining responsible control over the therapy process. We might have got to the root of this, but we might not have.

Experiential work of this intensity can only be safely done in the context of a structured program in which several therapists and a supportive peer group are consistently available. However, within such a setting, which is advantageous to patients for many reasons, cultivating a receptivity to and developing means to explore such feelings can often rapidly produce useful insights.

CONCLUSION

Women with eating disorders have turned away from relationships because relationships have failed them. Although desperately in need of connection to others, they have been unable to achieve connections that support a sense of self. And so they talk to themselves through the metaphors of ravenous binges, wrenching purges, and aching hunger. "Don't you see what we are doing?" one anorexic woman asked another. "We keep shrinking our world and soon it will vanish altogether." It is within the context of relationships that eating-disordered women can begin to reclaim the world and to reconstruct a relational self.

To recover, women with eating disorders have to find a new way to be with others, a way to experience authenticity within intimacy. As therapists, our contribution to this process consists in large part of our ability to extract meaning from the raw materials of interactional experience: the experience of the other, the experience of the self, the pushes and pulls toward and away from closeness, the magnetic fields of expectation exerting steady pressure toward predetermined patterns of feeling and response. Our patients can show us what is wrong with their relationships better than they can tell us. They need us to read the patterns and help them understand what has gone wrong, and then they need us to show them another way.

Anything that helps therapists amplify and articulate their experience of the therapeutic relationship is ultimately helpful. All too often the opposite occurs: The effort to understand and respond to the content overwhelms and suppresses awareness of these feelings. Nor do we have conventions by which, in discussing cases with supervisors or colleagues, we regard our reactions as being data as basic as what the patients say to us. For many of us there is still the fear of having the "wrong feelings." There is probably no way we can better support one another than to listen as each struggles to find words and concepts that can make of his or her experience with a patient a coherent and meaningful whole.

NOTE

1. The shorthand terms "anorexia" and "bulimia" are used throughout this chapter to refer to anorexia nervosa and bulimia nervosa as defined in the revised third edition of the *Diagnostic and Statistical Manual of Mental Disorders* (DSM-III-R).

REFERENCES

Chodorow, N. (1978). *The reproduction of mothering: Psychoanalysis and the sociology of gender*. Berkeley: University of California Press.

Deutsch, H. (1953). Occult processes occurring during psychoanalysis. In G. Devereux (Ed.), *Psychoanalysis and the occult* (pp. 133–146). New York: International Universities Press. (Original work published 1926)

Dinnerstein, D. (1976). *The mermaid and the minotaur: Sexual arrangements and human malaise*. New York: Harper & Row.

Freud, S. (1958). Recommendations to physicians practicing psychoanalysis. In J. Strachey (Ed. and Trans.), *The standard edition of the complete psychological works of Sigmund Freud* (Vol. 12, pp. 111–120). London: Hogarth Press. (Original work published 1912)

Freud, S. (1961). Some psychical consequences of the anatomical distinction between the sexes. In J. Strachey (Ed. and Trans.), *The standard edition of the complete psychological works of Sigmund Freud* (Vol. 19, pp. 243–258). London: Hogarth Press. (Original work published 1925)

Gilligan, C. (1982). *In a different voice*. Cambridge, MA: Harvard University Press.

Goodsitt, A. (1984). Self psychology and the treatment of anorexia nervosa. In D. M. Garner & P. E. Garfinkel (Eds.), *Handbook of psychotherapy for anorexia nervosa and bulimia* (pp. 55–82). New York: Guilford Press.

Heimann, P. (1950). On countertransference. *International Journal of Psycho-Analysis, 31*, 81–84.

Johnson, C. (1989, October 4–6). *Transference and countertransference: An open discussion*. Presentation given at the Eighth National Conference on Eating Disorders, Columbus, OH.

Johnson, C., & Connors, M. E. (1987). *The etiology and treatment of bulimia nervosa: A biopsychosocial perspective*. New York: Basic Books.

Kearney-Cooke, A. (1988). Group treatment of sexual abuse among women with eating disorders. *Women and Therapy, 7* (1), 5–21.

Klein, M. (1946). Notes on some schizoid mechanisms. *International Journal of Psycho-Analysis, 33,* 433–438.

Little, M. (1951). Countertransference. *International Journal of Psycho-Analysis, 32,* 32–40.

Miller, J. B. (1984). *The development of women's sense of self* (Work in Progress No. 12). Wellesley, MA: Wellesley College, Stone Center for Developmental Services and Studies.

Racker, H. (1957). The meanings and uses of countertransference. *Psychoanalytic Quarterly, 26,* 303–357.

Rich, A. (1976). *Of woman born: Motherhood as experience and institution*. New York: Norton.

Steiner-Adair, C. (1986). The body politic: Normal female adolescent development and the development of eating disorders. *Journal of the American Academy of Psychoanalysis, 14,* 95–114.

Strober, M., & Yager, J. (1984). A developmental perspective on the treatment of anorexia nervosa in adolescents. In D. M. Garner & P. E. Garfinkel (Eds.), *Handbook of psychotherapy for anorexia nervosa and bulimia* (pp. 363–390). New York: Guilford Press.

Tansey, M. J., & Burke, W. F. (1989). *Understanding countertransference*. Hillsdale, NJ: Analytic Press.

Tower, L. E. (1956). Countertransference. *Journal of the American Psychoanalytic Association, 4,* 224–225.

Winnicott, D. W. (1949) Hate in the counter-transference. *International Journal of Psycho-Analysis, 30* (2), 69–74.

·: *12* ·:

The Role of the Therapist in the Treatment of Eating Disorders: A Feminist Psychodynamic Approach

ANN KEARNEY-COOKE
Private Practice, Cincinnati

After working with eating-disordered patients for many years, I have come to realize that treatment progresses through three stages. These are not three distinct stages—since therapy is not like the baseball season, with an opening day and a final game—but a process whereby the patterns and issues are worked and reworked in each stage. This proposed stage model represents a generalization in which there are doubtless many exceptions, but it is useful as an organizing framework that cuts across personality styles and attempts to describe the therapeutic process for the heterogeneous group of women who struggle with eating disorders.

The stage model that I propose here draws from object relations theory and feminist theory. The outstanding contribution of the object relations approach is the emphasis on relationships and on working with unconscious processes such as projective identification and splitting. The important contribution of feminist theory is the recognition of gender as an organizing principle of all behavior, and of the way in which sexist social values and social structures become embedded in individual female psychology.

I begin with brief reviews of object relations theory and feminist theory, to provide a context for the discussion of this stage model. Then I describe key themes and interactional patterns that emerge in each stage, as well as the therapist's role in the healing process.

OBJECT RELATIONS THEORY

The core of every human being's development is the laying down early in life of a basic image and structure of the self, along with a basic sense of others and of the self in relation to others. Object relations theory is the body of psychoanalytic theory that addresses this aspect of development. The fundamental image of the self is referred to as the "self-representation"; the fundamental image of the other is called the "object representation." According to Althea Horner (1989), these mental structures become more complex over time and develop as a result of a combination of three factors: (1) the quality of the relationship with the primary caretaker, (2) the child's innate and constitutional physical and temperamental tendencies, and (3) the way in which the child experiences and ultimately conceptualizes his or her world. (The recognition of gender as an organizing principle of development that plays a major role in each of these factors is discussed later.) These inner representations of the self and the other, and the nature of their interrelationships in the mind, contribute significantly to the manner in which the self and the other are experienced in interpersonal relationships throughout the rest of one's life (Horner, 1989).

According to Cashdan (1988), the incorporation of relationships, beginning with the primary caretaker and extending outward to include other significant figures in one's life, forms the foundation of what ultimately becomes a self. Thus the child does not begin life with a self, but constructs one incrementally through engaging others socially. The relationships that people establish with one another are instrumental in maintaining a viable sense of self. Human beings engage constantly in self–other internalizations that complement and enhance their own and the others' respective identities. If people hope to retain an ongoing sense of who they are and where they fit in the world, they need to form meaningful relationships with significant others. It is the need for human contact that constitutes the primary motive within an object relations perspective.

Thus, the primary role accorded human relationships is the one dimension common to different schools of object relations theory. Within object relations theory, the mind and the psychic structures that constitute the mind are thought to evolve out of human interactions rather than out of biologically derived tensions. Instead of being motivated by tension reduction, human beings are motivated by the need to establish and maintain relationships. To understand what motivates people and how they view themselves, one must understand how relationships are internalized and how they come to be transformed into a sense of self (Cashdan, 1988).

Because the self is constructed interpersonally, the "mental disturbances," according to Cashdan (1988), are really disturbances in interpersonal relationships. Symptoms are construed in terms of one's representations of human relationships and their role in creating and maintaining present dysfunctional relationships. According to Kaiser (see Fierman, 1965), the patient suffers not from "symptoms" but from "contact disturbance." The focus shifts from seeing patients as suffering from an inability to reconcile inner impulses to seeing them as unable to engage others meaningfully in sustained and/or fulfilling relationships.

Using these ideas to conceptualize eating disorders, let us turn to theorists such as Johnson and Connors (1987) and Althea Horner (1989), who describe eating-disordered patients as being unable to engage others in gratifying relationships and turning instead to inanimate objects such as food and alcohol to meet their needs. Horner (1989) describes eating disorders as disorders of human relationships that have been displaced to the arena of food, appetite, and hunger. She sees the anorexic's denial of the need to eat as a metaphor for the denial of the need for any other person, because the anorexic experiences the "other" as psychologically toxic in some way.

The bulimic, according to Horner (1989), is less successful than the anorexic at denying her needs. The intensity of the patient's conflict between the need for her mother and father and the intense fear of closeness with them often leads to the fear that human contact will never be fulfilling for her. We often find that a bulimic woman has troubled relationships with both parents. The father seems to be overinterested in the daughter's physical appearance; he is as obsessively concerned with her weight and shape as she is. Often he is the one who made a comment about the eating-disordered woman's body at adolescence, which she remembers as the key motivating force for dieting and subsequent eating disorder. Many fathers also engage in inappropriate behaviors with their daughters, ranging from actual incest to sexually overstimulating behavior in which they describe their sexual relationships to their daughters, watch pornographic movies with their daughters, and the like.

Horner (1989) concludes that the daughter is in a bind: To turn to her father is to experience sexual dangers; to turn to her mother is to experience emotional abandonment and rage. She may try to deny needing either one of her parents, but may be unsuccessful in her attempt to remain safe. She is more likely to hide her true self and to behave in an adaptive, ungenuine, compliant manner with those on whom she must depend. Often she relates with a pseudocloseness that hides her emotional detachment and isolation. Though she feels drawn to others, her real self is frightened and does not let others in. She reaches out and then pulls back, allows others in and then gets rid of them. She stuffs herself with food and forces herself to vomit it out. Horner (1989) concludes that the "need yet fear of others" dilemma must be resolved if the individual is to recover from the eating disorder. She must give up the flight from relationships with others that the symptom also represents.

FEMINIST PERSPECTIVE

I view culture not merely as an influential element, but as crucial to understanding why women constitute such a large percentage of the eating-disordered population. By "culture," I do not mean only the societal pressures for females to be thin, but also the silencing of women that occurs through the socialization process. How does this silencing take place?

Woman as Body

Females in contemporary patriarchal societies still are identified fundamentally with their bodies. An eating disorder embodies very clearly the dilemma of "woman as body." In the problem of "woman as body," says Greenspan (1983), a woman suffers from an overexposure of physical visibility as a body, combined with impoverishment of genuine recognition as a person. As long as a woman is essentially defined by her body, she will continue to have a problem of feminine identity and an intense "charge" around her body.

In a feminist approach to the female body, women reclaim their bodies. Reclaiming the body means no longer seeing it through male eyes but through one's own. It involves changes in attitude, in which we celebrate the seasons of the female body as expressed through menarche, pregnancy, and menopause. Finally, it means that equality between the sexes is achieved not by women's making their body shapes lean, tubular, and masculine, but instead by according equal value to the curved, feminine body.

Silencing of Women

Females in our society are pressured to exclude a number of significant personal qualities or behavior patterns from their self-concepts in order to consider themselves feminine. Sexist thinking embodies the idea that women who take initiative, have needs for self-recognition (Walters, Carter, Papp, & Silverstein, 1988), or claim personal authority (Young-Eisendrath & Wiedemann, 1987) are unattractive, self-serving, and masculine. This aspect of female oppression deprives women of a sense of agency and of the capacity to be effective. This is acted out in the arena of "body," where even the location of curves and whether they should be excluded (1960s and 1970s) or exhibited (1980s) have always been determined by men. Women with eating disorders feel controlled by these beliefs; often they report their fears that if they give a voice to the parts of themselves considered unfeminine, they will lose other people. As they continually silence those parts of themselves, they feel hopeless and powerless. Losing others is especially frightening for eating-disordered patients, because they depend on others to fulfill functions that they feel they cannot fulfill for themselves.

Deprivation Model

Women are encouraged to accept the "deprivation model" as a way of life. This model is portrayed clearly in dieting, in which the "good woman" is able to survive on less nourishment than she really needs. The "never quite getting enough" syndrome teaches a woman that with willpower she can live without the food she needs, with earning less money than her male colleagues, and often with not receiving enough help at home. As Janet Surrey (1984) explains, within this deprivation model, a sense of effectiveness or agency for females comes to represent the ability to control oneself rather than to express oneself. This model must be replaced with a "fullness model," which encourages a woman to feed her body the food it needs and which frees her to ask for what she needs in relationships or work settings. In the fullness model, women are free to take up space in the world with their bodies or with their ideas, and to dress to express rather than to hide.

Idealization of the Masculine

The belief that all things masculine are of greater value than all things feminine has a profound effect on the psyches of females and often leads to feelings of shame and inadequacy. This tradition in Western civilization and most of psychology is one in which females are seen as inadequate males. This is highlighted in Freud's phallocentric model of development, where the biological inferiority of women is assumed on the basis of their lack of a penis (Freud, 1933/1965). Within this model, a woman is supposed to accept the "reality" of her castration, the "fact" of her organic inferiority; she is supposed to admit that the clitoris is actually a masculine organ—a rudimentary penis. Even childbearing is described as an expression of penis envy, according to Freud (Lee & Hertzberg, 1978). Although the bulk of empirical evidence does not support the theory of penis envy (Sherman, 1971), Freud's theory set the tone for the treatment of women and continues to be a major influence upon society in general.

This idealization of the masculine is evidenced in the devaluation of women's capacity to form relationships, to empathize, and to cooperate with others. These qualities are often regarded as weaknesses in our society and signs of women's inability to function on their own. Although intimacy and attachment are considered positive aspects of personal relationships, our culture bombards us with messages that contradict this view. Walters et al. (1988) state that even therapists often characterize these attachment traits as "intrusive," "controlling," or "overinvolved."

I believe that we need to adapt Walters et al.'s (1988) definition of adult maturity, which combines autonomy with connection. This definition of health is in contrast to the patriarchal splitting of these attributes, in which autonomy (actually separateness) is assigned to males and connectedness (actually dependency) to females. Feminist theorists such as Gilligan (1982) and Walters et al. (1988) state that such splitting leads us to mistake separateness or disconnection for autonomy (a valued sign of maturity), while connectedness is equated with dependency (a sign of immaturity) and thus is devalued. Again, I believe it is crucial that we appreciate the complexity of women's need to be both autonomous and connected, and that we as therapists assist female patients to integrate both needs into a sense of self.

In summary, the cultural issues I have discussed thus far attempt to explain why females are more at risk for the development of an eating disorder. The discussion of object relations theory enables us to see that the particular females at risk for the development of an eating disorder are those with characterological vulnerability resulting from early relationships. Using the ideas from both theories, therapists can assist females with eating disorders to examine their dysfunctional relationships, to explore their assumptions about the female body/self in a social context, and to redefine what it means to be an adult woman.

STAGE 1: DISRUPTING PREVIOUS EXPERIENCES OF SELF AND OTHER

Description

Most patients who come into treatment report that their eating is out of control. Often they are bingeing both in response to restrained eating and to overwhelming emotional states. They exhibit rigid attitudes toward food (e.g., designation of "good" and "bad" foods) and a disturbance in interoceptive awareness. "Interoceptive awareness," according to Bruch (1973), refers to an individual's ability to accurately identify and articulate a variety of internal states such as hunger, satiety, and affects. For example, initially when patients vomit, they report little pain or discomfort. Later in therapy they describe how their throats hurt and their eyes water during vomiting. In Stage 1, I think it is important for the therapist to assist patients in normalizing eating through food sheets and meal planning (Boutacoff, Zollman, & Mitchell, 1984), response prevention techniques (Rosen & Leitenberg, 1984), and handing out of psychoeducational materials (Garner, Rochert, Olmsted, Johnson, & Coscina, 1984). The goal of the food sheets is to help the patients see the connections among feeling states, events, and bingeing, and to help them undersand that some bingeing is a response to restrained eating (Weiss, Katzman, & Wolchik, 1986).

In the initial phase of treatment, patients also engage in much talk about their bodies. They exhibit body image distortion, body dissatisfaction, concern with body shape, and insensitivity to internal cues.

As we listen to eating-disordered patients describing vacillations in body image, it becomes clear that their body image has been formed insufficiently to sustain the stresses of developmental maturation; thus, it regresses in response to intense emotional states. Emotional states that are experienced as overwhelming (such as humiliation, depletion, depression, or rage) lead to changes in body image for eating-disordered patients (Krueger, 1989). At times of particular emotional turmoil, their body image becomes more distorted, vague, or irritating to them. Because of a lack of a cohesive, distinct sense of self, they achieve representation of the body through bingeing with foods, exercising excessively (an attempt to develop more definitive body boundaries), and starving to induce hunger pangs (Krueger, 1989). During this phase, it is important for the therapist to help patients to begin to decode their endless talk about their bodies and to begin to reconstruct their body image histories. At this stage the therapist also must help patients to uncover the various deeper meanings of different bodily shapes (e.g., fat and thin bodies), so they can be free to come to terms with their own shape and weight (Kearney-Cooke, 1989; Wooley & Kearney-Cooke, 1986).

As patients enter treatment, most are happy about the weight they have lost, but are concerned about the impact of their eating disorder on their lives. Thus in many ways the symptomatology is ego-syntonic (Rabinor, 1989). It is rare for a patient to enter treatment with an appreciation of the function that the eating disorder serves in her life. Only infrequently do patients enter therapy with an awareness of the deep level of isolation and deprivation they are experiencing. Many are involved on a superficial level in relationships, school, and careers, which distract them from the reality of their loneliness, powerlessness, and fear of dependence on others.

The Role of the Therapist

Women with eating disorders have developed a way of being with others that, to them, insures continued support and love. Thus a patient, beginning with the initial session, will attempt to figure out the needs of the therapist, the unwritten rules of therapy, and ways to keep the therapist interested in her (e.g., must she be seductive to keep the therapist's interest? Must she be funny and entertaining?).

It is the therapist's job in the initial phase of treatment to listen and to develop a relationship with the patient that is based on honesty, empathy, and compassion. The therapist must connect with the patient empathetically before the patient can establish herself as an observer of her own behavior and eventually of the therapist–patient dyad. It is crucial that the therapist set clear boundaries from the beginning, to let the patient know that this is a safe environment where meaningful work can be done. An initial therapeutic task is to help the patient to focus on herself, to elaborate on her experience, and to differentiate among internal states (as in distinguishing physical from emotional hunger, anger from sadness, and in some cases self from other). It is a time to listen to the way in which patients represent and perceive others. (Do they consistently see others as weak? potentially humiliating? omnipotent?) How do they represent or see themselves? (Do they often feel "small"? capable of destroying others?) Boskind-White and White (1983) emphasize the importance of recognizing the strengths that eating-disordered patients bring to treatment (e.g., the courage to begin therapy, to keep their jobs) and of discussing ways to expand them. It is a time for therapists to pay close attention to the way in which they are responding to the patients. (Are they doing more for a particular patient than for other patients? Are they feeling especially sad during a session?) Finally, it is a time to be aware of the way in which a patient attempts to connect with the therapist. For example, a woman who had been sexually abused as a child asked after each session to be hugged by the therapist. She also made it a point to discuss the explicit details of the sexual relationship with her boyfriend. The closer she felt to the therapist during the first few sessions, the more she attempted to connect in a way to which she was accustomed. Because of childhood abusive experiences she learned to eroticize closeness, which she acted out immediately in the relationship with the therapist. It is the therapist's job to be aware of this style of connection or avoidance of connection and eventually to help the patient see it.

In therapy, the woman who is struggling with an eating disorder continually describes relationships in which she cannot seem to connect with others in a way that is fulfilling for her. As the therapist "listens between the lines," it becomes clear that a key problem in the patient's relationships is her unconscious attempt to repeat relational patterns of the past. These patients, according to Cashdan (1988), are involved continually in the unconscious process of enlisting others to enact with them scenes from their internal object worlds. This process is acted out in relationships with others, both outside therapy and eventually in the therapeutic relationship. Let me describe an example of each relationship.

Case Example

Kristin, a 27-year-old anorexic patient who had been sexually abused by her father from the ages of 9 to 13, entered therapy and described her continual involvement with married men. In fact, she had never dated a man who was not "taken." As therapy progressed, she became increasingly dissatisfied with these types of relationships: She could never be seen in public, and the relationships took place at seedy bars or in her bedroom (the same place as with her father).

In the initial phase of therapy, Kristin decided to join a reputable dating service, which would enable her to engage in relationships with men who were available to her. After many dates, she met Joe; they seemed to like each other from the start. Initially she came into therapy excited, yet frightened about this good thing that was happening. It was new for her to be treated with respect—for a man to be genuinely interested in her and to follow through with promises to her. However, as the relationship progressed and as she became more panicked, she began to report fears that Joe was interested in her only as a "sexual object" and would leave her soon. She also shared that she was dieting again and was feeling fat. When the therapist explored her fear, she explained that she and Joe were doing less together in public and more in private in her home. When the therapist asked why this was happening, it became clear that Kristin was playing a major role in this change. She would tell Joe that she didn't like to go to dinner at restaurants; instead, she would suggest that they order carryout food, and would invite him to eat at her place and to watch often somewhat erotic movies. If he was not aggressive sexually, she assumed that he was not interested in her because she was fat. If he was sexually interested and responded to her sexually, she assumed that sex was his only real interest in her.

One way to look at this situation is that Kristin had lifted the unfinished abusive relationship with her father and deposited it onto her boyfriend. She was using powerful behaviors (dressing seductively, keeping the relationship out of public) to induce her boyfriend to behave as her father did. It was as if she was pushing him to play a role in the enactment of her internal drama—one involving a painful relationship with her father. Unfortunately, the receiver of this projection often leaves the relationship and validates the person's original fear that no one can ever really love her. Fortunately, in this case Kristin was able to see the role she was playing in repeating this drama and was able to stop. She had not picked a man like her father, and Joe was able to engage in a fulfilling relationship with her.

The therapist must be aware that sooner or later the interactions with a patient will take on the qualities of the patient's earlier relationships. Once the earlier, unfulfilling ways become part of the relationship, the therapist can respond in a manner very different from the patient's accustomed pattern. The therapist's atypical response to the patient's attempt to recreate old interactional patterns restores hope and allows change to occur.

Ogden (1982) invites us to imagine for a moment that the patient is both the director and one of the principal actors in the interpersonal enactment of an internal object relationship. Projective identification is the process by which the therapist is given the stage directions for a particular role. Ogden states that the therapist who has allowed himself or herself to some extent to be molded by this interpersonal pressure, and who is able to observe these changes, has access to a rich source of data about the patient's internal world—the induced set of thoughts and feelings that are experimentally alive, vivid, and immediate.

Case Example

Kate, a 24-year-old anorexic woman who was 6 months pregnant, came into a session describing how angry and hurt she felt that others were accusing her of not doing what she should to insure the baby's health. Her husband went so far as to say, "If anything is wrong with this baby, you'll know whose fault it is." Throughout the session Kate talked about drinking beer at parties, cutting down on calories because she was getting so fat, and working out at the health club to the point of exhaustion. The therapist found herself becoming increasingly concerned about the baby's health. She began to ask Kate questions about how much beer she was drinking and how many calories per day she was taking in. Kate began to look depressed. When the therapist asked her what she was feeling, she stated that she felt bad; the therapist didn't trust her either. The therapist acknowledged that after hearing her describe drinking alcohol, cutting down on calories, and exercising to the point of exhaustion, she had become concerned about the baby's health. When she realized what she was doing, the therapist suggested that they attempt together to understand what it meant that the therapist had become yet another person questioning Kate's behavior.

As they explored this issue, it became clear that Kate in fact was behaving in an appropriate way—eating properly and limiting alcohol intake—but was presenting herself to the world in such a manner as to induce feelings of concern and distrust. She was projecting a critical, nontrusting self onto the therapist (as well as onto others) and unconsciously was inducing others to act it out. She reported holding beer cans at parties (but drinking only a sip from each one) and eating small meals and drinking diet soda in public, while eating healthy meals when she was alone. Kate began to see the role she was playing in repeating an interactional pattern that was comfortable for her. She began to see how this pattern eventually led her to food. The pattern was that if she was criticized she failed, and if she failed she did not deserve to eat. She would restrain her eating and exercise vigorously. Growing up with a critical father and depleted mother, she had learned that she had to earn everything she received, even the basics (attention, nurturance, etc.). There was so little available in the family that she could only be recognized and given to when she performed well and was perfect. If she was less than perfect, she felt she must deprive herself, since she deserved nothing.

Summary of Stage 1

Throughout therapy, but especially in the initial phase, the therapist must be aware of re-emerging problems for the patient in relationships outside therapy, as well as in the therapeutic relationship. The therapist must be aware of the patient's attempts to induce him or her to engage in dysfunctional interactional patterns, and must avoid comforming to the role. In this way the therapist uses the relationship to begin to alter the patient's habitual and self-defeating ways of relating to others. In this process the patient begins to learn about her internal representation of others and how she repeats the corresponding interactional patterns in her present world, including the relationship with the therapist. In the second phase of treatment, patients have a chance to experiment with new ways of being in relationships with others, including expressing parts of themselves that they have hidden from others in the past.

STAGE 2: TESTING NEW EXPERIENCES WITH SELF AND OTHER

Description

Stage 2 is characterized by less binge-eating associated with starvation and instead restrained eating or bingeing signaling psychological difficulties. The patient begins to see the connection between her emotional states and her feelings about her body. Enough trust has developed between the therapist and the patient that the patient remembers and works through key experiences that affected body image (such as sexual abuse and shame).

Stage 2 also is characterized by a deeper connection between the therapist and the patient; the patient often acknowledges her growing dependency on the therapist. The therapist does more than merely help the patient to deal with inner objects; he or she becomes one of them. By allowing himself or herself to become part of the patient's projective fantasy and by rearranging the outcome of the relational scenario that ensues, the therapist becomes a powerful new presence in the patient's inner world. The therapist–patient dyad now becomes a subject for mutual observation and understanding. The patient uses the therapist to smooth the transition between letting go of painful relationships and incorporating more fulfilling relationships.

Patients whose identity was based on becoming what others wanted them to be or on becoming the opposite of what others wanted now must face their lack of identity. Internal feelings of emptiness and a lack of structure will come to the forefront in the second stage. This state often is accompanied by feelings of depression and by reactivation of symptomatology. Patients often must acknowledge that their present relationships repeat the unhealthy connections of the past, and must examine their role in this process (i.e., why they keep picking the same kind of people to be involved with or why they attempt to induce others to treat them as they are accustomed to be treated). Some of their present relationships will end; others will continue but will change.

Although an eating-disordered patient for the first time experiences glimmers of hope of satisfying connections in the future, she faces a tremendous challenge: Can she turn to others in a new, more satisfying way, so that her need for inanimate objects such as food or alcohol decreases? Can she begin to practice this new pattern in her relationship with the therapist? Can she tell the therapist how close she feels to him or her, or instead will she need to stop at the bakery after the session? Can she trust that the therapist is strong enough to hear her disappointments or doubts about him or her, or will she have to protect the therapist and leave empty-handed again? As the patient experiments in Stage 2 and gives a voice to the many parts of herself, will the therapist withdraw, judge, or humiliate her, or will he or she help her to integrate all these parts into a strong sense of self?

The Role of the Therapist

In this stage, it is important that the therapist respond empathetically both to the patient's more autonomous behavior and to her need for support and continued dependency. The therapist must send a clear, unambiguous signal that he or she will not participate in the relationship in the unfulfilling ways to which the patient is accustomed. There are several processes and a number of themes that evolve during Stage 2. In the interests of space, I only report on four and describe ways in which the therapist can provide a new experience of relatedness for the eating-disordered patient.

Case Example: Openness of Conflict

The therapist needs to communicate that he or she will not collude with the patient in her belief that the relationship will last only if they protect each other and never question or voice negative affect toward each other. That is, conflicts between the therapist and the patient are out in the open; the therapist's consistency and acceptance help the patient to develop the capacity to tolerate the feelings inherent in that process.

Mary, a 21-year-old bulimic with borderline features, began a session by describing a scene with her brother.

> MARY: I took my brother to California last week so he could meet my friends out there. On the plane coming home, he was quiet and looked real judgmental. I asked him what he was thinking and he said I wouldn't want to know. After much prodding, he finally said that he thought I was stuck in my life, that I wasn't going anywhere. I was so angry at him . . .
>
> THERAPIST: You seem stuck to me too. Let's try to understand what that's about.
>
> MARY: (Looks annoyed, says nothing.)
>
> THERAPIST: What are you experiencing?
>
> MARY: Nothing. I don't want to talk about the trip any more.
>
> THERAPIST: You look like you are feeling something. What's happening in your body?
>
> MARY: My heart's beating fast. I am nervous, scared. I mean, how dare you say I'm stuck? I can't believe you would have the nerve to say that to me. I would never imagine questioning you and

saying you are stuck with me. . . . I don't need this from you. This is bullshit. I'm leaving. *(Start to get up to leave.)*

THERAPIST: *(Stands at door.)* Please stay. We've worked out things before—we can work this out.

MARY: *(Sits down. Proceeds to tell the therapist the issues she has not helped her with.)* I never dreamed of questioning you.

THERAPIST: Why not?

MARY: You might get angry at me for making you feel incompetent or bad. Maybe you would feel so bad or mad that you would make up a reason not to see me. Then I would be left out there totally alone. I can't bear the thought of it. My stomach gets queasy thinking of that.

THERAPIST: I'm sure that is a frightening thought. But it sounds like you are alone with your struggles. You've been keeping them to yourself and protecting me.

MARY: Maybe that's why I feel real hopeless at times. . . . But it's still better than being totally alone, like if something happened to our relationship.

THERAPIST: So to keep this relationship, you feel you must never ask for anything that you're afraid I can't give you. You have to just live with not getting it.

MARY: I feel that way with everyone.

THERAPIST: My concern is that the end result is always the same: You end up with very little. Possibly if you asked you would get more. [End of session]

MARY: I still feel ugly, terrible. I'm afraid I'm going to ruin this relationship with you. It makes me not want to come back here.

THERAPIST: It takes a lot of courage to give a voice to the many parts of yourself—including your anger and disappointment with me. I want you to come back and keep working.

In these excerpts Mary revealed her unwritten rules for the relationship. One rule was that if she asked for something that she felt another could not give, she would be humiliated or abandoned by the other person. She believed that if she did not support the therapist's narcissism, she would be the recipient of the therapist's rage. This was the nature of Mary's interaction with both parents, and she brought it into treatment transferentially. Thus she was left with unfulfilled needs and experienced chronic feelings of deprivation and emotional hunger. The feeling of deprivation was one of the paths that led her to food. The world of food was under her control; she could go to it 24 hours a day; there was an endless supply where she could fill herself up temporarily.

It is also clear that as Mary came face to face with her anger, she felt that her only choice was to leave the relationship. In her words, "I'm going to ruin this relationship with you [because of it]." Initially she did not experience the expression of her anger as cleansing and empowering. For a long time, her anger had been expressed indirectly through the eating disorder symptoms and had never been quite released. It had piled up for so many years that she was afraid of it, afraid it would destroy the relationship. Mary feared that her anger, more than any other emotion, was a sign of her "badness" as a person. For this reason, it was crucial for the therapist to communicate that Mary's splitting off of "bad" parts of self (such as anger) was not grounds for abandonment, but needed to be experienced and integrated into herself. Mary needed to see that the therapist was genuinely interested in all of her, even her feelings of anger and disappointment toward the therapist.

Case Example: Intimacy without Acting Out

The therapist needs to communicate to the patient that intimacy can be accomplished without physically or sexually acting out. This requires the therapist to be clear enough about his or her own boundaries that the patient can struggle with her dependency needs without destroying the relationship. For example, Susan, a 21-year-old bulimic patient, came into an appointment wearing no underwear and sat in such a way that she was "flashing" the therapist. She had been sexually abused by her father from age 5 to 9. She would go into her parents' bedroom when she was scared; her mother would leave and sleep in Susan's room, and her father would molest her.

In Stage 2, Susan was asking: Would the therapist be like her father and not observe the boundaries, but base the relationship on sexuality and humiliation? Or would the therapist be like the mother and ignore the sexuality (i.e., not comment on the fact that she was flashing the therapist)? Would the therapist be able to assist her in translating physical feelings into words? Finally, would this be a safe relationship, where she could struggle with sexuality and find meaningful ways to express it as an adult woman?

Case Example: Encouraging Power and Competence

The therapist must encourage the patient to reclaim her power and competence, and must not collude with the patient's sense of lack of control of symptomatology. To do so, the therapist must assist the patient in understanding the sequence of behaviors that lead to disordered eating. For example, Carol, a 25-year-old bulimic patient, described her concerns about her new boyfried. The therapist listened, helped to clarify the nature of the concerns, and encouraged the patient to take these concerns seriously. In response to the therapy session, Carol went to her boyfriend's house and shared her reservations about the relationship with him. Then she went home, binged and purged until she was in a state of exhaustion, and fell asleep. She called the therapist and canceled the next appointment.

When Carol returned to therapy, she reported confusion about her behavior of the previous week: the exacerbation of symptoms and canceling the appointment. After the sequence of events was discussed, it became clear that Carol found something frightening about identifying and articulating to others her internal feelings or reactions. She felt effective and powerful, and was overwhelmed to the point that she needed to disempower herself through bingeing and purging. Thus the return of the symptoms was not merely a random recurrence of a bad habit, but was connected to her feelings' being taken seriously by the therapist and the boyfriend. She felt clear, separate, and effective; this feeling frightened her. She had developed a lifestyle in which she did not pay attention to internal states or consider it important to respond to them. This situation contributed to her chronic feelings of helplessness and confusion. She preserved this state by choosing others who responded so as to help her maintain this lifestyle; if they did not do so, she acted out (got drunk, missed appointments, purged, etc.). In such a case, it is crucial for the therapist to stay with the material and to communicate belief in the patient's ability to recognize and eventually to interrupt such a sequence.

Case Example: Validation of Personal Authority

The therapist needs to send a clear, unambiguous signal that he or she is able to handle the patient's growing sense of personal authority. A woman's ability to validate her own convictions of truth, beauty, and goodness in regard to her self-concept and self-interest is what Young-Eisendrath and Wiedemann (1987) call "personal authority." Self-confidence, personal agency, social functioning, body image, occupational functioning, sexual pleasure, and subjective self-assessment are all related to personal authority. Women in patriarchal cultures are discouraged from developing this quality. Through the therapeutic process, females with eating disorders begin to reclaim their sense of personal authority. It is crucial for the therapist to communicate that he or she can handle the patient's growing sense of authority and effectiveness and can encourage her to integrate it into her identity.

In one case, Barbara, a 26-year-old bulimic woman who attended graduate school and who had missed a previous session, entered therapy talking about how nice the therapist's office looked. After a period of superficial talk, the therapist asked her what was really going on. Barbara reported that she had read a chapter the therapist had written and felt very competitive with her for the first time. She thought she would like to write a chapter herself someday. Then she said that she thought she was actually capable of writing a better chapter than the therapist. After sharing this thought with the therapist, Barbara reported feeling guilty and scared that the therapist might be angry. She also stated that she felt big and fat, and that she was taking up "too much space" in the room. She reported feeling a break in the connection with the therapist.

The therapist talked about the difference between an enviable goal (the idea of Barbara's using envy to motivate herself to develop her ideas into a chapter) and feelings of envy, which left her feeling isolated from the other. The therapist also commented on Barbara's courage in bringing the issue of competition into the session and in opening the discussion about her growing sense of confidence and personal effectiveness. Barbara needed to know that as she developed a sense of personal authority, she could trust the therapist to honor it and to celebrate it with her, rather than punishing her through abandonment or rage.

Summary of Stage 2

By the end of Stage 2, patients begin to realize that their maladaptive ways of relating to the therapist are no longer viable. Instances of projective identification crop up now and then, but become less frequent and less intense as time goes by. This shift in the therapist–patient relationship marks the beginning of the final stage of therapy and signals a significant turning point in the treatment process.

Mary (the patient for whom therapy excerpts have been presented above) stated that her turning point occurred in the second stage of treatment. She said that it occurred on the day when she was angry and got up to leave, when the therapist stood at the door and said, "We've worked out things before—we can work this out." She realized that the therapist was genuinely interested in all of her even her anger and disappointment; the therapist would hang in there with her, as she had promised earlier in therapy. Mary was relieved to learn that her anger did not destroy the therapist, herself, or the relationship. They spent the session disagreeing and struggling, and both came out alive. From that moment, she reported, something changed in the therapeutic relationship and she began to see herself differently. Also for the first time, she had hope of overcoming her bulimia. In retrospect, Mary reported that that point signaled important changes in her relationship with others.

During Stage 2, a series of difficult interpersonal issues is addressed, and the patient sees that her needs can be met within a relationship. Confrontation has cleared the air; vulnerability has led to deeper connection, rather than abuse; the therapist and the patient know that their relationship is strong and that they can handle any potential struggle.

STAGE 3: CONNECTIONS THAT WORK

Description

Most patients are symptom-free by the third stage of the treatment. They no longer split cognitively around eating. For example, they no longer think that if they overeat at one meal, they have failed completely and so must overeat all day. They can see overeating at one meal for what it is, and can eat normally the rest of the day. There is usually some grieving for the symptom at this point. Patients recognize that the rituals around eating (whether bingeing, purging, laxative abuse, or restraining) had carried them through many difficult transitions in their lives. The symptom has been an important aspect of their identity and has made them feel special. For some patients, it may actually be useful to encourage bingeing and purging in the final phase of therapy to validate their ability to control it. Most patients now are able to see that cyclic bingeing in the future will be a sign of an intrapsychic or interpersonal issue that requires attention.

Most patients are experiencing a level of body acceptance. They have worked through most of the issues that left them feeling negative about their bodies. Just as they are able to view human relationships in more complex ways, they no longer view their bodies simply as the size of their thighs or how bloated their stomachs are; now health, body competence, and so on are part of body image. Patients see that attraction is not based solely on appearance, but on many other factors such as compassion, sense of humor, and intelligence.

In Stage 3, the eating-disordered patient continues in the process of forming a stable, integrated, cohesive experience of her body. This body image is composed of an accurate assessment of her body; clear, distinct body boundaries; and better acceptance of body shape and weight. Because most patients gain some weight, behaviors such as giving away the old wardrobe and buying appropriate-sized clothes are common.

Stage 3 also is characterized by reports that patients are engaging others in more fulfilling ways outside therapy and practicing new ways of relating to the therapist in therapy. Patients also are beginning to mourn the pending separation with the therapist. For the first time they exhibit the ability to tolerate the tension of opposites, differences in competing roles, and tension of growth. They recognize the mutual interdependence of self and other in all relationships. They show signs that treatment has repaired the early distortion of relationships, so they can proceed along the normal path of development.

At this time the therapist and the patient give each other feedback, including an assessment of how the patient has changed and of challenges that still need to be met. This stage also includes feedback on the therapist's work. The therapist encourages the patient to let him or her know what she found helpful in the way the therapist worked, as well as what was less helpful. The therapist then can use this feedback to enhance his or her work with future patients.

The Role of the Therapist

The separation process begins before the final stage of therapy. Throughout the therapy, a patient deals with the loss of the therapist in various forms: momentary failures in empathy by the therapist, actual separations due to illness or vacation, and moments when the patient realizes that she has nothing to talk about—that she has handled everything between sessions well and feels less need for the therapist's feedback.

Because the relationship is the healing ingredient in the therapeutic approach described here, the final stage, where separation is the major theme, is crucial for therapy. Separation, according to Cashdan (1988), is the culmination of a powerful internalization process that begins with the patient's incorporation of the therapist into a projective fantasy and ends with the patient's being able to use the therapist as a good object, which allows her to let go of feelings of badness and enables her to connect freely in fulfilling relationships with others. In the course of therapy, the therapist is incorporated within the patient's inner world and integrated into the patient's self as a healing object.

This internalization of the therapist creates a feeling of security, which enables the patient to experience aspects of early relationships as well as aspects of self that previously were split off. Significant others, experienced earlier as all good or all bad, now are seen in a more complex way. This perspective helps the patient to let go of the rigid, restrictive view that was nurtured by a highly polarized inner representation (Cashdan, 1988).

Case Example: Internalization of the Therapist

This internalization process (was exemplified) by Cathy, a 35-year-old nurse struggling with bulimia. She described the following experience after being assaulted physically at work:

> I was completely confused about how to respond to the assault by my patient. My initial response was to hit the candy machines in the hospital. But I remembered how we talked about delaying binges for a half hour. So I did. Then I thought "What should I say or do?" Each thought or plan of action that came to mind seemed wrong. But then

I asked myself, "What would [the therapist] do in this situation?" And then I talked it over with you in my head. I thought you would take action and press charges. So I did. Then I felt guilty, like I was a bitch pressing charges on this sick man. But I thought more about it and realized I wasn't a bitch. I was taking myself seriously and making a statement that being assaulted was not acceptable. I didn't even binge that day, although I considered it. I asked for support from the head nurse and then I called you. Both of you were there for me. That felt good; I felt strong but sad. I knew if I had called my parents they would have told me to forget it, that when you are a nurse sometimes these things happen and that I was making too big of a thing of this. But I did take action. It's freeing to take action and not always feel I have to put up with things.

Toward the end of therapy, Cathy reported an instance when she was asked to do more than her share at work. At this time she simply asked herself, "What would be the best way to handle this?" and decided to talk it over with her head nurse. Cashdan (1988) describes this progression to inner dialogue with oneself ("What's the best way to proceed?") as reflecting the progression from interaction with inner objects to interaction with the self.

This example also shows how, through the course of treatment, the therapist is "internally transmuted" into a source of worth and self-esteem. The growing sense that one is desirable and worthwhile forms the basis for the patient's restructuring of her inner world and for relationships in the outer world. A fortified self, strengthened by the incorporation of a good relationship, is the means by which object relations therapy allows the patient to give up the symptomatology and to engage in a healthier lifestyle.

As the therapist becomes more a part of the patient's inner world, the patient needs to rely less on the therapist's presence to feel secure. Thus separation and the ending of therapy become more imminent. To insure that the eating-disordered patient does not experience the termination of therapy as she experienced separations in the past, the therapist must engage the patient actively in the separation process. The therapist needs to acknowledge that he or she also has feelings about the separation; there is a loss for the therapist as well as for the patient. It is crucial for the therapist to express his or her many feelings about the therapeutic relationship coming to an end.

For example, the therapist may be excited that the patient has reached this juncture in her life, but also sad that she will no longer be an active part of the therapist's life. After going through so many experiences and feeling states together, it is difficult not to have strong feelings.

Working with these feelings of loss can lead to a termination that is growth-producing for both the therapist and the patient.

Case Example: Development of a Separation Ritual

Because a primary theme for Ellen, a 30-year-old bulimic woman, was the "deadness" she had experienced in relationships and in work, she and the therapist used this idea in planning a ritual to end therapy. The ritual was created around the Egyptian mummy theme. In the past, Ellen had silenced many parts of her true self and thus had felt emotionally dead throughout most of her life. Through individual and group therapy, she began to listen and to give a voice to her true self. She developed healthier relationships and felt fully alive for the first time in her life. She was able to give up the bulimic behaviors and to engage in relationships and activities that were more fulfilling to her. In describing this change, she often said that in the past she had lived a life of isolation and food, and through therapy had entered into a world of relationships and self-respect.

Just as the Egyptians placed gifts in the mummy case for the dead to take into their next life, Ellen and the therapist selected gifts that symbolized therapeutic work for Ellen to take to her life after therapy; these gifts represented femininity, self-respect, interdependence, resilience, and active struggling. Weeks were spent in planning the ritual and in discussing the meaning of each part. The ritual took place during the final session. Ellen brought music, and the therapist improvised with movement. Ellen brought two masks she had made out of tape. She painted one to represent herself; during the session she painted the other mask to symbolize the therapist. She painted as she asked the therapist questions about her personal life: her children, being a therapist, being a working mother.

Ellen read a final statement bridging her old life to life after therapy. She described her journey from isolation to connection with others, as well as her new relationship with her self. In turn, the therapist read a final statement to Ellen about the therapy. Ellen described the disappointments she had experienced in therapy, as well as the ecstasy of changes. She grieved for her obsession with food and body, and she grieved for other losses from her past (e.g., a grandmother who had died a year before therapy, a boyfriend with whom she had broken up). She talked about the new challenges ahead and the skills she had learned to deal with her symptomatology.

As this final stage of Ellen's treatment made clear, the therapist was no longer seen as a transformed version of figures in the past, but as a person in her own right. During this final session, the therapist and the patient had an opportunity to relate to each other in a new way.

GENERAL SUMMARY

The etiology of eating disorders is undoubtedly complex, involving an interaction of psychological, biological, and sociocultural determinants (Johnson & Connors, 1987). Because of the complexity and diversity of factors that initiate and sustain these disorders, Strober and Yager (1989) emphasize that the interventions required to treat them are quite varied. Goals for treatment may include the behavioral management of disordered eating, expressive therapies to correct body image disturbance, and a therapeutic relationship in which intrapsychic conflicts and interpersonal struggles can be worked through.

This chapter has focused primarily on the last-mentioned goal. The role of the therapist in the three stages of treatment has been described. The focus is on both the personal and the political—that is, the effects of early relationships on development, as well as how years of psychosocial gender conditioning leave females at risk for the development of an eating disorder.

The approach described in this chapter challenges the therapist to step out of the role of a silent expert and to struggle actively with the patient in the process of the "birthing of a self." This is not always a neat, structured process, but a dynamic one where there are many awkward moments. It challenges therapists to be clear about who they are and how they relate to others. It encourages therapists to be aware of their own struggles with shape and weight. It requires skills to assist patients in normalizing their eating and working through body image issues. Finally, as Steiner-Adair (1989) states, it demands an understanding of the cultural context in which an eating-disordered patient's struggle takes place, as well as the provision of a relationship where the patient can clearly experience herself as having an impact on others.

REFERENCES

Boskind-White, M., & White, W. C. (1983). *Bulimarexia: The binge purge cycle*. New York: Norton.

Boutacoff, L., Zollman, N., & Mitchell, T. E. (1984). *Healthy eating: A meal planning approach*. Eating Disorders Program, Department of Psychiatry, University of Minnesota.

Bruch, H. (1973). *Eating disorders: Obesity, anorexia nervosa, and the person within*. New York: Basic Books.

Cashdan, S. (1988). *Object relations therapy*. New York: Norton.

Fierman, L. B. (1965). *Effective psychotherapy: The contribution of Hellmuth Kaiser*. New York: Free Press.

Freud, S. (1965). *New introductory lectures in psycho-analysis* (J. Strachey, Ed. and Trans.). New York: Norton. (Original work published 1933)

Garner, D. M., Rockert, W., Olmsted, M. P., Johnson, C., & Coscina, D. V. (1984). Psychoeducational principles in the treatment of bulimia and anorexia nervosa. In D. M. Garner & P. E. Garfinkel (Eds.), *Handbook of psychotherapy for anorexia and bulimia* (pp. 513–572). New York: Guilford Press.

Gilligan, C. (1982). *In a different voice*. Cambridge, MA: Harvard University Press.

Greenspan, M. (1983). *A new approach to women and therapy*. New York: McGraw-Hill.

Horner, A. J. (1989). *The wish for power and the fear of having it*. Northvale, NJ: Jason Aronson.

Johnson, C., & Connors, M. E. (1987). *The etiology and treatment of bulimia nervosa*. New York: Basic Books.

Kearney-Cooke, A. M. (1989). Reclaiming the body: Using guided imagery in the treatment of body image disturbance among bulimic women. In L. M. Hornyak & E. K. Baker (Eds.), *Experiential therapies for eating disorders* (pp. 11–33). New York: Guilford Press.

Krueger, D. W. (1989). *Body self and psychological self*. New York: Brunner/Mazel.

Lee, D., & Hertzberg, J. (1978). Theories of feminine personality. In I. H. Freeze, J. E. Parsons, P. B. Johnson, D. N. Ruble, & G. L. Zellman (Eds.), *Women and sex roles*. New York: Norton.

Ogden, T. H. (1982). *Projective identification and psychotherapeutic technique*. New York: Jason Aronson.

Rabinor, J. (1989). *The process of recovery from an eating disorder: The use of journal writing in the initial stage of treatment*. Manuscript submitted for publication.

Rosen, J., & Leitenberg, J. (1984). Exposure plus response prevention treatment of bulimia. In D. M. Garner & P. E. Garfinkel (Eds.), *Handbook of psychotherapy for anorexia and bulimia* (pp. 193–209). New York: Guilford Press.

Sherman, J. A. (1971). *On the psychology of women: A survey of empirical studies*. Springfield, IL: Charles C. Thomas.

Steiner-Adair, C. (1989). Developing the voice of the wise women: College students and bulimia. *Journal of College Student Psychotherapy, 3* (2–4), 151–166.

Strober, M., & Yager, J. (1989). Some perspectives on the diagnosis of bulimia nervosa. *Journal of College Student Psychotherapy, 3*(2–4), 3–12.

Surrey, J. L. (1984). *Eating patterns as a reflection of women's development* (Work in Progress No. 83–06. Wellesley, MA: Wellesley College, Stone Center for Developmental Services and Studies.

Walters, M., Carter, E., Papp, P., & Silverstein, O. (1988). *The invisibile web: Gender patterns in family relationships*. New York: Guilford Press.

Weiss, L., Katzman, N., & Wolchik, S. (1986). *Treating bulmia: A psychoeducational approach.* New York: Pergamon Pres.

Wooley, S. C., & Kearney-Cooke, A. (1986). Intensive treatment of bulimia and body image disturbance. In K. D. Brownell & J. P. Foreyt (Eds), *Physiology, psychology and treatment of eating disorders.* New York: Basic Books.

Young-Eisendrath, P., & Wiedemann, F. (1987). *Female authority: Empowering women through psychotherapy.* New York: Guilford Press.

IV

INTEGRATIVE APPROACHES

∴ *13* ∴

Object Relations and the Family System: An Integrative Approach to Understanding and Treating Eating Disorders

LAURA LYNN HUMPHREY
Northwestern University Medical School
and Northwestern Memorial Hospital

A 20-year-old bulimic began to improve after more than a year of intensive treatment. As she made plans to move away for the next school term, her mother suddenly developed rheumatoid arthritis and needed the daughter to remain at home to care for her. In another family, the precipitous onset of multiple sclerosis in the mother coincided with her last child's attempt to individuate and to overcome her anorexia. Both of these families faced a painful, double-edged dilemma. If one member (in these two cases, the daughter with an eating disorder) shed his or her role as the "sick" or troubled one, it might have dangerous consequences for someone else (eventually a parent). This process of substituting one patient or problem for another in a family can be quite fluid. One family in the clinic had three teenage children, each with a severe addiction and self-destructive behavior. As soon as one child began to improve, another one would deteriorate until, finally, the father's alcoholism and the mother's suicidal depression could be addressed. Each of these families from my practice illustrates how integrally and inextricably involved family members are in a child's (usually a daughter's) eating disorder, and how her progress in treatment may have potentially serious implications for them as well. How are we to understand these complex, elusive, and unconscious processes in terms of current psychodynamic theories of anorexia and bulimia?

PRIOR FORMULATIONS OF THE FAMILY

Dynamic conceptualizations of anorexia and bulimia usually cite disturbances in the early mother–child or parent–child relationship that
predispose the child to developing an eating disorder during adolescence
(e.g., Bruch, 1973; Goodsitt, 1983; Masterson, 1977; Swift & Letven,
1984). The focus is on intrapsychic representations of these original
relationships in current life. Treatment then is directed at resolving the
developmental issues intrapsychically, through insight derived from interpretation and the relationship with the therapist. Yet clinical research
shows that such disturbed patterns in the family remain very much alive
and powerful in the ongoing interactions and relationship dynamics of
both anorexics and bulimics (see review by Strober & Humphrey, 1987;
see also Humphrey, 1988, 1989). For this reason, it would seem important to incorporate an understanding of the anorexic's or bulimic's family
in the present into our theories and treatment approaches. Unless this is
done, the daughter's own progress may be severely undermined by a
well-intentioned but unwitting family, or there may be serious casualties
among other family members, as illustrated by the cases above. The
purpose of this chapter is to develop such a family systems perspective on
anorexia and bulimia, but to do so within an essentially psychoanalytic
framework.

Systemic conceptualizations of the family to date have not been
primarily psychoanalytic in nature. Minuchin's structural approach taught
us about the many ways in which the anorexic child is needed by the
other family members in order to deny, and to detour them from confronting, other issues within the parents and their marriage (Minuchin,
Rosman, & Baker, 1978). This approach was the first to describe the
psychosomatic family as enmeshed, overprotective, and conflict-avoidant,
and as co-opting the anorexic daughter in alliances with one parent
against another, as in triangulation. Independently, Selvini-Palazzoli
(1978) made some very similar observations, and emphasized the importance of self-sacrifice, filial loyalty, and preserving appearances in
these families.

Also from a structural and strategic perspective, Schwartz, Barrett,
and Saba (1984) helped us to recognize the enormous impact of values,
roles, and customs through the generations in bulimic families. They also
elucidated the symbolic meanings of food for families with an eating
disorder. In her transgenerational view, Roberto (1986) described the
bulimic family legacies involving weight, eating, attractiveness, success,
and loyalty to the family before the self. Root, Fallon, and Friedrich
(1986) also emphasized the family life cycle and patterns surrounding food
and eating through the generations. They further classified bulimic fam-

ilies into "perfect," "overprotective," and "chaotic" subgroups, and for each one developed a specific conceptualization and treatment approach.

Each of these systemic formulations has been exceptionally rich and instructive in helping us to understand how the family operates as a whole, and how the eating disorder is vital in sustaining the overall balance and functioning of its members. What seems missing in these approaches is the integration of the family system dynamics with the intrapsychic and interpersonal elements of the members' relationships together. Object relations theory, expanded to incorporate the family system, seems very well suited to this task of integration, because its seminal intrapsychic constructs are interpersonal in origin (see Greenberg & Mitchell, 1983). This chapter, then, presents a conceptual formulation and an approach to treatment based upon an integration of object relations and family systems theories. It builds upon an earlier paper (Humphrey & Stern, 1988) in which we presented an integrative analysis of bulimic families from an object relations perspective, and is based in part on several related theoretical integrations of a more general nature (Gustafson, 1986; Pinsof, 1983; Scharff & Scharff, 1987; Slipp, 1984).

A set of working assumptions will facilitate this integrative formulation. First, I assume that the security and stability of the family as a whole is equal to or greater than that of each individual member. Second, there is a biopsychological press toward individuation, which emerges once the security needs of the family are met. Third, families are organized around central developmental issues that are transmitted intergenerationally. Finally, I assume that an individual's personality and behavior patterns fit and function perfectly in the family environment in which they evolved (see Humphrey & Stern, 1988, for more details). On the basis of these assumptions, which are themselves derived from object relations and family systems theories, let us now consider families with anorexia or bulimia.

There are two central organizing constructs from object relations theory that seem most relevant to families with an eating disorder. These are Winnicott's (1965) concept of the mother–infant "holding environment" and Klein's (1946/1975) conceptualization of early ego deficits at the level of part-object relations. Stern and I (Humphrey & Stern, 1988) proposed that families with an eating disorder have experienced certain failures in the early parental holding environment, and that these failures are transmitted through the generations. We believe that such failures lead to transgenerational, developmental adaptations, which result in relationships' being based on part-self and part-object relations, and on the use of primitive defenses that require others to complete the sense of self. These deficits and subsequent adaptations affect the quality and level of intrapsychic experience within individuals, as well as the interpersonal and systemic functioning of the family as a whole. Each of these processes is discussed in turn.

FAILURES IN THE HOLDING ENVIRONMENT

Winnicott's (1965) metaphor of the "holding environment" refers to the total empathic care that the "good enough" mother gives the infant during the first years of life. These maternal provisions include physical holding and affection; protection from injury; and providing the infant with a physical environment in which he or she can eat, sleep, learn, and grow to his or her potential. On a more emotional level, the holding environment includes nurturance, soothing, and containment of intense affect, normal grandiosity, and sexual impulses. "Holding" also refers to the mother's capacity to respond to the child's fluctuating states and needs in a nonmechanical, truly empathic way. Winnicott observed that it is through these holding functions that the child develops a fundamental sense of self and basic security. Once this is established, the child will begin to separate and become more playful, exploratory, and mastery oriented. The "good enough" mother enjoys this evolving individuation, but also remains available for the child to return to the mother when needed. As the mother responds to the infant's alternating needs for autonomy and dependency, the infant develops a resilient, cohesive, and enlivened sense of self.

The holding environment in anorexic and bulimic families fails them in (1) nurturance, (2) soothing and tension regulation, and (3) empathy and affirmation of separate identities. Parents and children alike are "starving" for nurturance, through emotional warmth and tenderness, and genuine unconditional affection for one another. This deficit in nurturance is compounded by an equally deficient capacity to tolerate and regulate tension and negative affective states. Families of anorexics and bulimics are unable to modulate frustration, anxiety, painful impingements from the environment, or overstimulation from either internal or external sources, so that these states interfere with their goal-directed functioning (see Gedo & Goldberg, 1973). This occurs because there is a profound absence of anyone in the family who can nurture, soothe, and sustain such overwhelming affects on a consistent enough basis.

Perhaps the most complex and demanding aspect of the family's holding environment lies in its capacity to empathize with each member's need to separate and individuate, which in turn enhances the structure and relatedness of the family as a whole. It requires that family members intuit and "mirror" each person's "spontaneous gesture" or "signal" (Winnicott, 1965) of emerging individuality, rather than imposing rigid expectations and roles from without. Unfortunately, in families with an eating disorder, these early and ongoing gestures are experienced as dangerous threats to the stability and well-being of the family, especially of the parents. This happens because the parents, were never mirrored in their attempts to separate from their own parents, so that they are still struggling with this developmental achievement themselves. Incomplete separation from the grandparents leaves the parents ill-equipped to facilitate this process in their own children.

Clinical experience with anorexic and bulimic families suggests that these failures in the holding environment are family-wide and multigenerational. They do not begin with the parents, nor will they end with the bulimic or anorexic daughter. Instead, the deficits in nurturance, soothing, and individuation reflect a transgenerational, developmental arrest or fixation that these families are trying desperately to master. It is an intergenerational legacy, if you will. The parents were never nurtured, soothed, or empathized with by their own parents, so that each parent is forever trying to master the deficits through re-enactments with their spouse and children. They impose their own preoccupations and unmet needs on their children, who in turn take care of the parents and sacrifice themselves; thus the pattern repeats itself (Humphrey & Stern, 1988).

Up to this point, I have emphasized the similarities between anorexic and bulimic families, but there are some striking differences as well. These differences are not so much in the underlying deficits with which they struggle, but rather in their particular adaptations to these deficits. In anorexic families, for example, nurturance can be lavished on the daughter, but only so long as she remains totally dependent and childlike. Once she begins to separate, she is negated, abandoned, or punished for doing so. The situation is different in bulimic families, where there is more likely to be a generalized experience of insatiable "hunger" for loving affection throughout the family. Another difference lies in the ways these two types of families attempt to regulate tension and dysphoric affects. The anorexic's family is quite constricted, superficial, and denying, just as she is herself. By contrast, the bulimic's family is more chaotic, hostile, and understructured—with the exception of the bulimic's mother, who fluctuates between intense neediness and being overwhelmed on the one hand, and cold, embittered denial and withholding on the other.

A parallel distinction can be observed in the ways each type of family responds to separation attempts. In anorexic families, the child's emerging self is enfeebled by invalidating and rejecting responses to separation, combined with solicitation of more dependent behavior (Masterson, 1977;

Minuchin et al., 1978; Selvini-Palazzoli, 1978). In bulimic families there is pervasive criticism, rejection, and self-preoccupation, even when the bulimic is enlisted in meeting the parents' needs. These clinical differences, along with the observed failures in the holding environment, have also received some empirical support (Humphrey, 1988, 1989; see review by Strober & Humphrey, 1987). Yet this is not the whole story in families with eating disorders. Klein's (1946/1975) contribution to object relations theory can enlighten us about these families as well.

DEVELOPMENTAL ADAPTATIONS THROUGH THE GENERATIONS

The ultimate result of the failures in the holding environment, repeated through the generations, is a family-wide developmental arrest at a stage before the emergence of a true self and nascent individuation. Family members remain fundamentally dependent on one another for their psychological integrity and stability. They are unable to maintain separate identities and self-contained personalities, so they must find some other means of adapting and surviving. In their attempt to insure the stability and security of the family as a whole, individual members act out their intrapsychic deficits and defenses through interpersonal relationships with one another. In families with anorexia or bulimia, the primary mechanisms involved in this process are splitting, idealization, and projective identification (Humphrey & Stern, 1988).

Klein (1946/1975) theorized that, in normal development, the young child initially experiences himself or herself and other people (i.e., self- and object representations, respectively) as split into all-good or all-bad "part-object" representations. The gratifying and powerful mother is all good; the frustrating and unavailable mother is all bad. The omnipotent self is all good, and the destructive self is all bad. During this stage of development, the child is unable to tolerate ambivalence, so he or she fears that the bad will destroy the good. In the language of defense mechanisms, the child splits its images of self and others into those who are loved, idealized, and introjected into the ego, and those who are hated, condemned, and projected outside the ego onto others.

Underlying this adaptive process is the unbearable burden of primary anxiety, primitive aggression, and fear of disintegration. Part-object defenses, in Klein's view, enable the child to maintain a vital sense of security, cohesion, and self-esteem. For this reason, then, the child is totally dependent on others, and even requires them to complete and stabilize the inner sense of self. Children who never progress beyond this stage of part-object relations remain fundamentally dependent on other people for their own psychological equilibrium. This is precisely the situation in anorexic and bulimic families. Also consistent with Klein's theory, there appear to be two primary mechanisms of adaptation operating: idealization and projective identification.

Idealization is the more conspicuous process in anorexic and bulimic families. There is a family-wide pressure to be "picture-perfect" and to conform to very high standards of achievement and physical appearance. Family members present a shallow, brittle facade of being successful, attractive, and "the picture of health" (Selvini-Palazzoli, 1978). Idealization can also operate in bulimic, and especially anorexic, families through the assignment of one member to the role of being the idealized object or the special one. Most often, this is the anorexic daughter in those families or a talented brother in the bulimics' families. The all-good object is expected to fulfill the parent's own fantasies for great success or achievement, or for the mothering and mirroring they never had. In return, the child receives affection, admiration, and a heroic self-image. In some families, these children are granted special privileges and a kind of pseudoseparation, so that they can go out into the world and fulfill their mutual dreams. If such a child begins to separate or fails to excel, then, very often, the failure is negated or denied. In this way, the idealized object is inextricably tied to the family system for psychological survival and a kind of pseudo-identity.

Projective identification is the more complex and elusive process operating in these families. Klein (1946/1975) first conceptualized projective identification as the splitting off of bad, unwanted parts of the self and projection of them into another person with whom one is in a dependent relationship. Since these bad projections are a fundamental aspect of the personality, they are experienced as a vital external extension of the projector's self. Slipp (1984) and Zinner and Shapiro (1972) extended Klein's formulation to the ongoing interpersonal dynamics among members of a family. Zinner and Shapiro (1972) first explained the essential elements needed to establish projective identification within the family: (1) The subject perceives the object as if he or she contained aspects of the subject's personality; (2) the subject can evoke parallel feelings in the object; (3) the subject can experience vicariously the behavior and emotions of the object; and (4) those in such dependent relationships are in collusion to maintain the mutual projections.

Based upon our experience with anorexic, and especially bulimic, families, it appears that projective identification is at the heart of their adaptation to the transgenerational failures in the holding environment. Parents project the unwanted parts of themselves into their child, then identify with those parts as extensions of the self. They perceive her, and she experiences herself, as greedy, demanding, incompetent, selfish, weak, dishonest, lazy, promiscuous, and so on. Through the projective identification, the parents and siblings are able to localize much of their warded-off anxiety and rage within her; they thereby maintain their own psychological equilibrium, and the stability of the family as a whole. The daughter accepts or identifies with these projections because she fears abandonment or rejection, and also because she is needed to fulfill a critical function for her family. For example, a father may unconsciously encourage and enjoy his daughter's acting out, but condemn her outwardly at the same time. A mother may be able to feel a kind of control over her own overwhelming feelings and needs by projecting them into the daughter, but remaining in close contact with her. Given this understanding of families with eating disorders, the bulimic or anorexic daughter emerges as both the victim and the heroine of the family. Effective treatment should incorporate a thorough appreciation of both these aspects of her identity, and her vital role in the stability of the family.

THE GENERAL APPROACH TO FAMILY THERAPY

Based on this conceptualization of anorexia and bulimia, family therapy will attempt to provide a "good enough" holding environment to promote whole-object relations and self-representations throughout the family system. This requires empathy, nurturance, containment of affect and projections, reasonable limits, appropriate boundaries, and support for separation–individuation. There is also a systemic assumption that whatever developmental patterns contributed to the need for the eating disorder will still exist, and remain vital to the family's equilibrium and security. These relational patterns will emerge in the complex transferences and processes of interaction among family members, and between the family members and the therapist(s).

The "good enough" therapist also conveys a healthy appreciation and respect for the family's developmental adaptation, without ascribing blame or pressuring the system to change. He or she treats the whole family as the "patient" in a sense, and considers each member's evolving role in the therapeutic process both in and out of sessions—for example, in phone conversations with the therapist. This is true even when a family member lives out of town, refuses to come in, insists that he or she is unnecessary, or the like. Everyone plays a role, so everyone is essential. In individual therapy too, it is often very helpful to involve the spouse, children, parents, and siblings at certain key points in treatment. This can consolidate the working-through process, promote separation, and avert or address other casualties as the family loses a critical, stabilizing function in the anorexic or bulimic member.

Therapeutic style and technique in this approach to family treatment are also consistent with an integration of psychoanalytic and family systems theories. The therapist's stance toward the family is friendly, respectful, active, and collaborative. The therapist is very real and natural in his or her affective responses to family members as well. This does not imply a loss of boundaries or poor role definition, but rather being truly, deeply involved in the family's psychological world. This insider's perspective enables the family to open up and trust the therapist, and it allows the therapist to use his or her own experience with the family to understand how the family members feel and function. This "realness" does not have to interfere with the unconscious and symbolic processes that operate in the family, such as primitive defenses and transferences. In fact, the opposite it true when the therapist can experience such relations at first hand.

In this integrative model of family therapy, the therapist moves easily between process and structural or strategic interventions as necessary. Process-oriented techniques include observing and interpreting for the family members how their ongoing interactions and transferences reflect developmental deficits and adaptations through the generations. For example, the therapist might interpret how the daughter's eating disorder represents the same wish for nurturance and separation that her mother cannot express to her grandmother. Exploration of dreams and fantasies within the family can also promote greater self-awareness and open disclosure of feelings to one another.

In contrast to process-oriented techniques, structural and strategic interventions are usually more confrontive and directive, and they do not rely on insight in order to be effective (e.g., Minuchin et al., 1978; Selvini-Palazzoli, 1978). These include such strategies as giving homework assignments, asking a child to move her seat in order to dislodge herself from the parents' marital conflicts, or prescribing the symptom. Such interventions can be extremely powerful and therapeutic when they are employed within the context of an empathic holding environment.

Certain aspects of the therapist's work with the family can be especially challenging in this open and involved approach. One of the most difficult of these is the therapist's function as a self-object for each parent. It is necessary so that the child can be freed from this vital but exploited position. Such a role can be tumultuous and disturbing in families with more primitive affects and wishes, as in the case of the bad object for a parental projective identification. Tolerating and mirroring the family's aggression and dependency are critical, yet they can also be very provocative for the therapist to experience. The "good enough" therapist must accept these unsettling projections and then return them to the family in a more ego-modulated form, without acting out the family's unconscious affects and fantasies.

This was needed of me in a bulimic family I saw recently. The daughter's impending separation stimulated her mother's paranoid fantasy that the father was going to leave her for a young divorced woman. My role was to contain the mother's overwhelming abandonment anxiety and rage, which had been projected onto the bulimic daughter. This was a very powerful experience for me, and I had to stay attuned to my own feelings of anger and mistrust toward the father, and fantasies of the family's abrupt, untimely termination of therapy. It helped considerably to understand how the projective identification had shifted from the daughter to me, and how it was therapeutic for me to tolerate it and mirror the abandonment anxiety for the mother.

As this case example illustrates, the specific content from session to session will depend primarily upon the family's own agenda, and whatever issues emerge as a result of the therapist's observations and interpretations. Usually the therapist would attempt to explore what the family is up against; what is at stake; how it operates and why; how the eating disorder is a misguided attempt to solve a problem; in what ways the anorexia or bulimia is the culmination of developmental deficits through the generations; and what is needed in order to free the system to move beyond its current adaptation, among other things. Regardless of the specific issues, however, the therapist's fundamental objective is to provide a nurturant, containing, and empathic holding environment. In this context, let us now consider the progress of therapy as it unfolds in the early, middle, and late phases of treatment.

THE EARLY PHASE: ESTABLISHING
THE HOLDING ENVIRONMENT

Family therapy begins with the first inquiry about treatment, whether this comes from another family member or from the patient herself. It is very common for a mother, a sister, or (less often) a father to make the first contact. The family member is concerned about the problem and genuinely wants to find help. Often, he or she has reached a point of desperation by this time and may need some information about the problem and suggestions about how to approach the issue with the anorexic or bulimic member. The initiating family member may also express a certain caution and skepticism about treatment, even though he or she realizes how serious the problem is. This initial conversation can provide the therapist with some important data about how the family operates under stress, and how its members relate to the eating disorder. Some families require a series of telephone contacts with the therapist before they are able to come in for a face-to-face meeting. One father I recently spoke to for the first time insisted that we not delve into the family relationships in order to treat his daughter's anorexia. He was quite fearful and mistrustful, and needed reassurance that I was not on a witch hunt.

Based on this first telephone conversation, the therapist can begin to formulate some working hypotheses about the family dynamics and roles, and can begin to establish some essential boundaries and alliances. It can also be the best opportunity to enlist the family members' involvement in treatment, because their motivation is highest at this point. Our experience suggests that the therapist does best to accept the family members where they are, and to try to respond with candor, warmth, and concrete information as it is needed.

The Initial Interview

Involving the family members in the first face-to-face interview lays the groundwork for their ongoing participation, and is helpful for several other reasons as well. At a practical level, it increases the likelihood that the anorexic or bulimic child will make the first appointment and follow up with the treatment recommendations. Sometimes the family's denial and ambivalence about therapy can be diminished by its involvement and reassurance. In addition, it seems very responsive to include anyone who has been in contact with the therapist by phone or who has encouraged the daughter to seek treatment. Involving other family members in the assessment process also improves the quality and depth of information obtained, especially when denial or shame makes the patient's report questionable or even unreliable.

At a more conceptual level, to exclude the family members from treatment or to collude with their resistance to treatment invites two types of repercussions. First, without the family's implicit consent, the child with the eating disorder may be unable to separate and get well. This is not surprising if one considers what a central and vital role her anorexia or bulimia plays in the family's equilibrium. When individual therapy begins to push for greater separation, the patient will feel that she is betraying her own parents if she aligns with the treatment team. Sometimes this is workable with interpretation alone, but too often the family needs some direct support in order to let her go.

The second kind of problem that can result from excluding the family from therapy is that another family member can become an unexpected casualty of the progress in individual treatment. It is almost inevitable either that another member will have to assume the anorexic's or bulimic's role as a self-object for the parent(s), or that the parents themselves will have to reintegrate the split-off or missing parts of their own personalities. Usually, another child will sacrifice himself or herself in order to protect the parents' fragile selves and relationships. Occasionally, though, it is a parent who will become suicidally depressed, have an extramarital affair, or develop a severe medical illness as a secondary consequence of the daughter's separation.

Once the face-to-face interview occurs, the therapist's role and opportunities broaden. It is usually best to meet with the anorexic or bulimic daughter alone first, and then to invite the family to participate in the remainder of the interview. Approximately 45 minutes are needed for each subgroup. During the meeting with the daughter alone, it is important to explore her developmental history and her feelings about her relationships with the other members of the family, in depth. In order for her to trust the therapist at all, and to be able to disclose these feelings to an outsider, the therapist must make the boundaries explicit between what she discusses in private and what can be shared with the parents. Sometimes there is a poor boundary to begin with between the individual and the family; in those cases, the therapist is making an intervention toward improving this self-definition. In other families, the daughter appreciates and responds well to the therapist's validation of her own private perceptions and feelings. In all cases, though, it is important for the therapist to define or preserve the boundaries between individuals and the family as a whole.

The initial meeting with the family will focus on gathering information and building rapport. The most important source of information about the family members is the therapist's observation of the process of their interactions together. In fact, in a study of family interactions in this population (Humphrey, Apple, & Kirschenbaum, 1986), we found that we could distinguish between bulimic/anorexic and normal families on the basis of a 10-minute discussion of the daughter's separation. Based on their process communications alone, we could differentiate successfully between the two groups over 80% of the time.

In addition to experiencing and observing the family's dynamics and roles, the therapist also inquires about the family members' developmental and psychiatric histories, their perceptions of how each member functions and relates in the family, the onset and evolution of the eating disorder, and their understanding of why this may have happened to them. It is important to focus on the daughter's eating disorder during the interview so that the family members feel understood and responded to, and so that they are not threatened too much by questions implicating them in the etiology. Most parents come into the first session feeling guilty and responsible for the daughter's problem, and this should be addressed directly. The therapist is not there to blame anyone or to pass judgment. Virtually all of these parents are well intentioned and have done the best that they could.

Inquiring about the family members' hypotheses of why the eating disorder began is often very revealing. They nearly always have some theory for understanding the eating disorder, and many of them will have read extensively before they ever meet the therapist. Some families are very guarded and defensive, and seem to externalize blame and responsibility. Other families only consider the more behavioral aspects of the disorder, but are able to link these to the daughter's poor self-esteem. Then there also those families that are more psychologically attuned, and can identify accurately some important developmental or family events that contributed to the anorexia or bulimia. Virtually no families, though, have a systemic understanding of how the daughter's illness serves an adaptive function for the family as a whole. The therapist can learn a lot more about the family members than just their implicit theories about the disorder by asking this kind of question.

Once the therapist has asked all of his or her questions, it is very important to give something back to the family. This includes answering the family members' questions, and also giving them a formulation of the eating disorder and recommendations for treatment. The therapist's conceptualization for the family of the nature and function of the anorexia or bulimia incorporates the family's hypotheses, matches the family members' level of development and insight, and teaches them something that they are open to learning. For example, I might suggest to a relatively uninsightful family,

> I agree with your observations about Cindy's condition, and I support your concern for her health and well-being. My impression is that Cindy developed her bulimia at a time when she felt unprepared for the new demands of high school and dating, in an attempt to slow down the clock and give herself some time to understand her changing body and feelings. As you pointed out, this was also a difficult time in the family because your father *(looking to Mom)* was ill, and your company *(to Dad)* was in a financial crisis. All of these pressures, and probably others that we aren't aware of, must have been overwhelming to Cindy and resulted in her turning to dieting and bulimia as a way to feel some sense of control and mastery.

This usually stimulates some discussion and questions from the family members, and they will often add their own new insights to the therapist's formulation. Then it is time to make the recommendations

about treatment and the need for family involvement. These recommendations grow naturally out of the therapist's stated understanding of
the problem and can be linked to it quite explicitly, so that the family can
stand behind the plan right from the outset. For the family above, I might
offer,

> So we would like to approach this bulimia from several angles. First,
> Cindy needs some education and support to improve her eating
> habits and reduce her binge-eating and vomiting. Second, she needs
> individual therapy to understand and work through her deeper feel-
> ings about her body, herself, and her relationships. Perhaps most
> importantly, Cindy needs her family's participation in therapy to
> help her with all of this, as well as to help you as she, and you, work
> through these painful problems. We would like to be there to sup-
> port and inform you as well as Cindy.

In all that the therapist says, the family members need to feel that he or
she respects them, enjoys them, and can truly understand them and be
helpful at this time of crisis.

The Early Sessions

The early phase of family therapy is devoted to establishing the holding
environment and setting the stage for deeper changes in the family's level
of object relations and self-structure. Providing nurturance, boundaries,
containment of affect, and support for individuation is at the heart of the
holding environment. Nurturance in this early stage consists of a warm,
comforting, active therapeutic stance. The family needs to know what the
therapist is truly made of, and what his or her deeper motivations may be,
so that trust may emerge in time. It requires that the therapist be willing
to gratify some of the self-object needs of the family members, as well as
to fill some of their deficits and longings. They are not able to utilize much
interpretation at this point, and instead need the therapist to provide
some of what has been missing. The eating disorder is almost always the
explicit focus in the early sessions. The therapist can address the eating
disorder directly, as well as conceptualizing it as a metaphor or behavior
sample for other levels of meaning and relating in the family.

The family usually begins the early sessions by asking the therapist
many questions, including, for example, "Should we stop buying snack
foods or lock the cabinets to keep her from bingeing?"; "How will we
know if she starts taking the laxatives again?"; "Can we still plan to go on
vacation in a few weeks?"; or "What will we talk about in family sessions?"
It is best for the therapist to answer some such questions frankly, but

to do so in a way that also encourages open communication and discussion. If the therapist avoids giving suggestions and advice altogether, the family members will see this as withholding and aloof, and they will become angry and guarded. On the other hand, if the therapist always tells them how to respond, they will find that intrusive and demeaning. The therapist has to strike a delicate balance in which he or she is guiding and teaching the family members how to really listen to and understand one another, so that their mutual disclosures and differences can be the basis of their negotiations.

The family's focus on the eating disorder also provides a good opportunity to work on the boundaries and roles with the family. Usually, the family has two simultaneous problems with its role structure: The boundaries inside the family are too fluid and lack appropriate generational hierarchy, and those relating to the external world are too closed and rigid. This has evolved in order to protect the family's fragile adaptation. It keeps outsiders out and insiders in. Those outside the family (including the therapist) are considered to be potentially dangerous threats to the family's stability and security. Inside the family, children are elevated to the role of parental confidants or allies on the one hand, but are also thwarted from pursuing age-appropriate relationships and activities beyond the family on the other. The family needs help from the therapist, as an "inside-outsider," to loosen and open the boundaries to the external world and to reinforce a firm but flexible structure within the family. At this stage of treatment, this is best accomplished through observations of these patterns shared with the family, and through structural interventions such as asking the children to sit together and listen quietly while their parents discuss a problem.

In addition to nurturance and boundaries, the therapeutic holding environment must provide the containment and regulation of affects and impulses. This is especially challenging in families with eating disorders, because they have deep, pervasive deficits in this aspect of holding. In families of anorexics, the therapeutic task is to help stimulate their awareness of their feelings and needs, and enable them to tolerate what has otherwise been extremely disturbing and overwhelming. Quite the opposite occurs in bulimic families. They experience and express their feelings and drives much more intensely. They are overtly conflictual, chaotic, and hostilely enmeshed. Holding these families involves titrating and modulating the unbearable intensity and neediness, and helping them to do so through nascent internal capacities and constructive external channels.

The therapeutic holding environment also encourages self-expression and tolerance of differences as steps toward separation. As both Minuchin (Minuchin et al., 1978) and Selvini-Palazzoli (1978) observed in their original formulations, family members in this population sacrifice their individuality for the greater good of the family. They speak for one another and negate or punish the expression of differences. At the very least, they cannot freely express themselves and trust that they will be accepted and understood. Early on, the therapist can promote self-expression and individuality by blocking their attempts to read one another's minds or thwart differences, in favor of speaking only for oneself and with candor and emotion.

These families feel so ambivalent and conflicted about revealing their true feelings that it distorts and undermines the clarity of their communication as well. Our research studies (e.g., Humphrey, 1989) have shown that families of both anorexics and bulimics use many more complex and confusing messages than do normal controls, and that there are even reliable differences between the two subtypes. They need help in tuning in to their true feelings and stating them directly and clearly, then accepting and negotiating their inevitable differences. Most families will work with relative comfort and interest on their communication problems, so this is often a productive focus in the early phase.

Regardless of how empathic and effective the therapist is in establishing all of these aspects of the holding environment, the family will need to test them again and again. These transference tests are an essential part of the therapeutic process, in that they enable the family members to learn, battle, reconcile, and eventually internalize the holding functions. Each family will undoubtedly choose the ones it needs most, but there are certain tests that are quite predictable for all families with eating disorders. One such test in bulimic families involves timing and affect containment. These families can easily entice an enthusiastic therapist into moving too quickly before the holding environment is sufficiently in place. They seem to be very expressive and motivated early on, and they may bring a very central issue into the treatment. This can be an unconscious test of the therapist's wish to change them and force separation before they are ready.

Another predictable test in bulimic and anorexic families involves mirroring the mother. It is usually the mother in these families who has the most intense and vital projective identification with the anorexic or bulimic child, and therefore has the most to lose if individuation occurs. Also by virtue of her role in the family, she often wields the most power in important decisions, including whether to remain in treatment. If the mother is going to allow her child and self-object to move away, she will need to feel that the therapist can step in to replace the needed functions. Most importantly at this stage, the therapist must be able to mirror the mother and help her to feel contained without making this explicit or conscious. If this fails and the mother feels too threatened, no one else in the family will challenge the inevitable termination.

A third type of transference test that the therapist can expect parallels the family's dilemma around separation. The family members will unwittingly tempt the therapist either to intrude on some aspect of their own responsibility, or to alienate them by becoming too distant and aloof, or both. This is precisely the challenge with which the anorexic or bulimic child presents her parents when she needs greater autonomy and self-sufficiency but is not really prepared to handle them, as demonstrated by her self-destructive and impulsive behavior. The family members need to feel and observe that the therapist can be trusted to respect their rights and boundaries without depriving them of some valuable new input and limits. If the therapist can provide these functions for the parents, then they can internalize them and offer the same to their children.

One other type of test that the therapist will inevitably face in the early phase of treatment with this population involves the family's narcissism. The family members present themselves as entitled, demanding, well informed, and socially and professionally well connected. Their busy schedules are more important than keeping their therapy appointments. They will test the therapist's patience and limits in this area many times. In addition to these devaluations, such families also need to idealize the therapist and the institution. This is necessary to mirror and fortify their own narcissistic vulnerabilities. The therapist's challenge is to contain and modulate these idealizations and devaluations without becoming too outraged, or inflated or deflated, by the experience.

Since families of anorexics and bulimics are unable to utilize interpretation during this early phase of therapy, the working through of these transference tests must be largely experiential and preconscious. However, the therapist can begin to set the stage for subsequent deeper analysis and interpretation all through the early sessions. This groundwork must be laid gently and carefully so that the family does not become even more defensive and suspicious. Several strategies have been particularly helpful with this. Perhaps most importantly, the therapist does not push the family members to explore their deeper feelings and issues, but rather listens carefully and responds to their own signals that they are relaxing their vigilant defenses. This incorporates Winnicott's (1965) construct of the "spontaneous gesture" during separation, in which the parent responds to the child's initiative rather than anticipating the child's needs for him or her.

As the family feels held, the parents will gradually begin to bring in more material from their own inner experience, from family problems other than the eating disorder, and even from relationships with the extended family. All of these topics, if approached delicately and slowly, will eventually begin to expose the underlying dynamics and deficits in holding and object relations. Once this process is initiated, the therapist can use these openings to explore the parents' roles and relations with their families of origin, and how these developmental patterns may make them more sensitive or vulnerable when they re-emerge in their new family. This is an iterative process of successive approximations toward ever more open disclosures of their deeper feelings and motivations. The family must also be allowed to turn back to their old defenses as they need to, and move forward as they seem ready. This requires that the therapist be available for "emotional refueling," as Mahler (1968) has described of the mother during the process of her child's moves between mastery and dependence.

Some families never progress beyond this early phase of treatment, and terminate as soon as the daughter's condition has stabilized. They may not need more than the educational, behavioral, and structural interventions of the early phase. For them, the holding provisions— combined with the work on boundaries and roles, communication, and problem solving, as well as support for the daughter's separation—may be all that is needed. For other families, the prospect of deeper change may be too threatening to continue once the crisis has passed. In either case, the therapist has no other leverage for continued treatment once the eating disorder has remitted and no one else has developed an obvious problem. The therapist can leave the door open or even suggest that the family come back in 2 or 3 months for a follow-up visit. It can also be helpful to predict the kind of patterns or problems that family members are likely to see if they need to return to treatment, such as the patient's depression or withdrawal, another child's health or school performance, a breakdown of communication, or the like. With all of the processes of the early phase in mind, let us now consider a case example of a family whom we will follow through each phase of treatment.

A Case Illustration

The Sterling family was referred for treatment by their family physician and a local hospital. The 18-year-old daughter, Lily, had been struggling with bulimia for almost 2 years, and had also dropped out of beauty school. The father worked as an attorney and was a partner in a large, successful law practice. The mother was a homemaker, with interests in gardening and collecting antiques. There was also a 15-year-old daughter, Iris, who was doing well academically and socially. Only the two grandmothers were still living; the paternal grandfather had died 4 years earlier of heart failure, and the maternal grandfather had had cirrhosis of the liver and died of complications of chronic alcoholism about 2½ years earlier. There were no other reported physical or emotional problems on either side. The family lived near both grandmothers, and all of the extended family were within a hundred miles.

The early phase of treatment with the Sterling family was fairly typical of this population. The family members were well meaning and engaging, and were willing to do anything that would help Lily. They attended their sessions quite reliably and seemed appreciative and relieved by our treatment protocol and expertise. The family idealized me and my male cotherapist, who was quite experienced in family systems therapy and almost finished with his dissertation. They responded well to our holding functions, especially affect containment and limit setting. They wanted to move too quickly for their own resources, and needed us to mirror them and titrate their overwhelming anxiety and frustration.

Mrs. Sterling at times would need constant nurturance and containment, and at other times would be the most insightful contributor. Mr. Sterling was like a third therapist, always trying to solve the problem and making helpful suggestions without exposing anything of himself. Lily was very tuned in to her mother, taking her cues from her mother's unstated but obvious needs. Sometimes she would provoke a conflict; other times she would be lighthearted and funny; and still other times she would be depressed and introverted—whatever her mother seemed to feel or need. Her sister, Iris, was the helpful, strong, cooperative child who could always be counted on to be responsible and cool-headed in a crisis.

The early sessions focused initially on understanding and managing the eating disorder. The family members learned to see fluctuations in the bulimia as signals that something was difficult for Lily and she could not express it any other way. We used this as a means to help them listen to one another's communications (both verbal and nonverbal) more carefully, and to reflect what they heard in their ongoing interactions. These sessions also addressed the need for a stronger generational boundary, so that the parents would confide in each other and the daughters could go their own way a bit more.

The family tested our holding capacity and our implicit agenda many times, usually through Lily's acting out. She got caught shoplifting clothes and was fired from a part-time job for failing to go to work, among other things. These crises followed a predictable pattern, some of which we were eventually able to observe with the family itself. A crisis would seem to happen at a moment of relative quiescence when some degree of separation was emerging. Lily would cause some disturbance that would bring everyone back together, angry and frightened, but full of intense emotion and commitment to the family. Each crisis enabled Mr. Sterling to troubleshoot and solve problems, as he emerged as a family hero. Mrs. Sterling was no longer panic-stricken about the loss and abandonment she feared would accompany separation. Lily herself felt some remorse and self-criticism, but these incidents only confirmed her self-image as an irresponsible loser. During this first phase, the family members were able to move away from their superficial understanding of the function of these crises and away from blaming Lily and her bad character. Through our observations of these repetitions, in the context of an adequate holding environment, they were gradually able to see that there was some adaptive purpose to these family emergencies and that everyone played a role in them. They tested our empathy for their separation anxiety, as well as our ability to set limits and be firm without intruding on their family boundary. This, of course, was the same test Lily gave her parents when she acted out.

There was not much discussion of the extended family at this point, but there was an unstated acknowledgment that we would need to discuss it in time. Occasionally, the relatives would be mentioned as part of another issue, and we would inquire casually about various people and their significance to the family. We were especially attentive to any mention of the two grandmothers, but did not pursue this material openly because this would have been too dangerous. We just listened and responded reflectively without pushing. It was more important that the family members begin to relax and trust us with this critical information about their object world. Meanwhile, Lily's eating disorder was improving, and the family was much more open and effective in their daily lives by the end of the early phase.

THE MIDDLE PHASE OF TREATMENT

Shifts in Process

Once the family members are willing to explore their deeper, more unconscious motivations and feelings, and the meaning and function of their adaptive mechanisms, then they have moved into the middle phase of therapy. The focus of these sessions is on identifying, observing, and exploring their unconscious motives and systemic processes, on both the *intra*personal and *inter*personal levels. Interventions during this phase become much more interpretive and symbolic, and they actively encourage separation and the development of healthier, more flexible defenses and boundaries. All of this work is possible only so long as the family members feel secure, nurtured, and contained enough in the therapeutic holding environment to allow them to trust the therapist and the ongoing relationship.

With the holding provisions in place, the therapist can begin to interpret the unconscious processes that operate among family members, as well as between all of them and the therapist. This begins to unfold as the therapist comments more on the here-and-now process of interactions between members, and what these interactions suggest about their underlying feelings and motivations. Usually, such ongoing interactions communicate many levels of meaning, both conscious and unconscious, to the observant therapist. Empirical research has also shown that interpersonal communications in families with anorexia or bulimia are replete with double messages and complex meanings, which are often beyond the families' awareness (Humphrey, 1989).

The family members may need help from the therapist as observer and interpreter of the unconscious in order to understand themselves and one another more fully. Initially, they receive this with some apprehension, because they are afraid of what they will learn. It is essential that the therapist not act as though he or she possesses some special knowledge about the family, but rather as if he or she is a kind of guide and interpreter in a foreign realm with a new language—that is, the unconscious world of the family. Gradually the family members themselves will learn to speak the language, and thereby bring this world into their conscious awareness. In my experience, family members come to share the therapist's fascination, appreciation, and respect for their unconscious life in time, and to see and hear those aspects of one another with greater clarity and empathy.

In a related vein, the therapist can help to shape the family members' self-expression and communication to reflect more of their true feelings and opinions, rather than what they believe they are expected to say. Such expectations are often based upon their roles and relations within the family, and are usually confining and oppressive to the sense of self and others. Simple inquiries by the therapist may be all that are needed at this point to prompt a deeper level of self-attunement and outward expression—for example, "Is there some other aspect of your feelings on this as well?"; or "Given what you told us earlier happened to you as a teenager, I wonder how you react when Sara misses curfew."

Another shift that occurs during the middle phase of therapy involves the incorporation of the extended family into the sessions, either in person or at least in discussion. Parallels and differences in family values and roles through the generations are explored, as well as their impact, both conscious and unconscious, on the family's current relationships. This seems least threatening if it begins with some developmental issue that has emerged with the identified patient, such as how decision making was done in each of the parents' families of origin. This discussion can greatly improve the parents' empathy for their daughter's wishes, as well as her understanding of their motivations and reactions.

Shifts in Content

The focus thus far has been on changes in the therapeutic process that occur during the middle phase of treatment; however, there are also important shifts in the content of the sessions. What might have been more educative or structural interventions during the early phase become more interpretive and transactional during this middle phase. Interpretation usually begins most easily with the function and meaning of the eating disorder. The anorexia or bulimia has unique meanings for each family, but its metaphorical significance at different levels is always compelling. For example, bulimia can express the daughter's ambivalence about autonomy because it is both an oppositional protest and a cry for help at the same time. Bulimia can also reflect the parents' ambivalence about her separation because it enables them to stay closely involved with her, while at the same time wishing that she would go. At a more systemic level, the bulimia might symbolize the family members' hunger for "good enough" mothering and mirroring, but fear of being deprived, and their false-self adaptation to this unconscious dilemma.

Usually, there is some kind of specific family legacy surrounding eating and physical appearance, which should be explored as well. For example, in each generation there may be a role reversal in which it is the daughter who nurtures and contains the mother, and not the other way around. For this generation, the bulimia is an expression of hunger and anger and confusion. For others, anorexia may be a metaphor for the lack of mirroring of the psychological self in favor of the physical and social self. In these families, anorexia reflects a degree of grandiosity, in which they deny their biological need for nourishment as an external representation of their shrunken, depleted emotional selves. With any such interpretations, the family members can usually accept observations about the "sick" member first, but gradually are more open to their own roles and contributions as well.

Exploring the adaptive function of the eating disorder is often an entry into the fundamental issue of separation within the family. Lack of separation is a central organizing deficit in families with eating disorders, at the level of both family structure and intrapsychic structure. Parents are not sufficiently separated from their own parents, from each other, or from their children. Therefore, much of the work of the middle phase of therapy is devoted to building separate identities within family members and for the family as a whole. Separation usually begins, as do most other developmental issues in these families, around the eating disorder. The family expresses its ambivalence about the daughter's separation through the eating disorder. She cannot freely move away from her dependence on the family without a wrenching process of coming and going. The parents and siblings, in turn, cannot bear to lose her even though they are exasperated, afraid, and angry.

Through the early work of the therapy, the daughter usually makes the first move toward separation by understanding and expressing her true feelings and differences within the family. The family members are both moved and frightened by this because it has serious implications for each of them. With their primary adaptation being challenged by the "sick" member, they are ungrounded and very anxious. The therapist must watch for casualties within the family system at this point, and try to hold the family in treatment until its members have readjusted their equilibrium. The first repercussion is usually that another child will replace the anorexic or bulimic as the focus within the family. Next, the mother's emotional fragility will emerge, along with her husband's unavailability and injured or depleted self. Marital problems are inevitable when there is so much internal and interpersonal turmoil. It is truly a dangerous time for the family, but it is also a time full of opportunity for change and hope.

What is the therapeutic response to this crisis? Holding. The therapist maintains his or her position as the good enough parent who provides and interprets exactly what is missing in the family itself—nurturance, containment, empathy, and support for individuation and self-fulfillment. At times, the needs of the family system will seem to be at odds with the developmental needs of the individual (see Stern, Chapter 5, this volume), but the therapist respects and encourages both. If the therapist neglects the family's press to remain enmeshed and undifferentiated, then the family members may feel betrayed and terminate treatment because they project that the therapist is trying to destroy their family. It is the most challenging time of all for the therapist because of the degree of chaos, primitive affect, and shifting transference and alliances.

Technically, the therapist relies on a balance between interpretive and structural or strategic interventions, and among intrapsychic, interpersonal, and systemic phenomena. Ideally, most processes within the family occur at all three levels, and these can be woven into the therapeutic experience for the family. Incorporating the extended family can also greatly facilitate the process at this point. For example, inviting each of the grandparents to describe how issues such as family loyalty, self-sacrifice, or success were dealt with as he or she grew up can be very enlightening. This might stimulate further discussion of how the grandparents' experiences shaped the decisions they made about their children, and how those in turn affected the anorexic or bulimic and her siblings. In the holding context, this kind of exploration is often experienced as poignant, intimate, and even ironic, in that what was initially intended to be some form of reparation or mastery of earlier deficits can result in an unforeseen repetition a generation or two later.

Once this process of separation begins throughout the family, the danger—but also the developmental progress—is geometric. The parents of the anorexic or bulimic child will begin to assert themselves to their own parents, who usually accept it more easily than they did the first time around. This enables the parents to solidify their own individuation, and therefore to empathize better with their anorexic or bulimic daughter's parallel efforts. At the same time, the therapist is helping the family to identify and analyze such issues through the transferences. One of the best means of unraveling these unconscious processes is through the use of projective identification, both between family members and between them and the therapist.

Klein's (1946/1975) construct of projective identification was originally conceived as an intrapsychic defense, but it has been expanded to encompass a family-wide adaptation (Zinner & Shapiro, 1972) and a therapeutic process (Tansey & Burke, 1989). Both are valid and valuable additions to the family treatment of eating disorders. As I have discussed earlier, families with anorexia or bulimia organize their self- and other representations around such part-object relations. The bulimic child is often the bad object, whereas the anorexic child is the idealized object. As the family begins to approach true separation, these projective identifications and idealizations will emerge, and the therapist will be brought into the experience as well.

The approach of true separation becomes more palpable to the therapist either because the family rigidly and unrelentingly clings to an unrealistic perception of the child despite growing evidence to the contrary, or because the therapist himself or herself begins to feel inordinately valued or devalued by the family. When the projective identification moves into the transference with the therapist, he or she begins to feel some of what the receiver experiences, but to a much lesser degree. For example, the therapist may become aware that the family has accumulated a large bill over the past few months, in part because of last-minute cancellations. When approached, the family may be quite entitled and devaluing toward the therapist and the work in treatment. The therapist may feel enraged but responsible for the whole problem, much as the bulimic daughter does. This kind of overreaction and hostile ambivalence in the therapist may signify the presence of a projective identification. Similarly, an introjected idealization can often be recognized when the therapist becomes overprotective and grandiose toward the family.

When a projective identification becomes a part of the transference, it can be addressed most effectively because it enables the therapist to understand more deeply how it operates; he or she can then help the family members to observe their own experience and try some new ways of relating. The therapist in the dilemma above might try an interpretation such as this:

I find that I am feeling somewhat angry and responsible about the unpaid therapy bills, and it reminds me of what Libby said earlier about her tuition payments. She felt that she had been blamed for your inattentiveness, but was not entitled to stand up for herself. I wonder if we all have allowed me to share in this experience with the family so that I might better understand what you are struggling with.

The case example of the Sterlings also illustrates how such processes operate in the middle phase of family therapy with eating disorders.

A Further Case Illustration

During the middle phase of treatment, the Sterling family began to explore their more unconscious motivations and feelings. They were somewhat less reliable about coming to sessions, and would sometimes send in subsets of the larger group. This was done ostensibly for some practical reason, but it always had some constructive, unconscious meaning as well. They were usually quite open to examining the significance of these subgroups, and seemed to use those sessions (as they did all the sessions) very productively. The emphasis shifted away from Lily's bulimia as she continued to work through her own issues in her individual therapy. Other members of the family were comfortable being the focus of discussion, and they did not seem to need to fall back on Lily's problems when things got heated.

Individual members and the family as a whole changed remarkably during this phase. Lily decreased her acting out and began to think and act for herself. This caused a lot of tumult initially. Her previously hyperresponsible sister was escorted home by the police on several occasions. The family attributed this to Lily's bad influence at first, but the cotherapist and I reframed it as Iris's attempt to be a normal teenager instead of everybody's referee and confidant. She found her way in time. Next, Mrs. Sterling began to attempt her own separation from her mother, Lily, and her husband. She was stormy and provocative toward all three of them, not unlike Lily. For example, she would call her husband while he was away on a business trip and tell him that Lily was driving her crazy, and that he had better come right home or she would have to leave or kick Lily out. She also told her mother that she held her responsible for the problems with Lily because of the emotional deprivation and cruelty she had felt as a child.

Mrs. Sterling gradually became more open to seeing her own individual therapist, at our suggestion. This was a breakthrough for her and for the family, because it meant that she would finally receive the kind of mirroring and empathy that she needed so desperately. Family sessions were quite often the stimulus for her own self-reflection, but her hunger was too pervasive and deep for us to satisfy along with everything else that would come up from week to week. The interface went smoothly, and each aspect of treatment enhanced the others. This additional support enabled Mrs. Sterling to work on her own developmental issues and to let Lily go. Lily, in turn, trusted that her mother was being held, so she could go on with her own individuation.

Not surprisingly, all of this turmoil surrounding the women's efforts to separate had a powerful impact on Mr. Sterling and the marriage as well. He was jealous, confused, shaken, and scared that he would lose his family. Until this point, it had always been Mr. Sterling who seemed rational, strong, and in control of a crisis. Now he was bewildered or anxious much of the time. At the heart of it, Mr. Sterling was afraid that his wife or Lily would leave the family or be injured or exploited by the harsh world outside, which only he had negotiated before. His wife was challenging everything, threatened to have an affair, refused to clean the house, and decided to begin a career outside the home at age 49. She and their daughters were trying to connect with him on a more emotional level, and for the first time were able to articulate that they felt that they did not really know him because he never shared his true feelings or motivations.

All of this work came to a climax when Lily decided to leave home and move in with her maternal grandmother. This was a remarkable solution to a number of separation issues. It was, in part, a collusion with her mother to give someone back to the grandmother as Mrs. Sterling tried to separate from her. It also enabled Lily and her mother to separate without really losing each other. For Mr. Sterling, this was the stimulus to finally express his fear and rage about all the intrusion and criticism from the grandmother over the years. Lily's move opened the door to inviting her grandmother into the family therapy directly, which we did.

Finally, with the grandmother's involvement, we were able to interpret and work through the multigenerational projective identification process. As Mrs. Sterling began to understand her own development more fully, she was able to observe her role as a bad object in her family of origin. She had had to sacrifice her own individuation to take care of her parents and to hold the family together. Much of this involved accepting her parents' projections of her as terribly inadequate, greedy, histrionic, seductive, and stupid. Mrs. Sterling internalized these projections of her, while her brother was the hero who could do no wrong. Once Mrs. Sterling became aware of her own rage and dependence as a result of this role, she was able to separate further, and also to see how she had needed to use Lily in the same way to rid herself of these unbearable introjections. Eventually, Lily heard this directly from her own mother with touching honesty and remorse.

THE LATE PHASE: RESOLUTION AND REBUILDING

Shifts in Process

As family members come to accept and appreciate their own and one another's deeper motivations and feelings, they can begin to resolve their underlying deprivations and longings and to rebuild their self-perceptions and relationships with one another. Much like the initial insights, this process of resolution and reconstruction is a progressive series of steps by the members toward greater awareness, mutual understanding, true acceptance of their family legacy, and then searching for their own unique solutions and readaptations. Although there are no discrete demarcations, this phase begins when the family is better able to provide its own holding environment, and the members are no longer so resistant and defensive about their intrapersonal and interpersonal worlds. Instead, they have become more truly self-directed and enthusiastic in their mission to explore and master their developmental legacy.

As the family internalizes the therapeutic holding functions, it becomes more nurturant, more self-containing and regulating, and more genuinely supportive of separation and individuation among its members. Parents turn toward themselves and each other when they feel lonely, inadequate, needy, injured, or angry; they are better able to communicate and connect with each other. They no longer need to rely on their children so extensively to help them to tolerate their own "bad" feelings and impulses (e.g., greed, aggression, and sexuality), because they can now better modulate these experiences intrapsychically and through mutual sharing and understanding. In turn, the children are freer to progress in their own separation efforts, and do not need to act out the family's unconscious conflicts and projections any longer. The generational boundaries have solidified, and those to the outside world have relaxed and opened.

This is an exciting and even joyful time in the therapy because the family feels its own strength and resilience again, and experiences the security and trust that something new and better will emerge out of all the confusion and pain. The members have not resolved every issue at every level, nor will they ever, but they have internalized the holding functions that will enable them to continue working toward this in their ongoing relationships. They have also established a pattern of relating to one another that incorporates truly listening to what is felt, expressing their feelings and thoughts openly, enjoying differences with one another, and appreciating more unconscious elements in their ongoing interactions. As a result of their earlier discussions, family members also have a greater respect for, and sensitivity about, specific issues and vulnerabilities that stimulate turmoil and reactivity in the family.

Inherent in this new way of relating together is an advance in the developmental level and object relations of individual members and the family as a whole. They no longer need to rely on primitive defenses such as projective identification and idealization in order to sustain a vital sense of integration and esteem. This has changed fundamentally at both the intrapsychic and interpersonal levels, so that each member now has a self-contained and differentiated sense of self and other. Family members can tolerate and regulate intense affect and even ambivalence without needing to project, deny, split off, or act out as they used to. All of these gradual changes have enabled them to begin to truly know themselves and one another as autonomous individuals connected through affectionate, understanding relations with one another.

During the late phase of therapy, the role of the therapist also changes considerably, in response to the family's emerging strength and capabilities. They have internalized the therapist and many of his or her holding functions, and now can provide these for themselves and one another. The therapist steps back from the process of their work together and establishes a new boundary between himself or herself and the family. The role is a more symbolic one in which the therapist represents all of the work and functions that were provided earlier, but are no longer needed for the most part. It is analogous to the role of a parent for an adult, individuated child—that is, as an object representation who is whole, differentiated, available, and empathic, but unnecessary as a self-object.

Shifts in Content

The content of the therapy sessions will have changed too by this time. Parents and children alike will identify much more with the therapeutic process, and even verbalize how important and valuable the experience is for them personally. They can observe complex sequences of events within the family and recognize how they are related dynamic, and systemic processes. Family members will make their own insightful interpretations about how emotional events and interpersonal transactions may be expressions of intrapsychic or even systemic operations. Parents will often request sessions without the children to discuss marital issues, and will sometimes also decide to work actively on relationships with their own parents. They openly acknowledge that they are benefiting too from the family therapy, and often express surprise at how far they have been able to come.

It becomes a matter of course to discuss the impact that grandparents, aunts, and uncles have on the emotional life of the family, both historically and presently. The family members usually progress through a phase in which they want to shut out the extended family; then later, when they feel more consolidated, they want to renegotiate new roles and relations. This process can be greatly enhanced by involving such people directly in the family sessions while this reconstruction is occurring. Children learn a great deal from watching their parents work through parallel issues with each other and their own parents.

Over the course of the family members' evolution, they have also begun to develop new, more constructive, self-fulfilling, and robust adaptations to their transgenerational legacy. Each family, once freed of the old adaptation, will construct a unique solution perfectly suited to its particular history, experiences, and personalities. It is fascinating and gratifying for the therapist to witness this process unfolding in a family that was once so anxious and defensive. It is a creative and intimate exchange between family members that somehow transforms the vulnerabilities and deficits of past generations into a vital, loving, and individuated family of the present. These new adaptations may range from the anorexic or bulimic daughter's emergent identification with her mother as a strong, lively, and ambitious woman, to a father's decision to get off the fast track in his career so that he can have more time with his family and pursue his lifelong dream of traveling around the world. Most readaptations involve dramatic changes for the family, but at this point they are usually eager and excited at the prospect. Truly fundamental changes in the family system reverberate throughout the generations. Let us now follow along with the Sterling family's progress in the late phase of therapy.

A Final Case Illustration

The late phase of therapy with the Sterling family was truly a time of resolving old issues and rebuilding their world. Much of the focus initially continued to be on Mrs. Sterling, who was going through a metamorphosis before our eyes. Instead of projecting her own hunger, impulsiveness, and inadequacy onto Lily, and her rage and idealization toward her parents onto her husband, Mrs. Sterling was containing these within herself and working them through. She began to set goals for herself and her life as Lily and Iris needed less time from her. She lost weight and recovered her girlish figure and energy, and began to make specific plans for a career outside the home.

Mrs. Sterling also shifted away from provocations and accusations toward her parents, and instead was genuinely assertive and expressive of her feelings and needs. This led initially to a withdrawal from the extended family, especially her mother. She decided to spend the Thanksgiving and Christmas holidays with the immediate family only, for the first time ever. She explained herself to her mother and siblings without sulking or blaming, or speaking through Lily or her husband; she simply asserted her own needs and wishes. Her intention was to act in accord with her true feelings and needs, and not out of a sense of duty or role. She allowed her daughters to maintain their own relationships with the grandmother, but was no longer willing to do it for them, such as by buying gifts or sending cards in their behalf.

With their mother working on her own individuation, Lily and Iris were free to pursue theirs. Lily made steady progress with her bulimia and became more cooperative and communicative at home. She started working at a new job full-time, and traveled to and from work with her father each day. This gave them a chance to talk and to get reacquainted after all their conflicts and mutual withdrawal. They also began working on a project together in which Lily was trying to learn more about setting goals and following through, which was her father's forte. At one point Lily became aware of her anger that her mother's feelings and issues were dominating the therapy sessions, and that she felt jealous of all the attention her mom was getting from the therapists. This was interpreted as also reflective of her anger for having had to stifle her own development because her mother's needs had come first.

Iris too was separating. She did not need to act out or shut out her family in order to feel separate and self-determined. She was reconnecting with the family without assuming her old parentified role. Iris and Lily were good friends, but also had their own separate social networks. Iris had been boycotting family sessions for a while, saying that she had her own life to live (not unlike her mother's attitude toward her family of origin), but she started participating in them again as well.

Mr. and Mrs. Sterling had to work through the effects of her new growth and strength. It was very difficult for Mr. Sterling to accept these changes at first, mostly because he was afraid that he would lose her and the family would dissolve. He had a very tough time trying to keep up with her and with the aftershock of her sometimes wild fluctuations in mood and behavior. He could see that everything was at stake, and this mobilized his efforts to open up and express his deeper feelings and thoughts. Mr. Sterling also changed positions in his law practice so that he would not have to travel or work such long days. He helped out much more around the house and especially with Lily and Iris. This involvement with them further contributed to their separation from their mother, and to their selection of more promising boyfriends. Every member of the family was finding the balance between pursuing his or her own personal development and needs and sustaining a feeling of closeness and connectedness within the family. Gradually, they phased out of regular family and individual therapy sessions, but at this writing they still keep in touch.

Based on our experience with this family and many others, it seems important, if not essential, to include spouses, parents, siblings, and grandparents in the treatment of anorexia and bulimia. In the case of the Sterling family, the mother, the sister, and the marriage would all have been in serious jeopardy as Lily improved, had they not been integrally involved in the treatment as well. Lily herself would not have been able to separate and progress if she had not trusted that her family would be well cared for in her absence. Without the context of a "good enough" holding environment, and a safe forum to analyze and modify the family's developmental adaptations, Lily or someone else in the family would surely have had to sacrifice his or her own individuation for the sake of the larger group. Individual progress in anorexia or bulimia can be quite at odds with the transgenerational press for repeating the old patterns in the family, again and again.

The Sterling family also illustrates how the application of techniques based on object relations and family systems theories can be integrated into a coherent, mutually informative approach to the treatment of eating disorders. As it often happens, the family system functioned to contain and regulate intrapsychic processes within family members, as well as the expression of those self-deficits and conflicts through their interpersonal relationships. Lily's bulimia and acting out functioned as stabilizing adaptations for the family at both the intrapsychic and systemic levels. Had we focused exclusively on any one aspect of the family's experience, we might have risked treatment failure or even another casualty during the process. Each level of a family's experience mirrors and ripples through the others, and that is what this approach to integrative therapy attempts to do.

REFERENCES

Bruch, H. (1973). *Eating disorders: Anorexia nervosa, obesity, and the person within*. New York: Basic Books.

Gedo, J. E., & Goldberg, A. (1973). *Models of the mind*. Chicago: University of Chicago Press.

Goodsitt, A. (1983). Self-regulatory disturbances in eating disorders. *International Journal of Eating Disorders, 2*, 51–60.

Greenberg, J. R., & Mitchell, S. A. (1983). *Object relations in psychoanalytic theory*. Cambridge, MA: Harvard University Press.

Gustafson, J. P. (1986). *The complex secret of brief psychotherapy*. New York: Norton.

Humphrey, L. L. (1988). Relationships within subtypes of anorexic, bulimic, and normal families. *Journal of the American Academy of Child and Adolescent Psychiatry, 27,* 544–551.

Humphrey, L. L. (1989). Observed family interactions among subtypes of eating disorders using structural analysis of social behavior. *Journal of Consulting and Clinical Psychology, 57,* 206–214.

Humphrey, L. L., Apple, R. F., & Kirschenbaum, D. S. (1986). Differentiating bulimic–anorexic from normal families using interpersonal and behavioral observation systems. *Journal of Consulting and Clinical Psychology, 54,* 190–195.

Humphrey, L. L., & Stern, S. (1988). Object relations and the family system in bulimia. *Journal of Marital and Family Therapy, 14,* 337–350.

Klein, M. (1975). Notes on some schizoid mechanisms. In *Envy and gratitude and other works, 1946–1963*. New York: Free Press. (Original work published 1946)

Mahler, M. S. (1968). *On human symbiosis and the vicissitudes of individuation*. New York: International Universities Press.

Masterson, J. F. (1977). Primary anorexia nervosa in the borderline adolescent— an object relations view. In P. Harocollis (Ed.), *Borderline personality disorders* (pp. 475–494). New York: International Universities Press.

Minuchin, S., Rosman, B. L., & Baker, L. (1978). *Psychosomatic families: Anorexia nervosa in context*. Cambridge, MA: Harvard University Press.

Pinsof, W. M. (1983). Integrative problem-centered therapy: Toward the synthesis of family and individual psychotherapies. *Journal of Marital and Family Therapy, 9,* 19–35.

Roberto, L. G. (1986). Bulimia: The transgenerational view. *Journal of Marital and Family Therapy, 12,* 231–240.

Root, M. P., Fallon, P., & Friedrich, W. N. (1986). *Bulimia: A systems approach to treatment*. New York: Norton.

Scharff, D. E., & Scharff, J. S. (1987). *Object relations family therapy*. Northvale, NJ: Jason Aronson.

Schwartz, R. C., Barrett, M. J., & Saba, G. (1984). Family therapy for bulimia. In D. M. Garner & P. E. Garfinkel (Eds.), *Handbook of psychotherapy for anorexia nervosa and bulimia* (pp. 280–311). New York: Guilford Press.

Selvini-Palazzoli, M. (1978). *Self-starvation: From individual to family therapy in the treatment of anorexia nervosa*. New York: Jason Aronson.

Slipp, S. (1984). *Object relations: A dynamic bridge between individual and family treatment*. New York: Jason Aronson.

Strober, M., & Humphrey, L. L. (1987). Familial contributions to the etiology and course of anorexia nervosa and bulimia. *Journal of Consulting and Clinical Psychology, 55,* 654–659.

Swift, W. J., & Letven, R. (1984). Bulimia and the basic fault: A psychoanalytic interpretation of the binge–vomiting syndrome. *Journal of the American Academy of Child Psychiatry, 23,* 489–497.

Tansey, M. J., & Burke, W. F. (1989). *Understanding countertransference: From projective identification to empathy.* Hillsdale, NJ: Analytic Press.

Winnicott, D. W. (1965). *The maturation processes and the facilitating environment.* New York: International Universities Press.

Zinner, J., & Shapiro, R. (1972). Projective identification as a mode of perception and behavior in families of adolescents. *International Journal of Psycho-Analysis, 53,* 523–530.

·· *14* ··

Disorders of the Self in Anorexia Nervosa: An Organismic–Developmental Paradigm

MICHAEL STROBER

*School of Medicine, University of California at Los Angeles
and UCLA Neuropsychiatric Institute and Hospital*

Anorexia nervosa has long been considered a model for illustrating how mental and biological processes become inseparably joined in disease. But as frequently as this point has been reaffirmed in the literature, the nature of this interface has been little explored. Undoubtedly among the reasons is the great complexity of the illness. Its somatic and psychological aspects certainly encompass a wide and puzzling range of phenomena, each of which has been analyzed on several different levels from a diversity of theoretical viewpoints. And on the clinical front, the available knowledge has yet to support any one method of treatment as unequivocally more valid or efficacious than the next. It may be because of the lack of absolute sureness of approach that clinicians sometimes push theoretical biases to their extreme in order to feel certain in their actions, especially when faced with the many challenges these patients present. This is understandable, maybe even commonplace, yet it still has the disadvantage of an uncompromisingly one-sided approach to the patients' mind–body pathology.

Indeed, as it becomes increasingly clear that human afflictions cannot be reduced to simple paradigms, there is greater willingness to build conceptual bridges between once disparate fields of study in the hope of arriving at a more complete understanding of their fundamental nature and causes. Reflecting this rapprochement, biologically oriented workers are beginning to urge that broader recognition be given to certain core psychoanalytic ideas, just as an increasing number of psychoanalysts now reject as too doctrinaire the idea that biological data are largely irrelevant to the methods and assumptions of psychodynamic theory and practice (Kandel, 1979; Grotstein, 1987; Reiser, 1984).

The present chapter aims to apply such a collaborative framework to the phenomenology of disordered self-functioning in anorexia nervosa. Rather than attempting a detailed critique of the promises or limitations of other approaches to this issue (Geist, 1989; Goodsitt, 1984), I address how several closely related findings in modern developmental psychology, psychobiology, and personality genetics offer new understanding of the processes and adaptive mechanisms by which symptom patterns and other important clinical phenomena emerge. The findings to which I refer are as follows: (1) The emerging self, rather than a passive recipient of outside influences, actively structures experiences in the sensorimotor, perceptual, and affective domains from early in life; (2) the manner in which affectivity organizes self-experience and self-object functions throughout development is greatly affected by endogenous regulators of arousability and other adaptive behaviors; and (3) the limits within which particular behavior styles and coping patterns are expressed dynamically in normal and pathological functioning are set largely by heritable personality traits and the biological structures presumed to underlie them. In the interest of clarity of exposition, these ideas are discussed first. The final section of the chapter illustrates their heuristic relevance by recasting the phenomenology of anorexia nervosa in essentially organismic–developmental terms.

ORGANISMIC REGULATION OF EARLY SELF-EXPERIENCE

The emergence of selfhood has long been a central overriding interest of psychoanalysis and developmental psychology. Recently, the subject has received active attention from developmentalists representing a wide range of theoretical positions, whose scientific efforts have generated a substantial new basis for understanding the processes by which selfhood is gradually formed during ontogeny. One by-product of this knowledge explosion is a fuller appreciation of the complex pathways along which experiential and organismic factors interact in normal growth and development, and in pathogenesis. A complete account of these findings is well beyond the scope of this chapter; however, the reader can find excellent summaries elsewhere (Lichtenberg, 1983; Stern, 1985). Here, I highlight selectively some major points that bear on the clinical focus of this volume.

It is undeniable that environmental influences play an important role in psychological development. However, the origins of social experience are now understood to be more complex and dynamic than once thought. Whereas traditional developmental theory viewed the infant as an essentially passive assimilator of environmental events, recent evidence (Stern, 1985) culled from sophisticated video recording of mother–child interactions shows that the actions of each are unusually well synchronized in the dimensions of time and space. The rhythmical form and adaptive harmony of these exchanges have led modern researchers to conclude that the emerging self is biologically capable of organizing and schematizing early encounters with the environmental surroundings in ways that traditional theory never deemed possible. Thus, just as it surely is the case that the caregiver's mirroring and attunement are crucial early nutrients of the infant's self-experience, it is equally apparent that the developing self makes active use of predesigned structures to initiate, facilitate, and regulate these actions.

In Stern's (1983, 1985) view, the exchanges between infant and caregiver are essentially focused along three lines—namely, "mental state sharing," "self–other complementing," and "state transformation." Each is assumed to have quite specific implications for structure formation. The main element of mental state sharing is commonality, or isomorphism, of experience; it is achieved when self or caregiver induces a similar action or experiential state in the other, thereby blurring self–other boundaries. Stern postulates that state sharing is a rudimentary form of subjective intimacy—an awareness of the extent to which affect intensity is "interexperienced"—that lays down the foundation for later self-esteem. By contrast, in self–other complementing self and caregiver engage in distinctly different but complementary actions, the effect of which is to demarcate self–other boundaries more sharply. And third, state transformation involves shifts in level of consciousness and neurobiological arousal following gratification of needs or drives. Stern likens this to the relationship of self to an anaclitic object and considers it essential to the development of physical intimacy. It will not escape the notice of some readers that these ideas correspond to other theoretical formulations—for example, Fairbairn's (1944) psychology of dynamic structures; Atwood and Stolorow's (1984) concept (extended from that of Kohut, 1971, 1977) of intersubjectivity; and Tomkins's (1962) notion of innate affect-regulating programs, which attune the self to changes in the intensity properties of stimuli.

Temperament and Affectivity

Few of us would question the great diversity and uniqueness of emotional experience. That people vary widely in their threshold and intensity of response to states of pleasure and distress, as well as in the ability to tone down or modulate affect states, has been known since the advent of psychoanalysis and figured prominently in Freud's early thinking about psychic conflict and defense. In developmental psychology as well, individual differences in reactivity have been viewed as exerting significant impact on the course and quality of psychological adjustment (Thomas & Chess, 1977). It is a fact of nature that some human beings are unusually resilient, weathering the most stressful challenges with little more than minor and transient distress, whereas others suffer immensely in the face of far less urgent or pressing demands; such is the nature and impact of temperament.

Interest in the developmemtal ramifications of temperament first surfaced during the 1930s and 1940s, prompted by growing evidence that infants respond in characteristically different fashion to common patterns of parental care (Thomas & Chess, 1977). Temperament has since been conceptualized as unlearned, biologically driven, and unconsciously motivated dimensions of affect and motor behavior, encompassing the following: the regularity of biological functions; patterns of approach–withdrawal to novel stimuli; adaptability to change; intensity of reactivity; threshold sensitivities; the prevailing tone and quality of mood; and attention span and persistence (Thomas, Chess, & Birch, 1969). Many of these dimensions are quite stable over time and moderately to strongly heritable (Plomin & Rowe, 1977); however, temperament is by no means immutable, nor is it uninfluenced in its expression by environmental factors. Nonetheless, from its conception as a predisposing structure that regulates drive expression and affect response, it has been surmised that extremes of temperament are not an uncommon source of conflict with the caregiving environment and an antecedent cause of pathological adjustments. Indeed, during the course of their landmark study of temperament and behavior disorder, Thomas and Chess (1977) found that it was in temperamentally "extreme" individuals that difficulties in development were most prominent. More recently, this work has been extended further by giving attention to the role played by temperament in the quality of early attachments and other aspects of social experiences (Goldsmith & Campos, 1982).

The implications of this view of the child's relationship to his or her world for understanding normal and deviant ontogeny of self-experiences are not trivial. For if it is granted that certain instinctively organized mechanisms regulate intrapersonal and intersubjective states in unique ways, then attention to the nature of individual differences in organismic processes is obviously essential to an understanding of the affective qualities predominating in self-development, as well as the conditions under which they are altered. This being so, I would argue that we can conclude little about effects of the caregiving environment on psychological deviance until an organismic perspective is added.

In short, the concept of individual temperaments is an observation of considerable theoretical and clinical significance. It is the observation that the impact of environmental events, whether of a positive or negative emotional valence, is neither fixed nor predictable; rather, because we are uniquely predisposed in our response to appetitive, pleasure-arousing, and anxiogenic experiences alike, diverse outcomes are bound to arise. Such being the case, temperament is not simply descriptive, but explanatory of certain adaptive and psychopathological variations in personality (Goldsmith & Campos, 1982; Thomas et al., 1969). To repeat an earlier point, this must not be taken to imply that social influences are largely irrelevant to pathogenesis. It only suggests that it is impossible to gain an adequate conception of how the individual and his or her social environment evolve in mutual adaptation, or maladaptation, without reference to organismic factors that regulate and structure developmental processes. As I discuss next, these ideas are central to reformulated theories of personality conceived on a basis of dynamically operating biological structures.

A Neuroadaptive Model of Personality

The study of personality historically reflects a number of very different theoretical and scientific traditions that have remained fairly well insulated from one another. In this section I briefly sketch out a newly developed organismic point of view, outlined in a series of integrative papers by Cloninger (1986, 1987, 1988), from which many of the ideas in this chapter are derived. A thorough account of the material on which Cloninger's ideas are validated is impossible to attempt here, so only the major points are highlighted. These may be summarized briefly as follows:

1. The foundations of personality comprise three bipolar dimensions—namely, behavioral activation and novelty seeking; behavioral inhibition and harm avoidance; and behavioral maintenance and reward dependence. Each dimension is a superordinate structure in its own right with highly specific steering and modulating functions.

2. These dimensions are the outcome of genetic, constitutional, and learning factors; however, contrary to popular belief, the total body of evidence at hand indicates a far greater influence of genes than of environment in the foundation of these personality traits (Plomin, 1986).

3. The generality of these three dimensions is quite significant; this

is to say that their behavioral correlates are highly routinized and stable within individuals and across environmental situations to a remarkable degree.

4. Finally, individual differences in learning history, in the nature of response to environmental demands, and in the expression of psychopathological behavior derive from, and are readily predicted by, knowledge of the covariation of these dimensions within individuals. The distinctive features of these three dimensions, based on Cloninger's (1987) account, are now considered.

"Behavioral activation and novelty seeking" refer to modulation of the intensity or excitability of response to novel, rewarding, or aversive stimuli. At one extreme on this dimension are individuals who characteristically avoid sameness, monotony, and frustrative nonreward, and who actively search out excitement, stimulation, and complexity in their environment. In contrast, individuals low in novelty seeking express a preference for a stable, invariant, and emotionally temperate environment. When they are clinically disturbed, individuals high in novelty-seeking traits are likely to be impulsive, intolerant of routines, thrill-seeking, and erratic. On the opposite side, low scorers on this dimension will be seen as emotionally restrained, slow to change interests, excessively methodical, and rigidly persistent.

"Harm avoidance" refers to the intensity of response to aversive stimuli and situations that convey uncertainty or threat. One extreme on this dimension reflects heightened anticipation of discomfort or displeasure in spite of supportive reassurance; extreme worry, even over minor issues; poor adaptability to change; and slow recovery from emotional stress. At the opposite extreme are confidence and optimism; extreme resilience; and ease of adjustment to stressful challenge and changes in usual routine. Behaviorally, individuals who score high on this dimension are obsessive worriers prone to anxious, dysphoric mood; they are inhibited and cautious when confronted with the unfamiliar; and they are overaroused by excited, appetitive, or stimulating situations. In contrast, individuals low in harm avoidance are lacking in inhibition, prefer excitement, and bounce back quickly from injury or discomfort.

Last, "reward dependence" refers to the tendency to condition easily to signals of reinforcement—in particular, succor, approval, and sentiment. Extremes on this dimension are marked on one end by dependence on others for emotional support, hypersensitivity to signs of approval and rejection, and persistence even in the face of nonreward; and on the other by nonconformity and self-determination, lack of shared intimacy, and insensitivity to social pressures. At the clinical level, high scorers are self-sacrificing and excessively deferential, unusually sensitive to the feelings and needs of others, and prone to highly driven and repetitive reward-seeking behavior even when frustrated or disappointed. In contrast, extremely low scorers are socially detached, dispassionate, and motivated strongly by immediate gratification.

In this model, the likelihood of suffering maladjustive tendencies is explained not so much in terms of individual levels of a trait as in terms of their relative equilibrium. This is because each dimension plays a role complementary to the other in determining the repertoires of behavior evoked by different situations. Thus, individuals with normative adjustment are predicted to be evenly balanced on these dimensions (what Cloninger terms the "intermediate adaptive optimum"), whereas risk of pathological development is assumed to be highest in individuals who are extremely deviant on different trait combinations. Whether any one pattern ultimately confers advantage or disadvantage in the individual case may also depend partly on social factors (e.g., qualities of the home environment, experiences of loss or rejection, parental marital status, social class, etc.). But in view of how the relative strengths of novelty seeking, harm avoidance, and reward dependence influence the morphology of behavior at so many levels, it is only logical to extend the scope of this influence to psychopathological expressions as well. In simple terms, one would not expect the development of reckless, impulsive, antisocial conduct in individuals who by nature are harm-avoidant and resist novelty, any more than we would anticipate the occurrence of chronic anxiety or rigidly obsessive behavior in individuals in whom novelty seeking and low hard avoidance are pre-eminent. So it is that personality structures account for consistencies in the form of behavior in normal and pathological states.

In summary, the convention of viewing human behavior solely in dynamic, environmental terms and of dismissing theories of biological causality as too mechanistic and dispassionate are simplifying distortions. The merit of this organismic paradigm is simply that it enables us to better appreciate, and explain more parsimoniously, how individuals maintain a stable and distinctive phenomenology of relating to the outside world. Early experience most surely influences behavior in the psychodynamic sense; yet the nature of the individual's adaptation to nurturing and pathogenic events is to a significant degree bounded—constrained or dictated, if you will—by biologically regulated processes that organize specific patterns of functional behavior. Therefore, at the very least, these ideas bridge to psychodynamic theory by drawing attention to lawful principles by which the self maintains constancy, develops structures of meaning, and forms patterned styles of normative and psychopathological adjustments to environmental challenge.

DISORDERS OF THE SELF FROM AN ORGANISMIC–DEVELOPMENTAL VIEWPOINT

The nature of self-experience has also gained distinction recently as a subject of theoretical and clinical discussion in contemporary psychoanalysis. These efforts have been of great value in studies of psychopathology and have altered the foundations on which psychodynamic treatment have been based. Although space does not permit extensive discussion, the major elements are summarized here so that the importance of the preceding ideas of psychoanalytic thinking about self pathology can be brought into full relief.

Many streams of influence have fostered present inquiries on the self in psychoanalysis; however, the largest intellectual debt is owed to the seminal writings of Kohut (1971, 1977), and later extensions of his theories by Stolorow and colleagues (Stolorow & Lachmann, 1980; Atwood & Stolorow, 1984; Stolorow, Brandchaft, & Atwood, 1987). Common to all writings within this framework is the overarching emphasis, theoretically and clinically, on the phenomenology of self-experience. In their eloquent account of this perspective, Atwood and Stolorow (1984) describe the self as a "psychological structure through which self-experience acquires cohesion and continuity, and by virtue of which self-experience assumes its characteristic shape and organization" (p. 34). It is from such a focus that the paradigmatic concept of "self-object," upon which Kohut laid so much emphasis, derives its significance. The self-object is, in brief, a set of psychological functions experienced subjectively as necessary for the maintenance, restoration, and transformation of self-experience (Stolorow et al., 1987). The concept has broad significance and clinical application, insofar as it highlights a fundamentally important aspect of self and object—namely, that their relationship constitutes an indissoluble, dynamically organized psychological system within which experiences are patterned and structured over time (Atwood & Stolorow, 1984; Stern, 1985; Stolorow et al., 1987). It is from this extension of self-psychological theory that we have come to better appreciate how the "intersubjective context" (Atwood & Stolorow, 1984) is importantly associated with harmonious and disharmonious aspects of psychological development.

On this point, self psychology has drawn from empirical observations of child development in describing the phases through which self-experience achieves increasing differentiation, coherence, and regularity, and how actions taken by the caregiver make such growth in the complexity of self-structure possible (Stolorow et al., 1987). Succinctly stated, the most important of these actions are (1) differential responding to the child's feeling states, which aids the formation and increasing demarcation of self–other boundaries; (2) balancing, or synthesis, of the child's discrepant emotional states, which allows for the eventual integration of self-experiences; (3) toning and modulation of intensely felt affect states, which enables the child to exprience new emotions without disruption; and (4) cognitive/verbal articulation of the child's feeling states, through which affect is desomatized and the content and personal meaning of self-experience become further enlarged and more richly textured.

There are several notable implications of this framework for understanding the genesis of psychopathology. One is the pervading assumption that all psychopathological behavior is rooted in an intersubjective context; from this view, the most crucial determinant of regressive symptomatology is the incomplete development, rupturing, or distortion of vital self-object ties. Elaborating on this point, Grotstein (1986, 1987) suggests that all primitive mental states can be viewed holistically in terms of the relative lack of coherence among various elements of self- and interactional (intersubjective) regulation. The corresponding extension of this idea is that symptomatic states are also restitutive in important ways; as they are activated in different emotional settings, they serve adaptively as instruments of regulation, or, conversely, as compensations for dysregulation. As Grotstein (1987) puts it,

> Dysregulated states of alarm or tension threaten catastrophe to the organism and consequently precipitate symptoms that reflect this . . . or seem to screen it through secondary symptomatology, offering a "makeshift floor" under, or container around, a fragmenting self to protect it from disintegrating catastrophe. (p. 349)

Thus, a myriad of symptomatologies, psychosomatic states included, can be seen as developmentally pre-emptory modes of affect expression that serve to mitigate experiences of meaninglessness, formlessness, and dissolution when self-object ties are threatened (Grotstein, 1986, 1987; Stolorow et al., 1987). Under this conception, they become in a very real sense vital to the subjective well-being and integrity of the self, no matter how horrific or self-defeating they may seem to others.

At this juncture, we are drawn to consider the synthesis of these viewpoints. As stated previously, the parochial attachment to dynamic versus organismic constructs in developing models of psychopathology inevitably hinders a broader, theoretically balanced understanding of clinical phenomena. But there is in fact ample justification for paying more than lip service to organismic–developmental factors when studying disorders of the self, to which ample reference has been made in recent literature (Plomin, 1986; Scarr & McCartney, 1983). This is because individual differences in response to dynamically important events are dictated to a very large extent by genetic variations that drive and restrain behavior and that influence responsiveness to environmental challenges and opportunities in unique ways (Scarr & McCartney, 1983). From this position, the question of the relative importance of deficiencies or trauma in early experience versus underlying biological handicap now gives way to a consideration of their compound and reciprocal influence on self-development. The value of this synthesis is that it offers a theory-guided understanding of how genetically extreme temperaments and personality traits can predispose an individual to a lower-than-optimal threshold for experiencing inner tensions and to a correspondingly greater sensitivity to disruption of self-object ties; when such individuals are inclined by nature to avoid novelty and harm and are possessed of an unusual responsiveness to environmental cues, they will inevitably experience a more pressing intrapsychic need to maintain unwavering control over threatening affective states. The long-term implications of these tendencies for self-structure have been noted by Grotstein (1990), who suggests that it is the inability to fend off threatening and unpleasant emotions at times of developmental change that underlies self-experiences of shame and humiliating weakness. This perceived deficiency, he asserts, is at the core of the diminished sense of initiative and efficacy that pervades primitive mental states—a legacy of "defectiveness" and "powerlessness" wherein "the hapless patient consciously and/or unconsciously experiences his or her limitations as defects (deficits or deficiencies) and consequently conducts his or her life in a manner tha militates against the irruptive expression of these weaknesses" (Grotstein, 1986, p. 103).

Thus, it is when anxiety is persistently attached to affective experience, or reactivated when new adaptations are required, that the self becomes liable to feelings of denigration and contempt, which all too often are construed as a failure of "character." It is small wonder, then, that with individuals in whom this sense of "defectiveness" is present, the withholding of mental contents—the felt necessity of secrecy (often mistakenly labeled as alexithymia)—is so common an occurrence (Grotstein, 1987). To this I add the following point: that it is particularly in individuals with heritable tendencies to worry and brood excessively (harm-avoidant characteristics) that residues of dysphorogenic experiences— states of diffuse unease or unpleasure—linger on and eventually permeate all levels of self-identity and psychological functioning. This, I believe, is the organismic–developmental foundation on which vulnerabilities to fragmentation, feelings of meaninglessness and ineffectiveness, and intolerance of affect are based. But it is from the knowledge of how regressive states also restore threatened self-object ties, whether to maintain feelings of safety, esteem, or distinctiveness, that we ultimately come to appreciate their deeper personal significance.

ORGANISMIC MEDIATORS OF REGULATION
IN THE INTERSUBJECTIVE CONTEXT

What applies to the regulation of affect experience by the self applies also to the interpersonal environment. In the same way that the concept of temperament has been applied in developmental psychology and psychoanalysis, it has been recognized that each family exhibits highly individual behavioral traits that are the correlates of underlying temperamental properties of its members. As Steinglass (1987) puts it,

> These traits, in turn, are the behavioral manifestations that clinicians focus on when they use descriptive phrases like "high-energy versus low-energy" families, "hot versus cool" families, "flexible versus rigid" families (high versus low tolerance for novelty) and so forth. (p. 45)

It follows naturally that just as individual psychological health reflects a balance in personality structures regulating harm avoidance, novelty seeking, and reward dependence, homeostasis of the family cannot be understood fully without taking account of structures used by its members to manage potentially destabilizing forces in the environment. It is to be acknowledged accordingly that families will inevitably differ, says Steinglass (1987), in "predilictions for types of regulatory mechanisms, optimal behavioral ranges, and relative rigidity or flexibility" (p. 43). Considering this point, the intersubjective nature of self pathology may now be formulated in the general idea that child and caregivers mutually and interactively make use of biologically patterned structures of adaptation (or maladaptation, as the case may be) in managing their internal and external environments. This being so, pathogenic situations are as likely to arise when the personality structures of each are markedly and irreconcilably disparate as when they share highly similar patterns of extreme tendencies.

Consider, for example, the implications for self-development when child and parent share (by virtue of heredity) traits of harm avoidance, low novelty seeking, and reward dependence (an uncommonly frequent scenario in anorexia nervosa, as I discuss more fully later on). In this instance, each is disposed to orderliness in daily routines, to distress when affectively alarmed, and to easy motivation and conditioning by reward. The clinical implications may be summarized to this effect: The regulation of affectivity in child and parent is so similarly contoured that opportunities for mastering the unsettling aspects of developmental change—and, with the transition from childhood to adolescence, for enlarging self-experiences beyond the comforting security and boundedness of the familial environment—are sharply restricted. In essence, each party perceives the other as that party experiences himself or herself (recall here Cloninger's description of these personality types)—that is, as exquisitely sensitive to psychological injury. Each accordingly is unusually susceptible to avoidance behaviors that tone down, or prevent the irruption of, unacceptably arousing emotional states. It can thus readily be understood that as the range of allowable feelings of *dis-ease* narrows and the preference for stability and familiarity strengthens, the child's potential for achieving differentiated and consolidated self-feelings of autonomy, vigor, and initiative is hindered. The problem lies not only in subtle derailments in mirroring, but also in the fact that the extreme symmetry of genetic avoidance tendencies among family numbers compromises the development of mature self-object ties and shapes a view of self as unsteady, unprepared, and easily menaced by new challenges and stresses.

Clinical implications of a disharmony among harm-avoidant, novelty-seeking, and reward-dependent traits can also be considered in a somewhat different light—one that concerns the manner in which self-experiences are restructured at times of developmental change. Sandler (1983) has hypothesized that when parent and child share the capacity to tolerate negative affect, a state of "open-space equilibrium" will exist that allows the child to disengage more readily from habitual patterns and to explore novelties in the environment actively; to adjust to discrepancies in emotional state; and to integrate new affective experiences without feelings of threat or restraint by caregivers. This point gives further insight into why for some individuals developmental change is an impetus for differentiation and expansion of self-experiences, but for others it is a signal of impending, inexorable calamity. It is when the inherent capacities for affect modulation and structure transformation are limited that maturation (and, by extension, selfhood) becomes the embodiment of dreaded psychological contents and unwelcome physical change.

I have now drawn on data from several areas to suggest that biological structures of experience provide a frame of reference for understanding the pathogenesis and maintenance of self-deficits. The application of these ideas to the problem of anorexia nervosa is now considered.

THE PHENOMENOLOGY OF SELF-EXPERIENCE IN ANOREXIA NERVOSA

Few researchers would dispute the idea that anorexia nervosa arises from a multifactorial continuum of causal factors. For this reason, the premorbid developments of young people (primarily young women) at risk are not exactly comparable. At the same time, it is difficult to miss some very compelling similarities.

Interest in the causal relationship of personality to anorexia nervosa has a long history, beginning in 1694 with Morton's observation that states of nervous atrophy (phthisis nervosa) appear to occur more often in individuals with "violent passions" of mind. Nearly two centuries later, Gull (1874) and Lasegue (1873) similarly noted how anorexia nervosa receives its impetus from "mental perversities" and "concealed emotions." More recently, Casper (1983) posited that instability of self-concept is formative in predisposing certain vulnerable adolescents to employ thinness misguidedly to regulate emotions and enhance feelings of esteem and autonomy. And, concerning the maturational context in which anorexia nervosa arises, Crisp (1980) writes,

> She may feel "out of control"—inflicted first with the physiological fact of puberty and then by its psychological and social consequences. No solutions offer themselves personally or socially; the intensifications of dieting with its early effect on newly acquired adult reproductive processes is circularly reinforced until biological regression is complete . . . the individual is safe experientially, but totally unsafe biologically. (p. 19)

The effects of malnourishment and general biological regression on personality are not insignificant, to be sure; however, even in the weight-recovered state, young women with anorexia nervosa are significantly more self-doubting, submissive, deferential to authority, compliant with outside demands, and stimulus-avoidant than their peers (Strober, 1980, 1981). But it is in the phenomenology of self-experience, as it is revealed through intensive psychotherapy, that the struggle between conflicting psychological influences is most compellingly depicted. It is from the detailed investigation of the patient's inner world that we learn of the omnipresent fear of seeming weak, inadequate, and average; the inability to take pleasure in leisure; a reluctance to confront risks and novelty, to engage in uninhibited spontaneous action, or to assert feelings; and the experiencing of impulses and desires as wasteful distractions to achieving higher moral objectives.

How, then, do we relate these characteristics back to the points discussed earlier? Most importantly, they suggest that it is in extreme tendencies toward avoidance of harm, low novelty seeking, and reward dependence that the epigenetic core of anorexia nervosa lies. By this, I mean that this particular configuration of personality is what renders these individuals vulnerable to the many complex emotional demands and challenges of puberty. In short, it is the organismic–developmental foundation of self-experience as lacking a strong, resilient core. In my view, the dissonance in selfhood that puberty lays bare, which we see reflected in a myriad of ways in the phenomenology of anorexia nervosa, may be formulated as a conflict between personality structures that reinforce conformity, allow little deviation from routine, and maintain close checks on affectivity on the one hand, and developmental imperatives of a fundamentally different sort on the other. Because individuals with anorexia nervosa are by nature excessively dependent on environmental structure for security and affirmation of worth, and rather poorly suited to change and emotional arousal, their experience of puberty is that of a transition for which they seem hopelessly ill prepared. It is nothing short of a menacing, affectively uprooting somatopsychic event that reveals their humiliating susceptibility to states of *dis-ease* and impingement by outside forces.

It is important to realize here that the very neuroadaptive traits underlying this vulnerability also lay down the structure for behaviors that are set in motion to protect and fortify the self. As we have seen, individuals who shun harm and novelty will characteristically mitigate feelings of threat by maintaining fixed, highly patterned, and compulsively ritualized actions—and there can be no doubt that such biological predilections are carried to extreme lengths in the anorexic's self-imposed starvation and unrelenting exercise. To carry this point further, I would submit that the symptoms of anorexia nervosa can take hold and endure so assiduously *only* in individuals in whom the heritable tendencies of harm avoidance and low novelty seeking are present to a greater degree.

It can thus be readily understood that in most cases anorexia nervosa, rather than being a flirtation with death, is an indefatigable struggle to exist, but to exist within the most narrow of perimeters—where there is conclusive assurance that complex needs and emotions are absent, that the family is not perturbed, and that expectations for the individual's behavior are well demarcated. Indeed, the key somatopsychic formulas in anorexia nervosa are "survival on less" and "avoidance of change." In illustration of these points is the case of a highly verbal 14-year-old female who described her present situation in these terms:

> I feel different from my friends; I'm just not interested in the things they are. I like being home with my parents and little sister and doing schoolwork.

However, as her therapy progressed she came to speak of feeling perplexed and unsettled by the emergent impulses and emotions of adolescence, and of wishing she could retain the safety and predictability of childhood when she felt her parents always understood her needs. Yet, over the course of her therapy, she came to detest those very aspects of her personality so admired by others. She voiced hatred of her compliance, her reluctance to explore the new and unfamiliar, and her sensitivity to others; indeed, it was at this juncture that her behavior became decidedly more unpleasant. It was soon after this change emerged that her parents began to lament the fact that their daughter was beginning to behave more like other teenagers with each passing day.

It is thus of great psychological and adaptive significance that as symptoms of illness unfold, we see in patients a new and uncharacteristically stubborn self-sufficiency and rejective attitude toward others—taken to extreme in the refusal to nourish their bodies. Their friends and families react with alarm and bewilderment, yet for the patients the narrowing of their experiential and biological state of being—the elimination of affectivity, instinctuality, and neediness—becomes a matter of the greatest psychological importance. True, the physiological effects of starvation and exercise engender ritualized, obsessive thinking and a dulling of emotion to the point where life is sterile and drab; however, the effects are no less comforting, insofar as they neutralize developmental changes that now threaten a previously stable and more ordered existence. In effect, the patients' frenetic activity and preoccupation with weight, shape, and the minutiae of food intake—symptoms of their disease—are new adaptive "arrangements" serving to maintain a selfhood increasingly plagued by emergent states of *dis-ease*. Thus, for these young women the control of bodily functions becomes the new "makeshift floor" (Grotstein, 1987) on which their weakened self-structure comes to rest.

By no means am I suggesting that this is a causal mechanism by which to explain the peculiar distortions of body shape characteristically associated with anorexia nervosa; the nature of this phenomenon remains, in my view, poorly understood. What I am implying is that for these young women the experience of puberty is one of betrayal—an embarrassing and psychically threatening exposure of their weaknesses at coping. I believe that such experiences are akin to the states of boundarylessness and humiliation considered by Grotstein (1990) to be universally present in all primitive mental disorders; in anorexia nervosa, they are eventually concretized in anxieties over body shape and the suppression of physical urges and needs. Only when its symptoms are viewed in these terms can the paradox of anorexia nervosa—how it can be functionally restitutive in the dynamic sense, while seeming so sadistically hostile and devitalizing—be fully understood.

Of course, the fears roused by puberty extend to the family environment as well. In this regard, it can be said that the defects in coping referred to above lie at the interface of individual and familial temperaments. As Crisp (1985) put it,

> A young child's natural dependency and undifferentiated characteristics may be enhanced by overprotective family attitudes . . . and rewarding of compliant behavior. The potential for avoidance behavior may be reinforced as natural fearfulness of the outside world by the parents' own enmeshed relationship and their associated fear of outside influences. This latter fear will be much enhanced in them as well as in their child when she reaches puberty. (p. 9)

Sandler's (1983) previously discussed notion of "open-space equilibrium" is apposite here, for clinical experience shows how the enmeshments that characterize many anorexic families compromise the development of autonomy and the readiness to adjust to novel and affect-inducing changes in the environment. It is in such families that individuals with coping deficits are apt, under the pressures of change, to retreat from opportunities to broaden self-experience and to merge defensively with each other, thereby perpetuating maladaptive self-object ties. Here again, the way in which these regressive mergers are played out in the phenomenology of the illness is self-evident.

Several points deserve further comment in this regard. Just as the anorexic struggles experientially, she is now equally certain of being a burden to those on whom the need to depend is so great, but whom she perceives as similarly ill equipped to manage developmental change. But what is so extraordinary about the pathogenesis of anorexia nervosa is that it ultimately brings about the very dependence on environmental supports that the patient so detests. Indeed, this is unavoidable, since human beings are incapable of enduring long periods of deprivation without their intrapsychic life becoming increasingly dominated by object hunger and the intense drive to gratify unmet needs. Thus, it is in direct proportion to the patient's disavowal of biological need that parents, loved ones, and helping professionals alike are mobilized into that most basic of caregiving tasks: to feed and protect, so the child does not perish. Of course, despite all protests to the contrary, this is precisely what the patient longs for: to be insulated from menacing and ill-understood maturational changes and self-experiences of incompleteness and defect. Even so, it remains baffling how such obviously destructive avoidance symptoms persist so tenaciously; however, I would suggest that it may partly reflect the tendency for individuals with extreme harm avoidance to acquire strong conditioned responses to aversive stimuli and to remain hypervigilant in estimating potential risks in ordinary circumstances (Cloninger, 1986). The circumstances here are the emergence of puberty—as represented symbolically, if not metaphorically, in the changing contours of body shape—and the threat it portends for the anorexic's vulnerable self-structure.

Thus it is crucial to understand that anorexia nervosa, in all its varying degrees of severity, always reflects a condensation of two seemingly irreconcilable aims: an assertion of separateness (or, more accurately, the repudiation of need and desire), and the reinstatement or perpetuation of archaic self-object ties. Indeed, how to renounce ties to others and assert personal control while at the same time appearing in such obvious need of protective care constitutes a challenge even for those patients with the greatest capacities for rationalization and self-deception. Said one 18-year-old woman during the third month of her hospital treatment,

> I hate the idea of needing or wanting anything. But the thing is, my needs keep getting stronger; this is what scares me. You tell me that to need is to be normal. But I feel helpless, because I feel and want so much!

So it is that the vicious spiral set in motion by anorexia nervosa is unavoidable, biologically as well as intrapsychically. For as starvation and withdrawal from others progress, the felt intensity of vital needs grows. The attitude of the patient may seem that of noninvolvement—a life emptied of meaningful emotion, feeling, or passion—yet she is forever on the alert lest she be tempted or aroused in some way. Her greatest fear is the abandonment of restraint and the giving in to feelings and needs that by now have become, in her mind, even more devouring and insatiable, though rarely do patients understand how their state of biological deprivation comes into play here. Hence, food, hunger, the body, and affect experiences in general become even more alluring as the control to which they are subjected becomes more unyielding. The patient thus feels greater urgency to withhold and deny so as not to expose the humilating "legacy of defectiveness" she and her family share alike—their collective inability to tolerate and manage strong displays of unpleasant emotion and uncertainty.

Relevant to this point are the following comments of a 23-year-old woman in the fourth year of her treatment:

> My appetite for so many things seems out of control. I hated it when I thought of nothing more than what I weighed and how much I ate, but I felt safe. Now I feel that if I let myself go I'll do everything with such drive that people will feel smothered.

This young woman was, from early in her childhood, unusually well mannered, poised, and sensitive. Her parents considered her to be immune from stress and conflict, as she seemed to manage life so effort-lessly and with such little protest. What the patient never revealed to them was her virutally constant worry and tension about the most trivial matters. So great was her *dis-ease* that she vowed never to let it surface for fear that no one could possibly comprehend its origin, and because she feared it would be too much for her gentle and mild-mannered parents to bear.

The point illustrated in this brief closing vignette is how the unsteady and defective sense of self in anorexia nervosa so often reflects a corre-sponding difficulty in the family's effort to accommodate the need for change and for tolerating dissonance—a problem that reveals, at its very core, vicissitudes in the organismic–developmental constituents of self-experience.

CONCLUDING REMARKS

The ultimate test of any theory's utility is the extent to which it broadens our comprehension of human functioning. As stated at the outset, an-orexia nervosa is so complex and puzzling an illness that no single theoret-ical approach can be complete in itself. The particular advantage of the approach taken here is that it informs our knowledge of the unique and distinguishable aspects of self-experience in normal, as well as psy-chopathological, development. In spite of strong historical resistance to recognizing the contribution of organismic factors to psychoanalytic un-derstanding of disease, nothing in the present chapter outwardly disputes the importance of psychoanalytic insights. To the contrary, the sub-stantive advantages of the organismic–developmental paradigm are (1) that it can serve as a general framework in which to amplify and integrate other clinical and theoretical data; and (2) that it takes account of a growing consensus that genetics, biology, and psychology are closely interrelated aspects of the total phenomenology of self-experience. In these terms, anorexia nervosa comes to be seen as a problem of how individuals struggle to preserve unity of the self under the impact of developmental changes that seem so fundamentally at odds with their basic nature. It is in response to this unfolding tension and "discontinuity of being" (Grotstein, 1990) that they feel compelled to wage a self-exhausting struggle to maintain a life of ritual and mastery of inner and outer experience. In consideration of the "how" and "why" of symptom formation and the essential nature of psychological risk, the organismic–developmental paradigm addresses questions that traditional psy-chodynamic theories leave unexplained.

REFERENCES

Atwood, G. E., & Stolorow, R. D. (1984). *Structures of subjectivity: Explorations in psychoanalytic phenomenology*. Hillsdale, NJ: Analytic Press.

Casper, R. C. (1983). Some provisional ideas concerning the psychologic structure in anorexia nervosa and bulimia. In P. L. Darby, P. E. Garfinkel, D. M. Garner, & D. V. Coscina (Eds.), *Anorexia nervosa: Recent developments in research* (pp. 387–392). New York: Alan R. Liss.

Cloninger, C. R. (1986). A unified biosocial theory of personality and its role in the development of anxiety states. *Psychiatric Developments, 3,* 167–226.

Cloninger, C. R. (1987). A systematic method for clinical description and classification of personality variants. *Archives of General Psychiatry, 44,* 573–588.

Cloninger, C. R. (1988). A unified theory of personality and its role in the development of anxiety states: A reply to commentaries. *Psychiatric Developments, 6,* 83–120.

Crisp, A. H. (1980). *Anorexia nervosa: Let me be.* New York: Grune & Stratton.

Crisp, A. H. (1985). Nature and nurture in anorexia nervosa: A study of 34 pairs of twins, one pair of triplets, and one adoptive family. *International Journal of Eating Disorders, 4,* 5–28.

Fairbairn, W. R. D. (1944). Endopsychic structure considered in terms of object relationships. *International Journal of Psycho-Analysis, 25,* 70–131.

Geist, R. A. (1989). Self psychological reflections on the origins of eating disorders. In J. R. Bemporad & D. B. Herzog (Eds.), *Psychoanalysis and eating disorders* (pp. 5–28). New York: Guilford Press.

Goldsmith, H. H., & Campos, J. J. (1982). Toward a theory of infant temperament. In R. N. Emde & R. J. Harmon (Eds.), *The development of attachment and affiliative systems* (pp. 161–194). New York: Plenum Press.

Goodsitt, A. (1984). Self psychology and the treatment of anorexia nervosa. In D. M. Garner & P. E. Garfinkel (Eds.), *Handbook of psychotherapy for anorexia nervosa and bulimia* (pp. 55–82). New York: Guilford Press.

Grotstein, J. S. (1986). The psychology of powerlessness: Disorders of self-regulation and interactional regulation as a newer paradigm for psychopathology. *Psychoanalytic Inquiry, 6,* 93–118.

Grotstein, J. S. (1987). The borderline as a disorder of self-regulation. In J. S. Grotstein, M. F. Soloman, & J. A. Land (Eds.), *The borderline patient* (Vol. 1, pp. 347–383). Hillsdale, NJ: Analytic Press.

Grotstein, J. S. (1990). Invariants in primitive mental disorders. In L. B. Boyer & P. L. Giovacchini (Eds.), *Master clinicians on treating the regressed patient* (pp. 139–164). Northvale, NJ: Jason Aronson.

Gull, W. W. (1874). Anorexia nervosa (apepsia hysterica, anorexia hysterica). *Transactions of the Clinical Society of London, 7,* 22–28.

Kandel, E. R. (1979). Psychotherapy and the single synapse: The impact of psychiatric thought on neurobiologic research. *New England Journal of Medicine, 301,* 1028–1037.

Kohut, H. (1971). *The analysis of the self.* New York: International Universities Press.

Kohut, H. (1977). *The restoration of the self*. New York: International Universities Press.

Lasegue, C. (1873). On hysterical anorexia. *Medical Times Gazette, 2*, 265–266.

Lichtenberg, J. (1983). *Psychoanalysis and infant research*. Hillsdale, NJ: Analytic Press.

Morton, R. (1694). *Phthisiologica; or a treatise of consumptions*. London: Smith & Walford.

Plomin, R. (1986). *Development, genetics, and psychology*. Hillsdale, NJ: Erlbaum.

Plomin, R., & Rowe, D. (1977). A twin study of temperament in young children. *Journal of Psychology, 97*, 107–113.

Reiser, M. F. (1984) *Mind, brain, body: Toward a convergence of psychoanalysis and neurobiology*. New York: Basic Books.

Sandler, L. S. (1983). To begin with—reflections on ontogeny. In J. Lichtenberg & S. Kaplan (Eds.), *Reflections on self psychology* (pp. 85–104). Hillsdale, NJ: Analytic Press.

Scarr, S., & McCartney, K. (1983). How people make their own environments: A theory of genotype–environment effects. *Child Development, 54*, 424–435.

Steinglass, R. (1987). A systems view of family interaction and psychopathology. In T. Jacob (Ed.), *Family interaction and psychopathology: Theories, methods, and findings* (pp. 25–66). New York: Plenum Press.

Stern, D. (1983). The early development of self, other, and "self with other." In J. Lichtenberg & S. Kaplan (Eds.), *Reflections on self psychology* (pp. 49–84). Hillsdale, NJ: Analytic Press.

Stern, D. (1985). *The interpersonal world of the infant*. New York: Basic Books.

Stolorow, R. D., Brandchaft, B., & Atwood, G. E. (1987). *Psychoanalytic treatment: An intersubjective approach*. Hillsdale, NJ: Analytic Press.

Stolorow, R. D., & Lachmann, F. M. (1980). *Psychoanalysis of developmental arrests*. Madison, CT: International Universities Press.

Strober, M. (1980). Personality and symptomatological features in young, nonchronic anorexia nervosa patients. *Journal of Psychosomatic Research, 24*, 353–359.

Strober, M. (1981). A comparative analysis of personality organization in anorexia nervosa. *Journal of Youth and Adolescence, 10*, 285–295.

Thomas, A., & Chess, S. (1977). *Temperament and development*. New York: Brunner/Mazel.

Thomas, A., Chess, S., & Birch, H. G. (1969). *Temperament and behavior disorders in children*. New York: New York University Press.

Tomkins, S. S. (1962). *Affect, imagery, consciousness: Vol. 1. The positive affects*. New York: Springer.

∴ *15* ∴

The Integration of Psychodynamic and Behavior Therapy in the Treatment of Eating Disorders: Clinical Issues versus Theoretical Mystique

DAVID L. TOBIN
The University of Chicago

CRAIG L. JOHNSON
*Laureate Psychiatric Clinic and Hospital, Tulsa
and Northwestern University Medical School, Chicago*

With the exception of one very notable book by Wachtel (1977), questions regarding the integration of psychodynamic and behavior therapy have remained largely unexplored (see also Wachtel & Wachtel, 1986). Several books have suggested the possibility of common factors (e.g., Frank, 1973; Goldfried, 1982), but these efforts tend to dilute rather than synthesize the advantages of different models. Wachtel (1977), on the other hand, does a careful job of evaluating the divergent components of psychodynamic and behavior therapy and examines how differences in the two approaches might complement each other. The purpose of this chapter is to examine these questions with specific reference to treatment for eating disorders.

This may seem to some readers an unnecessary exercise—either because one is unwilling to consider alternative models, or because one assumes that similar issues and concerns are already addressed in both models. The latter attitude is characterized by the comments of an anonymous reviewer of a previous paper on integration (Johnson, Connors, & Tobin, 1987), who suggests "that most treatment approaches, implicitly at least, already make such an integration between psychodynamic and behavioral approaches and the old debate is somewhat passé. On the other hand, I have not yet seen anyone specifically discuss this need for integration and, as such, this type of observation may be needed."

This kind of confusion may explain why there has been almost no published work in the area of integrating psychodynamic and behavior therapy for the treatment of eating disorders. This can be particularly frustrating when it is apparent that competing camps discuss very similar clinical issues, have similar points of view regarding clinical strategies, and yet strive to differentiate their particular models of treatment.

A good example of this can be found in a chapter on the cognitive–behavioral treatment of anorexia by Garner and Bemis (1984). They suggest that "the [therapeutic] relationship becomes a key source of data for the assessment of beliefs," and further note that "The patient frequently makes specific inferences about the therapist' feelings towards her, and these may emerge as themes that re-emerge in therapy" (1984, p. 111). Although Garner and Bemis note that this sounds "dangerously close to a traditional 'transference' interpretation," they assure us that "there are substantial distinctions in theoretical frameworks and modes of conducting therapy that make the parallel between approaches [psychodynamic vs. cognitive–behavioral therapy] very limited" (1984, p. 111). Thus, even when there is common ground between Garner and Bemis's cognitive–behavioral approach to treatment and psychodynamic approaches, they reject a direct comparison. Such attitudes make rapprochement between the two approaches very difficult.

Though Garner and Bemis might disagree, divergent approaches to working with difficult patients have resulted in treatments that closely resemble each other, in practice if not in theory. For example, Swenson (1989) argues that despite theoretical differences, both Kernberg (e.g., 1975) and Linehan (e.g., 1987) intervene in a number of similar ways with their borderline patients. Furthermore, recognition of the inadequacy of short-term, focused cognitive–behavioral therapy for personality-disordered patients has led behavioral therapists to emphasize the importance of focusing on the client–therapist relationship (Kohlenberg, 1987). Other cognitive–behavioral therapists have integrated cognitive therapy with interpersonal and experiential therapy (Greenberg & Safran, 1987; Safran, 1984), resulting in a triadic view of treatment that functionally approximates several important aspects of psychodynamic psychotherapy. Similarly, psychodynamic therapists have found it necessary to incorporate behavioral therapy into their approach to working with eating-disordered patients (Johnson et al., 1987). Thus, whether it is acknowledged or not, desegregation is occurring in practice if not in theory. We feel that this is happening because therapists and patients struggle with each other in similar ways, regardless of the therapists' theoretical orientation.

This chapter is intended to be a "how-to" manual for both behavioral and psychodynamic therapist, so that practitioners who are familiar and comfortable with a particular model can appreciate how another perspective may increase the efficacy of treatment. In addition, concerns about how integration might interfere with the practice of psychotherapy are addressed. The following pathway to such an understanding is proposed: (1) Brief outlines of the respective treatment approaches are presented; (2) common ground is explored; (3) concerns regarding integration are considered; and (4) a model for integration is proposed.

Obviously, this chapter cannot fully represent the considerations and richness of either psychodynamic or behavioral approaches. The outlines of these respective techniques may seem superficial. Nevertheless, they are presented in order to familiarize readers with our experience and perspective, so that readers have a context to explore their own concerns regarding integration. References are provided that outline specific techniques more thoroughly.

BEHAVIOR THERAPY

There are two primary sources for the behavioral treatment of eating disorders, both of which have cognitive components in their treatment packages. One is a chapter on cognitive–behavioral therapy for bulimia by Fairburn (1984), and the other is on the chapter cognitive therapy for anorexia by Garner and Bemis (1984). Because the first component of Garner's treatment usually involves hospitalization, Fairburn's approach probably gives the practitioner of individual psychotherapy a more comprehensive guide to conducting outpatient treatment. Both approaches are derived from more general cognitive–behavioral models (e.g., Beck, Rush, Shaw, & Emery, 1979; Guidano & Liotti, 1983; Mahoney, 1974; Marlatt & Gordon, 1978; Meichenbaum, 1974), and both offer the reader a much more comprehensive model for conducting cognitive–behavioral treatment of eating disorders (see also Johnson et al., 1987) than does the current discussion. Rosen and Leitenberg's (1982) combinations of exposure and response prevention is another behavioral approach to the treatment of bulimia, but it is not clear that adding this component increases the efficacy of behavioral approaches to treatment (Agras,

Schneider, Arnow, Raeburn, & Telch, 1989; Buckley, 1987; Leitenberg & Rosen, 1989).

Behavioral approaches to treatment are symptom-focused. In the treatment of eating disorders, target symptoms include restricting behaviors, binge-eating, purging behaviors, and the thoughts and feelings that are thought to mediate performance of these behaviors. The cognitions that have most frequently been targeted include drive for thinness and body dissatisfaction (e.g., Garner & Bemis, 1984). Affective targets that are most frequently described include the anxiety and depression that are thought to accompany being out of control with food (e.g., Rosen & Leitenberg, 1982).

Most current behavioral approaches to treatment of eating disorders incorporate cognitive therapies and are grounded in social learning theory (e.g., Bandura, 1977). Most involve training in self-management skills (e.g., Kanfer & Scheft, 1987; Rehm & Rokke, 1988; Tobin, Reynolds, Holroyd, & Creer, 1986), meaning that the patient is expected to play a very active role in the treatment process. Training in self-management includes such skills as self-monitoring of thoughts and behaviors (Beck et al., 1979) and self-instructional training (Meichenbaum, 1977).

Although not all behavior therapists agree on the best way to change disordered eating, there are enough common elements to warrant a generalized description of the treatment process. Treatment usually begins with a didactic, educational phase, in which the therapist provides information that is pertinent to the behavior or symptoms that are to be controlled. Concurrently, the therapist and patient collaborate to identify the target symptoms to be self-managed. This identification process can go through many stages of refinement, but with an eating disorder patient, a general picture of the patient's eating patterns is a desirable place to start. The patient is then asked to self-monitor factors that influence eating patterns and difficulties. After a representative sample of the patient's eating patterns have been collected, any of a variety of self-regulatory skills are taught, and homework assignments are given to promote generalization of behaviors learned in the clinic.

We find Fairburn's (1984) cognitive–behavioral approach to outpatient treatment of bulimia nervosa particularly appealing for the following reasons. First, there is a relatively simple, semistructured protocol for therapists and patients to follow. The simplicity means that skills training can be easily accomplished, and a semistructured format is particularly suited to integration with psychodynamic work. Second, Fairburn accurately assesses, we believe, the relative value of behavioral self-management training over cognitive therapy, which is more difficult to accomplish. Fairburn suggests that many patients do not need or will not be able to benefit from the cognitive component of his treatment.

Thus, he begins with the following eight components of psychoeducation and self-management training: (1) the establishment of a sound therapeutic relationship; (2) the disruption of habitual binge-eating, self-induced vomiting, and laxative abuse; (3) the introduction of a pattern of regular eating; (4) education about the physical consequences of binge-eating, self-induced vomiting, and laxative abuse; (5) education about the "effectiveness" of vomiting and laxative abuse to control weight; (6) weekly weighing; (7) examination of the "function" of binge-eating and self-induced vomiting; and (8) the enlistment of cooperation from friends and relatives (Fairburn, 1984, p. 167). We are particularly pleased with Fairburn's self-monitoring form (1984, p. 170), which is structured enough to help patients gather important information and yet simple enough to promote compliance with self-monitoring.

This simplicity also allows therapist and patient considerable flexibility in what they decide to record. Fairburn uses the back page of the monitoring sheet to do cognitive work, which he teaches patients in great detail (if they need it) during the second stage of treatment. The second stage of treatment involves the following six steps: (1) the establishment and maintenance of a pattern of regular eating; (2) reduction of dietary restraint; (3) identification of circumstances that tend to result in binge-eating; and helping the patient cope more effectively with these circumstances; (4) the identification of and challenging of thoughts, beliefs, and values that perpetuate eating difficulties; (5) helping the patient's difficulties with body image; and (6) initiating the termination process (1984, p. 176).

Finally, Fairburn tapers the session frequency in the third stage of treatment down to three interviews at 2-week intervals. The third and final stage focuses on maintenance and strategies to manage relapse. It should be again noted that readers unfamiliar with Fairburn's work should look at his detailed description of this treatment process.

We believe, and there are considerable data to suggest, that many patients will be helped by this and similar approaches to treatment (for review, see Johnson & Connors, 1987, Ch. 12). But these findings also suggest that a significant percentage of patients do not benefit from behavioral approaches to treatment (or any other treatment approach). Although the exact figures vary somewhat from study to study, the percentage of treatment failures roughly coincides with the percentage of eating disorder patients who present with concurrent personality disorders (e.g., Gwirtsman, Roy-Byrne, Yager, & Gerner, 1983; Johnson, Tobin, & Enright; 1989),—somewhere between one-half and one-third of patients.

It is our clinical experience, and there are preliminary data to suggest (Johnson, Tobin, & Dennis, in press), that eating disorder patients who present with concurrent personality disorders need a considerable "dose" (Howard, Kopta, Krause, & Orlinsky, 1986) of psychodynamically oriented treatment added to skills training in self-management before they are able to achieve self-regulation of their eating habits. This is a unique finding, because no previous studies have tried to combine treatment approaches or looked at the impact of personality disorders on treatment outcome for eating disorder patients. Other interventions, including family therapy, pharmacological therapy, support groups, impatient hospitalization, and day hospital, may also be helpful (Tobin, Johnson, & Franke, in press); however, there therapies are often employed in support of the individual psychotherapy component of treatment.

PSYCHODYNAMIC PSYCHOTHERAPY

In sharp contrast to behavioral approaches to treatment, psychodynamic psychotherapy is not symptom-focused. Treatment involves a frequent and lengthy course of psychotherapy, such that the issues underlying a patient's eating symptoms emerge in a transference to the therapist. It is thought that once the transference is understood by the therapist, interpreted to the patient, and worked through in the therapeutic alliance, eating symptoms will spontaneously remit. Most psychoanalytic work that is specific to eating disorders has attempted to demonstrate the presence of conflictual material common to a specific set of symptoms (e.g., Schwartz, 1988; Wilson, 1983).

Research has virtually eliminated the possibility that eating-disordered patients, even within a symptom subgroup, are faced with a common developmental difficulty or have followed an inevitable pathway to the onset of symptoms. Empirical work suggests that eating-disordered patients face a wide range of developmental difficulties, and that character difficulties and level of depression or anxiety are relatively uncorrelated with the severity of eating symptoms (Garner, Moldofsky, & Garner, 1980; Gwirtsman et al., 1983; Johnson et al., 1989, in press; Steinberg, Tobin, & Johnson, 1990; Levin & Hyler, 1986; Pope, Frankenberg, & Hudson, 1987; Swift & Stern, 1982). Thus, psychodynamic theorists who write either about the range of developmental difficulties that may face eating-disordered patients or about a kind of developmental difficulty that is commonly found in eating-disordered patients have more closely reflected the empirical findings of clinical researchers than either those psychodynamic theorists who hypothesize a specific underlying conflict or those biological and behavioral theorists who specify some other unidimensional pathway to the onset of symptoms.

Several papers on clinical practice have taken the former approach. Goodsitt's (1984) paper on self psychology and the treatment of anorexia nervosa is an excellent example of a description of a type of developmental deficit and appropriate intervention that is common to many (but not all) anorexic patients. Stern and Humphrey (Humphrey & Stern, 1988; Stern, 1986; see also Humphrey, Chapter 13, this volume) have evolved an approach to working with anorexia and bulimia that is based on object relations theory and that integrates psychodynamic and family systems work. Utilizing the notion that therapy shares characteristics of the mother–infant holding environment (e.g., Winnicott, 1965), the therapist is expected to intervene in such a way as to appropriately meet the patient's level of ego functioning and type of developmental deficit. Patients are understood to present with a wide range of developmental difficulties, so that different patients may require different intervening strategies. Similarly, it is hoped that a patient's developmental needs will change over time, requiring the therapist to adjust strategies, much in the same way a parent is expected to meet the changing needs of a developing infant (Mahler, 1968).

This kind of developmental perspective is not always seen in psychoanalytic theory. Kernberg (1988) and Kohut (1971), for example, have each emphasized a particular kind of developmental difficulty, and the difficulties do not significantly overlap. As a result, they prescribe quite different clinical interventions. But other psychoanalytic theorists have incorporated these more specific models (e.g., Adler, 1985; Pine, 1985) into a developmental model (e.g., Mahler, 1968; Winnicott, 1965) that accommodates changing developmental needs. These more encompassing models, along with the work of Humphrey and Stern, have served as one of the foundations for the psychodynamic components of our treatment philosophy.

In addition to incorporating object relations and developmental theory into the treatment process, the other key ingredient to our approach to psychodynamic treatment is the notion that the therapeutic relationship is a social one (Gill, 1982; Hoffman, 1983; Strupp, 1989; Sulivan, 1953). This conceptualization represents a radical departure from classical psychoanalytic theorizing about the treatment process, though it is not clear that it represents much of a departure from the way in which Freud himself actually practiced psychotherapy. The traditional notion that the analyst functions as a blank screen allows the assertion that transference is a distortion, that it is purely a re-enactment of the patient's history. However, there are a number of problems in this assumption, many of which have been outlined by Hoffman (1983). Foremost of these, from our perspective, is the notion that the therapist is able to and must maintain neutrality through a very passive involvement with the patient. Obviously, the introduction of behavioral therapy into a psychodynamic therapy must contaminate and invalidate such a frame (e.g., Langs, 1982).

Although it is possible (perhaps even likely) that Hoffman would balk at the extent to which the introduction of behavioral therapy would violate the process of psychoanalytic psychotherapy, his arguments vis-à-vis the social nature of the therapeutic relationship are applicable. The implication of these arguments is that to withhold education and skills training from a patient with disregulated eating habits creates an interpersonal relationship re-enacting the inadequate parenting that has predisposed the patients to develop eating difficulties in the first place. This view is highly consistent with that of the Wachtels (Wachtel, 1977; Wachtel & Wachtel, 1986), who hypothesize that in addition to the patient's history, there are re-enactments in the patient's present experience that continuously recreate the patient's former object world. Thus, if disregulated eating habits are employed to that purpose, they must be challenged outside of the sessions in the same way that distortions of the therapist must be challenged within the session.

Although it is even more difficult to capsulize psychodynamic approaches to treatment than behavioral approaches, the following recommendations by Strupp (1989) provide a heuristic for treatment that is consistent with our own conceptualization. It will be noted that these recommendations contradict the need for behavioral intervention. However, they apply only to the psychodynamic component of the treatment process, and do not comprise the whole treatment we are describing:

> 1. Nothing is more important than the transactions between patient and therapist in the here and now of each therapy hour, and precedence must always be given to the patient's current experience, particularly the affect accompanying it.
> 2. The therapist's primary activity should be empathetic listening, with a minimum of interference (e.g., small talk or self-serving comments). Except in rare instances, he or she should desist from giving advice, guidance and the like. According to this principle, empathetic and respectful listening (with the exception of the clarifying comments as I will show) provide the optimum support and help a therapist can and should give. It also provides the patient with the greatest opportunity (not always welcomed) to become aware of his or her experience and to develop autonomy, which in turn permits interpersonal intimacy (as opposed to enmeshment). This recommended stance also leaves the field as uncontaminated as possible and provides a vacuum as it were, into which the patient's experience can flow.
> 3. Attempts to clarify the patient's experience, with particular emphasis on metacommunications about the patient–therapist relationship, should be clear, concise, free of jargon, and relate as closely as possible to the contemporaneous transactions that both can observe. . . .
> 4. By all odds, the greatest challenge facing the therapist is the skillful management of enactments that often put the therapist on the defensive, evoke boredom, irritation, anger, hostility and in other respects put "pressure" on the therapist to behave in ways that are in-

compatible with his or her stance as an empathetic listener and clarifier. Feeling manipulated, controlled, or imposed on are typical examples. These are precisely the maneuvers that get the patient into trouble in his or her interactions with significant others in the present, and they constitute the "illness" the therapist is called on to cure. (Strupp, 1989, p. 719)

This description of psychodynamic treatment is as concise and as free of jargon as any we have seen, and yet it captures much of what we believe to be the fundamental task of psychodynamic psychotherapy. As the reader may have noted, however, Strupp is inconsistent in the presentation of his model as social on the one hand, and the extent to which he feels it is possible and necessary to maintain a neutral frame vis-à-vis the process of empathetic listening on the other. Strupp would constrain us from introducing behavioral interventions, on the grounds that they would contaminate the listening process. However, in a social paradigm as discussed by Hoffman (1983), empathetic listening alone can be inadequate, both in terms of the disregulated eating habits and in terms of the patient's characterological needs. For example, a very disturbed patient (e.g., one with borderline personality disorder) may experience the therapist as withholding and unconnected if the majority of the therapy hour is spent listening to the patient. With a patient from this (large) subgroup, the therapist must be considerably more active than is suggested in Strupp's description. Even the use of "small talk" and self-disclosure can be occasionally justified if it facilitates the patient's experience of being responded to by the therapist (Greenberg, 1986).

Despite this inconsistency, we are in agreement with Strupp's premise that the therapist's commitment to understanding the "metacommunications" about the patient–therapist relationship is central to psychodynamic psychotherapy; we believe that it is a critical component of an integrated approach to treatment as well. This means that the therapist needs to understand how the actions and reactions between patient and therapist contribute to the maintenance of the patient's difficulties, and to find some way of educating the patient about this process (e.g., interpretation). While part of this educational process involves linking up the patient's current experiences to previous ones (e.g., how the patient's current experience of his or her spouse reflects previous experience of his or her mother or father), such recounting is not accomplished at the cost of the patient's experience in the here and now. Important events often occur in therapy that have no clear historical predecessor, and these need to be appreciated in the context of the current relationship between patient and therapist.

Strupp's description of analysis of transference provides a useful heuristic for understanding how the therapeutic relationship is helpful to patients. Although we do not feel that Strupp's lack of active intervention (e.g., training in self-management) is optimal for patients with eating disorders, we acknowledge that combining psychodynamic and behavior therapy presents technical difficulties. For example, patients cannot free-associate when their therapist is checking for compliance with homework assignments. Given that asking about homework is sometimes necessary, an approach such as Strupp's offers the therapist a psychodynamic "home base" for observation, reflection, and the generation of hypotheses regarding transference and countertransference.

INTEGRATION

The following is a model for integrating psychodynamic and behavior therapy in the treatment of eating disorders. The model recognizes that there are overlapping dimensions in both kinds of treatment, but also recognizes significant differences. While we want to be as straightforward as possible in describing an integrated treatment approach, clinical decisions about when to utilize one approach as opposed to another can be complicated. The rest of the chapter explores some of these considerations and, finally, presents an outline for an integrated approach to treatment.

Strupp's (1989) and Fairburn's (1984) descriptions of their respective treatment approaches provide a base for describing the components of an integrative approach. This includes (1) a behavioral component with psychoeducation and skills training to promote the patient's self-management of eating habits; and (2) a psychodynamic component that emphasizes empathetic listening and uses the therapist–patient dyad as a model for understanding and resolving the patient's intrapsychic and interpersonal difficulties.

The factor that distinguishes most clearly between psychodynamic and behavior therapy also presents the greatest challenge to integrating the two approaches. This involves when, where, and how the therapeutic process is thought to be most helpful. For behavior therapy, the emphasis is on the acquisition of new behaviors (or the extinguishing of old behaviors) that affect symptoms in the patient's everyday life. Though new behaviors may be introduced in the clinic, the primary focus of treatment is in their performance outside of therapy. In contrast, psychodynamic therapy is thought to be most helpful when the patient changes behavior or experiences a change in affect, insight, attitude, or relatedness during a session. Changes outside of therapy are thought to follow. Consequently, the therapist may focus on the patient's behavior, thoughts, or feelings in quite different fashion, depending on which therapy component is being emphasized at a particular point in time.

Both psychodynamic and behavior therapy include methods for correcting distorted attitudes and beliefs, and these methods tend to diverge along the same lines as the rest of treatment. Behavioral treatment typically uses what happens outside of the session as a mechanism for challenging distorted beliefs, whereas the psychodynamic treatment uses what happens during the session (between the therapist and patient) as a way to challenge distorted beliefs. Adherents of both approaches tend to regard the challenging of beliefs as among the most difficult of therapeutic tasks to accomplish.

The heuristic above starkly contrasts the two approaches to treatment, but clinical practice does not always leave psychodynamic and behavioral colleagues on such divergent paths. For example, either type of therapist would want to know what brought the patient to seek treatment. Both would be interested in getting to know the patient and in trying to understand the patient's day-to-day experiences. Both psychodynamic and behavior therapists are likely to appear empathetic and concerned about the patient's difficulties (variations in this dimension have more to do with individual therapist differences than theoretical orientation). These activities are likely to comprise the significant part of any therapeutic endeavor and have been identified as nonspecific or common factors (Frank, 1973; Goldfried, 1982). These common therapeutic activities facilitate integration, but are not sufficient to comprise it.

Integration involves not only carrying out what is common to the two modalities, but also modulating the time spent in divergent activities. Our approach to this aspect of integration is partially derived from previous clinical and research experience in the development of minimal-contact cognitive–behavioral treatments for other disorders (e.g., Holroyd et al., 1988; Tobin, Holroyd, Baker, Reynolds, & Holm, 1988). Tobin and his colleagues (1988) found that chronic tension headaches could be effectively treated with a cognitive–behavioral regimen similar to the one described by Fairburn (1984), except that the entire treatment was delivered in only three clinic sessions. These sessions were administered over a period of 2 months, with patients having extensive homework assignments between sessions. Every patient in the cognitive–behavioral treatment achieved a least some benefit, and most patients achieved a substantial reduction in their headaches. One of the factors that undoubtedly contributed to the treatment's efficacy was artifactual to the study but is central to the premise of this chapter. Though patients in the study demonstrated wide variability in the severity of their headaches, with some patients demonstrating almost constant severe pain, there was a screening process that probably eliminated patients who demonstrated significant character pathology. Thus, patients with severe tension headache but no characterological difficulties could learn to control their headaches in only three clinic sessions.

Another lesson from this study was that behavior change could be quite circumscribed and still have a significant impact on symptoms, as there was only one clinic session that was devoted to either a problem-solving or a cognitive restructuring intervention. The therapist and patient collaborated in devising one specific behavioral (or cognitive) goal that might have an impact on the patient's headaches. One of the guidelines for maximizing the effectiveness of such limited therapist contact was the following question: "What is the smallest change in behavior that will make a significant impact on this patient's symptoms?"

The implication of this study is that eating-disordered patients without personality disorders are also capable of quickly learning and effectively performing self-management strategies to control their eating. Several lines of evidence support this contention. First, there is evidence to suggest that eating symptoms are independent of depression and personality deficits in clinical populations (Johnson et al., 1989; Tobin, Johnson, Steinberg, & Dennis, 1990). Moreover, 1-year follow-up data suggest that the eating symptoms of bulimic patients without personality disorders are likely to remit in fewer than 30 sessions, while bulimic patients with borderline personality disorder are likely to need upwards of 100 sessions to achieve control over their eating (Johnson et al., in press). The length of these respective treatments meant that the non-character-disordered patients received primarily cognitive–behavioral interventions, while the borderline patients received significantly more psychodynamic, relationship-oriented work.

These findings suggest that eating-disordered patients who are relatively free of characterological difficulties may benefit from a brief treatment that focuses on the acquisition of a few self-management skills. Also, because it is not always clear how personality-disordered patients will respond to self-management training unless given the chance, we typically begin treatment with psychoeducation and self-management training similar to these elements of Fairburn's treatment package. Bulimic patients without personality disorders have little trouble complying with the task of self-monitoring and are often able to quickly introduce three meals a day, which helps break the diet–hunger–binge–purge cycle. Body dissatisfaction and drive for thinness are likely to be in a range that is within normal limits for young women (Johnson et al., 1989) and that presents little impediment to remission of symptoms. Thus, the cognitive therapy component of Fairburn's treatment is usually not necessary or is relatively easy to carry out with this patient subgroup. Also, episodes of bingeing and purging are likely to be experienced in an ego-dystonic fashion and to increase these patients' level of depression (Steinberg et al., 1990). Without the social–biological impetus of restrictive dieting to deregulate a patient's eating, binge–purge episodes become self-extinguishing by virtue of the self-inflicted (and unsought after) dysphoria. With the eating symptoms quickly under control, therapist and patient have the opportunity to explore the patient's other concerns, which are likely to reflect developmental issues normative to the patient's age group. The remission of symptoms leads to either the exploration of these other issues and the renegotiation of a more psychodynamic framework, or the ending of treatment.

This relatively straightforward course of treatment does not characterize work with bulimic patients who suffer from chronic personality disorders or with more severely anorexic patients. For patients with borderline (e.g., Adler, 1985; Johnson & Connors, 1987; Kernberg, 1988) or narcissistic (e.g., Goodsitt, 1984; Kohut, 1971) personality disorders, a broadly defined interpersonal and intrapersonal context in which the eating symptoms serve an adaptive function is likely to interfere with the acquisition of self-management behaviors. For borderline patients, symptoms are used to manage separation–fusion anxiety (Summers, 1988) and to deny or soothe severe depression (Steinberg et al., 1990). For narcissistic patients, symptoms are used to isolate and protect ego ideals, to soothe narcissistic tensions, and to seek idealization from others (Goodsitt, 1984). There is little "hard" evidence but some anecdotal evidence (Johnson & Connors, 1987; Tobin, Johnson, & Franke, in press) to suggest that chronic anorexic patients can present with even more serious character difficulties, such as a paranoid character structure. In order to help these patients achieve self-regulation of their eating-related difficulties, it is often necessary to meet the self-regulatory needs of the patients' object world through psychodynamic psychotherapy. Obviously, resolving characterological difficulties can take a long time, but some progress in this area is often necessary before a patient is able to "collaborate" in developing self-management skills.

Several examples may help to illustrate this point. A narcissistic patient with bulimia had great difficulty performing the simplest of self-monitoring tasks. She bristled at even the mention of her inability to perform homework assignments. Though several months of treatment provided some interesting insights into the patient's family relationships, she still had not changed one aspect of her behavior. Finally, in one session she was able to reveal how degrading she found the work related to her eating symptoms. Her experience of receiving a homework assignment was similar to criticism she received from her family: "Quit feeling sorry for yourself and just do it." Once this aspect of her experience with the therapist was appreciated and interpreted, she was able to decrease her bulimic symptoms immediately.

Another patient demonstrated symptoms of both anorexia and bulimia. She was very undifferentiated from her very borderline mother, who was in turn very undifferentiated from the patient's grandmother. Individual treatment focused on the daughter's eating symptoms and the rage she felt over her mother's use of her as a self-object. Family treatment was also necessary to help manage both the patient's and the mother's anxiety regarding the daughter's separation–individuation. The patient often refused to consider homework assignments, especially trying new foods. The therapist was then drawn into letting go of the behavioral component of treatment, because the patient would experience homework assignments as intrusive and punitive. Subsequently, however, she would then experience the abandonment of the behavioral component as a repetition of the neglect she experienced with her mother—which triggered anxiety and rage over separation. Acknowledgment of the therapist's cyclic collusion with this dynamic, and confrontation of the patient's setting up of this re-enactment, were necessary before she would undertake any new self-management tasks.

Unless the therapist understands the transference and countertransference implications of a particular behavioral intervention, or what Strupp describes as the metacommunications about the patient–therapist relationship, a characterological patient who is noncompliant can quickly become a treatment failure. While a behavioral therapist will endeavor to find a nonresistant path to promoting collaboration, theoretical bias risks obscuring a significant source of information: the therapeutic dyad. In addition, the behavior therapist is also left without the benefit of many years of observation and documentation (albeit mostly nonexperimental) of therapist–patient behavior and the possible ways in which the patient's developmental history might influence the therapeutic dyad.

Although the description above suggests some of the complexity involved in the integrated treatment of eating disorder patients, it does not provide much in the way of straightforward guidance of when to do what. This remains a complicated question, and we defer to another source for guidance. Gustafson (1986) describes a "method of methods" for integrating diverse psychoanalytic and systemic practices, which is applicable to our goal of integration (again, we cannot do justice to the complexity of this approach, and the reader is encouraged to consult the original source). Gustafson builds his model on a very brief psychotherapeutic encounter—as little as a single session. Thus, he also attempts to create the maximum benefit with the fewest words (or the least amount of homework).

Gustafson initiates the session by listening to what the patient tells him about their current dilemma. Starting with what seems most obvious, Gustafson explores solutions to the patient's presenting problem while being sensitive to the "opposing currents" that impede the obvious solutions. Gustafson succeeds in this by allowing the patient to "decenter" him; this is a process by which the patient disrupts the stated collaborative exercise for a new and compelling, yet previously unstated, goal.[1]

There are two primary "decentering" maneuvers that are salient to our present discussion. The first maneuver occurs when the patient has significant difficulty with behavioral homework. If the patient has the necessary skills to perform the homework (e.g., the ability to self-monitor meals), noncompliance is frequently a communication by the patient that the therapist does not understand the broader context serving to maintain symptomatic behavior. Behavior therapists, especially radical behavior therapists (e.g., Hayes, 1987), would also be interested in understanding this broader context. However, psychodynamic theorists have done more work in the area of listening and trying to understand how a broader context may reveal a previously unstated agenda (e.g., unconscious motives, embarrassing wishes). When the patient signals to the therapist that such a misunderstanding exists in the treatment, a shift must take place in which the patient takes over structuring the session agenda. The patient must begin the session, and the therapist must make every effort to follow whatever material the patient generates. Sometimes the therapist must educate patients on when this shift needs to occur and the purpose for the change in session process, so that they do not experience abandonment. Other patients will quite naturally take the lead in attempting to present their difficulties. This shift in treatment can be a most difficult one for therapists who are primarily behavioral.

The second maneuver by patients that can decenter the therapist occurs after the initiation of a more psychodynamic frame, when patients regain interest in behavioral work. This renewed interest is easily understood when the patients understand why they had difficulties with homework in the first place. However, patients often want or need behavioral work even without the benefit of an appreciable increase in insight. At this point the distinction between behavioral and psychodynamic intervention can become murky, as one must simultaneously attempt to understand the metacommunication of the request (often expressed as a complaint) and to assess how best (or whether) to resume the behavioral work. The distinction between approaches can become murkier still if the therapist decides to use behavioral techniques to achieve traditionally psychoanalytic goals (e.g., using self-monitoring or cue control to promote object constancy; Johnson & Connors, 1987). If a patient remains symptomatic, regardless of whether or not the insight is achieved, it is important for the therapist to reintroduce behavioral techniques at some point. This can be difficult for therapists who are primarily psychodynamic in their orientation.

The longer the course of treatment, the more complicated doing or not doing a particular intervention can become. This can be particularly true for character-disordered patients who use massive avoidant defenses (e.g., Adler, 1985) to obscure what is important to them. The eventual path to some clarity about when to do what and what it means to the patient when the therapist does anything is in understanding and appreciating the patient's transference as it emerges in the treatment. When this occurs, the patient's strong affects regarding important material can illuminate what direction to take. An often important precursor to the emergence of the transference is the therapist's countertransference experience of the patient's projected identifications (Kernberg, 1988). Being able to manage, interpret, and empathize with these affects—so painful they are projected off—is often the first step to helping patients connect with important parts of themselves that are invested in maintaining symptoms. The more clearly the therapist understands the intrapsychic and interpersonal context in which the symptoms occur, the more accurately he or she can make decisions.

There are many nuances to this process, such as the ability to differentiate countertransference reactions that are unique to the therapist from those reactions triggered by the behavior of the patient. Similarly, it is important to distinguish those reactions of the patient that are distortions and reflect transference from those that are reasonable responses to the therapist (e.g., Hoffman, 1983. This is particularly important in an integrated approach to treatment, because the therapist will be, to some degree, usurping the patient's initiative and imposing on the patient's wishes through the introduction of skills training and homework assignments. However, this is often less problematic than depriving patients of skills that would help them self-regulate their eating behavior. Moreover, the complexity that behavioral interventions introduce to the analysis of a patient's transference is not only manageable but useful, as we have found that offering symptom management strategies can help to focus transference issues quickly.

A HEURISTIC FOR INTEGRATIVE TREATMENT

Having emphasized the potential complexity of an integrative approach to treatment, we now provide the following set of guidelines:

1. Patients who are relatively free of character pathology may be initiated in brief, once-a-week individual therapy. Patients with very severe eating symptoms but no character pathology may need twice-a-week treatment to help overcome the maintaining effects of the diet–hunger–binge–purge cycle. Patients with character pathology usually

need twice-a-week psychotherapy, regardless of the severity of their eating symptoms (Johnson et al., in press).

2. The initial focus of treatment for all patients can be primarily psychoeducational and self-management oriented. Areas of information that can be particularly helpful to patients include basic nutrition, the ways that dieting can promote weight gain, sociocultural and feminist perspectives on concern for physical appearance, and the idea that purging is not an effective way to limit calories. The self-management task that is fundamental and often sufficient to helping patients remit bingeing and purging is self-monitoring of foods eaten and eliminated through purging. The other simple yet powerful self-management strategy is to help patients eat three meals a day. Patients rarely need more than one additional behavioral intervention to help them promote these goals. This third intervention must come from understanding the unique difficulty a given patient has in regulating eating. To help identify this intervention, the therapist must try to identify the smallest possible change in behavior that will help a patient regulate eating.

3. If the psychoeducational and self-management therapy becomes derailed by the patient's difficulty and noncompliance with homework assignments, the therapist and patient must explore a broader context in which the patient's symptoms are serving an adaptive function. We have tried to outline what some of the contingencies affecting patient noncompliance might be in Figure 15.1. Though patient difficulties are not always divided so straightforwardly, we have separated three domains of non-compliance/resistance that should be explored: environmental contingencies, intrapersonal contingencies, and transferential contingencies.

This exploration may lead the focus of treatment not only away from the behavioral self-management of symptoms, but away from discussion of symptoms at all. The therapist's primary task is to come to a greater understanding of patients' experience, not only in terms of their attempts to manage symptomatic behavior, but also their experience of other aspects of themselves, their experience of others, and their experience of the therapist as well. The therapist must listen for the possibility of unspoken agendas that interfere with patients' attempts to self-regulate their eating (e.g., does changing eating behavior interfere with a patient's sense of security by increasing the opportunity for involvement with others?). This process may take many months, and it may be that these unspoken agendas can never be verbalized by the patient (or the therapist) until they emerge in the therapy relationship itself; in such cases, some (or considerable) analysis of transference is likely to be necessary before the patient will be able to proceed with managing symptoms.

It should be noted that analysis of transference can be necessary even when a patient is able to comply with homework assignments. If the

ASSESSMENT

(e.g., eating symptoms, personality disorder,
depression, patient concerns).

COLLABORATIVE GOAL SETTING

(e.g., reduce binge-eating)

EDUCATION/SKILLS TRAINING

(e.g., teaching self-monitoring)

HOMEWORK

(e.g., self-monitoring)

UNDERSTANDING NONCOMPLIANCE/RESISTANCE

Environment Contingencies	Intrapersonal Contingencies	Transferential Contingencies
• Interpersonal (e.g., will lose defense against involvement with others)	• Knowledge Deficit (e.g., didn't understand the assignment)	• Transference (e.g., felt coerced into performing task)
• Familial (e.g., change would disrupt family equilibrium)	• Biological Deficit (e.g., patient has concentration difficulties due to depression)	• Countertransference (e.g., therapist is acting out patient's projected rage by asking unreasonable goals)
	• Attitudes/Beliefs (e.g., patient will become obese the moment he or she gives up dietary restraint)	
	• Difficulties in Object Constancy	
	• Narcissistic Deficit	
	• Neurotic Conflict	

INTERPRETATION

(e.g., communication of an
understanding of the patient's difficulty)

COLLABORATIVE GOAL SETTING   ANALYSIS OF TRANSFERENCE

FIGURE 15.1.   Understanding patient noncompliance/resistance.

patient feels manipulated, or experiences the need to please the therapist without addressing his or her own concerns, then compliance with "collaborative goal setting" may only serve to maintain maladaptive attitudes and behavior. This process is analogous to the analysis of patients with "false-self" personality (e.g., Kohut, 1971; Winnicott, 1965), where the patient adapts to meet the needs of the therapist. This problem, in particular, underscores the therapist's need to listen for the metacommunications (Strupp, 1989) between patient and therapist.

4. Ideally, when something new about the patient's difficulty with change is understood, or a renewed interest in managing symptoms is expressed by the patient, the therapist can reintroduce the prospect of behavioral goals. Less ideal circumstances require the therapist to reintroduce behavioral goals even without increased insight. These less-than-ideal circumstances may involve prolonged or deteriorating symptomatic behavior, or symptoms that interfere with progress in other aspects of the therapy. Whenever the therapist switches from behavioral to psychodynamic strategy, he or she must be sensitive to the patient's experience of the change and implications for the transference. Behavioral goals should remain simple and be used sparingly. Picking the right goal at the right time maximizes the possibility that the patient will experience success in managing symptoms.

5. Because there are common techniques in psychodynamic and behavior therapy, it is important that the therapist acknowledge and signal the patient that a change in orientation is occurring. This can be accomplished with the simplest and most basic of techniques from both orientations. When a therapist wants to signal the implementation of psychodynamic work, he or she should allow the patient to begin the session. If a session has already begun, the therapist can ask questions that reflect concern for the patient's experience (e.g., "How did you feel when I asked you to monitor your eating?") When behavioral work is to be initiated, the therapist should begin the session by asking about the patient's success with homework assignments and review self-monitoring forms. As previously noted, it is extremely important for the therapist to be sensitive to the patient's experience of these shifts in the therapeutic process.

CONCLUSIONS

While there is little empirical work to support the effectiveness of combining psychodynamic and behavior therapy in the treatment of eating disorders, there is preliminary evidence to suggest that integrative treatment is necessary for some eating disorder subgroups. Johnson et al. (in press) found that the presence of borderline personality disorder impeded treatment outcome of bulimia, depending on whether or not an adequate "dose" (Howard et al., 1986) of psychodynamic therapy was added to cognitive–behavioral treatment. While the bulimic symptoms of most patients without borderline personality disorder remitted with only cognitive–behavioral therapy, bulimic patients with borderline personality disorder needed an average of 100 sessions (twice a week for 1 year) before their bulimic symptoms remitted.

We hope that the reader has gained some appreciation for the complexity, the necessity, and most of all the feasibility of integrating psychodynamic and behavior therapy. Mixing theoretical models that are as divergent as these two approaches increases the complexity of conducting psychotherapy. This complexity presents technical problems for the therapist, some of which we have tried to address. Despite these difficulties, we believe that an integrative approach can facilitate treatment of eating disorders. We have provided some guidelines for deciding how best to initiate an integrative treatment process, as well as how to introduce and reintroduce divergent components of treatment.

For clinicians who are not inclined toward an integrative approach, the process of modulating divergent approaches to treatment may introduce unwanted confusion into the treatment of eating disorder patients—a treatment process that can be challenging with many such patients. However, therapist confusion is not always negative, and can be viewed as one of many opportunities for the patient to communicate to the therapist that something is missing from therapy or is being misunderstood by the therapist. Not knowing what direction to take with patients is the dilemma that sometimes faces all therapists, regardless of theoretical orientation. This confusion may be resolved in the minds of some therapists by adherence to a particular orientation. However, this strategy runs the risk of abandoning the experience of patients. In this case, theoretical orientation serves the needs of the therapists and not the patients. Integration allows therapists to abandon theoretical constructs in favor of maintaining a connection to the patients' experience.

NOTE

1. Gustafson defines four general "currents" that can oppose each other in individual psychotherapy, leaving the patient (and therapist) without solutions. His method for handling decentering by the patient is quite germane to our discussion of integration, but the reader is also encouraged to explore the specific content areas described by Gustafson: (1) difficulties with the expression of needs and instincts, (2) difficulties with a constant attitude, (3) interpersonal difficulties that

comprise security operations, and (4) difficulties with the family system. Because Gustafon wrote about brief therapy, he does not emphasize the emergence and utilization of transference in the therapy dyad, but his principles can be extended to the context of longer-term treatment. Stern (Chapter 4, this volume) also discusses the "opposing-currents" approach.

REFERENCES

Adler, G.A. (1985). *Borderline psychopathology and its treatment*. Northvale, NJ: Jason Aronson.

Agras, W. S., Schneider, J. A., Arnow, B., Raeburn, S. D., & Telch, C. F. (1989). Cognitive–behavioral treatment with and without exposure plus response prevention in the treatment of bulimia nervosa: A reply to Leitenberg and Rosen. *Journal of Consulting and Clinical Psychology, 57*, 778–779

Bandura, A. (1977). Self-efficacy: Toward a unifying theory of behavior change. *Psychological Review, 84*, 191–215

Beck, A. T., Rush, A. J., Shaw, B. F., & Emery, G. (1979). *Cognitive therapy for depression*. New York: Guilford Press.

Buckley, P. A. (1987). *Exposure plus response prevention in the short-term group treatment of bulimia*. Paper presented at the annual meeting of the Association for Advancement of Behavior Therapy, Boston,

Fairburn, C. G. (1984). Cognitive–behavioral treatment for bulimia. In D. M. Garner & P. E. Garfinkel (Eds.), *Handbook of psychotherapy for anorexia nervosa and bulimia* (pp. 160–192). New York: Guilford Press.

Frank, J. (1973). *Persuasion and healing*. New York: Schocken.

Garner, D. M., Moldofsky, H., & Garner, D. M. (1980). The heterogeneity of anorexia nervosa. *Archives of General Psychiatry, 37*, 1036–1040.

Garner, D. M., & Bemis, K., (1984). Cognitive therapy for anorexia nervosa. In D. M. Garner & P. E. Garfinkel (Eds.), *Handbook of psychotherapy for anorexia nervosa and bulimia* (pp. 107–146). New York: Guilford Press.

Gill, M. M. (1982). *Analysis of transference: Vol. 1. Theory and technique*. New York: International Universities Press.

Goldfried, M. (1982). *Converging themes in psychotherapy*. New York: Springer.

Goodsitt, A. (1984). Self psychology and the treatment of anorexia nervosa. In D. M. Garner & P. E. Garfinkel (Eds.), *Handbook of psychotherapy for anorexia nervosa and bulimia* (pp. 55–82). New York: Guilford Press.

Greenberg, J. (1986). The problem of analytic neutrality. *Contemporary Psychoanalysis, 22*, 76–86.

Greenberg, L. S., & Safran, J. D. (1987). *Emotion in psychotherapy: Affect, cognition, and the process of change*. New York: Guilford Press.

Guidano, V. F., & Liotti, G. (1983). *Cognitive processes and emotional disorders*. New York: Guilford Press.

Gustafson, J. P. (1986). *The complex secret of brief psychotherapy*. New York: Norton.

Gwirtsman, H. E., Roy-Byrne, P., Yager, J., & Gerner, R. H. (1983). Neuroendocrine abnormalities in bulimia. *American Journal of Psychiatry, 140,* 559–563.

Hayes, S. C. (1987). A contextual approach to therapeutic change. In N. S. Jacobson (Ed.), *Psychotherapists in clinical practice: Cognitive and behavioral perspectives* (pp. 326–378). New York: Guilford Press.

Hoffman, I. Z. (1983). The patient as interpreter of the analyst's experience. *Contemporary Psychoanalysis, 19,* 389–422.

Holroyd, K. A., Holm, T. E., Hursey, K. G., Penzien, D. B., Cordingly, G. E., Theotonous, A. G., Richardson, S. C., & Tobin, D. L. (1988). Recurrent vascular headache: Home-based behavioral treatment versus abortive pharmacological treatment. *Journal of Consulting and Clinical Psychology, 56,* 218–223.

Howard, K. I., Kopta, S. M., Krause, M. S., & Orlinsky, D. E. (1986). The dose–effect relationship in psychotherapy. *American Psychologist, 41,* 159–164.

Humphrey, L. L., & Stern, S. (1988). Object relations and the family system in bulimia: A theoretical integration. *Journal of Marital and Family Therapy, 14,* 337–350.

Johnson, C., & Connors, M. (1987). *The etiology and treatment of bulimia nervosa: A biopsychosocial perspective.* New York: Basic Books.

Johnson, C., Connors, M., & Tobin, D. L. (1987). Symptom management of bulimia. *Journal of Consulting and Clinical Psychology, 55,* 668–676.

Johnson, C., Tobin, D. L., & Enright, A. B. (1989). Prevalence and clinical characteristics of borderline patients in an eating disordered population. *Journal of Clinical Psychiatry, 50,* 9–15.

Johnson, C., Tobin, D. L., & Dennis, A. B. (in press). Differences in treatment outcome between borderline and nonborderline bulimics at one year follow-up. *International Journal of Eating Disorders.*

Kanfer, F. H., & Scheft, B. K. (1987). Self-management theory and clinical practice. In N. S. Jacobson (Ed.), *Psychotherapists in clinical practice: Cognitive and behavioral perspectives* (pp. 10–77). New York: Guilford Press.

Kernberg, O. F. (1975). *Borderline conditions and pathological narcissism.* New York: Jason Aronson.

Kernberg, O. F. (1988). Object relations theory in clinical practice. *Psychoanalytic Quarterly, 57,* 481–505.

Kohut, H. (1971). *The analysis of the self.* New York: International Universities Press.

Kohlenberg, R. J. (1987). Functional analytic psychotherapy. In N. S. Jacobson (Ed.), *Psychotherapists in clinical practice: Cognitive and behavioral perspectives* (pp. 388–443). New York: Guilford Press.

Langs, R. (1982). *Psychotherapy: A basic text.* New York: Jason Aronson.

Leitenberg, H., & Rosen, J. (1989). Cognitive-behavior therapy with and without exposure plus response prevention in treatment of bulimia nervosa: Comment on Agras, Schneider, Arnow, Raeburn, and Telch. *Journal of Consulting and Clinical Psychology, 57,* 776–777.

Levin, A. P. & Hyler, S. E. (1986). DSM-III personality diagnosis in bulimia. *Comparative Psychiatry, 27*, 47–53.

Linehan, M. M. (1987). Dialectical behavior therapy for borderline personality disorder. *Bulletin of the Menninger Clinic, 51*, 261–276.

Mahler, M. S. (1968). *On human symbiosis and the vicissitudes of individuation: Vol. 1. Infantile psychosis*. New York: International Universities Press.

Mahoney, M. J. (1974). *Cognition and behavior modification*. Cambridge, MA: Ballinger.

Marlatt, G. A., & Gordon, J. R. (1978). Determinants of relapse: Implications for maintenance of behavior change. In P. Davidson (Ed.), *Behavioral medicine: Changing health lifestyles* (pp. 410–452). New York: Brunner/Mazel.

Meichenbaum, D. (1974). *Therapist manual for cognitive-behavior modification*. Waterloo, Ontario: University of Waterloo Press.

Pine, F. (1985). *Developmental theory and clinical process*. New Haven, CT: Yale University Press.

Pope, H. G., Frankenberg, F. R., & Hudson, Is bulimia associated with borderline personality disorder? A controlled study. *Journal of Clinical Psychiatry, 48*, 181–184.

Rehm, L. P., & Rokke, P. (1988). Self-management therapies. In K. S. Dobson (Ed.), *Handbook of cognitive–behavioral therapies* (pp. 136–166). New York: Guilford Press.

Rosen, J., & Leitenberg, J. (1982). Bulimia nervosa: Treatment with exposure plus response prevention. *Behavior Therapy, 13*, 117–124.

Safran, J. D. (1984). Some implications of Sullivan's interpersonal theory for cognitive therapy. In M. A. Reda & M. J. Mahoney (Eds.), *Cognitive psychotherapies: Recent development in theory, research, and practice*. Cambridge, MA: Ballinger.

Schwartz, H. J., (Ed.). (1988). *Bulimia: Psychoanalytic treatment and theory*. Madison, CT: International Universities Press.

Steinberg, S. L., Tobin, D. L., & Johnson, C. (1990). The role of bulimia behaviors in affect regulation: Different functions for different patient subgroups. *International Journal of Eating Disorders, 9*, 51–55.

Stern, S. (1986). The dynamics of clinical management in the treatment of anorexia nervosa and bulimia: An organizing theory. *International Journal of Eating Disorders, 5*, 233–254.

Strupp, H. H. (1989). Psychotherapy: Can the practitioner learn from the researcher? *American Psychologist, 44*, 717–724.

Sullivan, H. S. (1953). *The journal of psychiatry*. New York: Norton.

Summers, F. (1988). Psychoanalytic therapy of the borderline patient: Treating the fusion–separation contradiction. *Psychoanalytic Psychology, 5*, 339–355.

Swenson, C. (1989). Kernberg and Linehan: Two approaches to the borderline patient. *Journal of Personality Disorders, 3*, 26–35.

Swift, W. J., & Stern, S. (1982). The psychodynamic diversity of anorexia nervosa. *International Journal of Eating Disorders, 2*, 17–35.

Tobin, D. L., Holroyd, K. A., Baker, A., Reynolds, R., & Holm, J. (1988). Development and clinical trial of a minimal contact cognitive–behavioral treatment for tension headache. *Cognitive Therapy and Research, 12,* 325–339.

Tobin, D. L., Johnson, C. L., & Franke, K. (in press). Development of an eating disorder program. In J. J. Sweet, R. H. Rozensky, & S. M. Tovian (Eds.), *Handbook of clinical psychology in medical settings*. New York: Plenum.

Tobin, D. L., Johnson, C. L., Steinberg, S. L., & Dennis, A. B. (1990). Multifactoral assessment of bulimia nervosa: *Support for a biosychosocial model*. Paper presented at the 11th annual meeting of the Society of Behavioral Medicine, Chicago.

Tobin, D. L., Reynolds, R., Holroyd, K. A., & Creer, T. L. (1986). Self-management and social learning theory. In K. A. Holroyd & T. L. Creer (Eds.), *Self-management of chronic disease* (pp. 29–55). Orlando, FL: Academic Press.

Wachtel, E. F., & Wachte, P. L. (1986). *Family dynamics in individual psychotherapy*. New York: Guilford Press.

Wachtel, P. L. (1977). *Psychoanalysis and behavior therapy: Toward an integration*. New York: Basic Books.

Wilson, C. P. (1983). *Fear of being fat*. New York: Jason Aronson.

Winnicott, D. W. (1965). *The maturational processes and the facilitating environment*. New York: International Universities Press.

Index

Printed in the United Kingdom
by Lightning Source UK Ltd.
131901UK00001B/102/A